Brief Mental Health Interventions
for the Family Physician

Springer
New York
Berlin
Heidelberg
Barcelona
Hong Kong
London
Milan
Paris
Singapore
Tokyo

Brief Mental Health Interventions for the Family Physician

Michael V. Bloom, Ph.D.
Director of Behavioral Science
Sioux Falls Family Practice Residency
Sioux Falls, South Dakota

David A. Smith, M.D., C.M.D.
Professor of Family Medicine
College of Medicine
Texas A&M University;
President
Geriatric Consultants of Central Texas
Brownwood, Texas

With a Foreword by Macaran A. Baird, M.D., M.S.

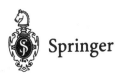 Springer

Michael V. Bloom, Ph.D.
Director of Behavioral Science
Sioux Falls Family Practice Residency
Sioux Falls, SD 57105

David A. Smith, M.D., C.M.D.
Professor of Family Medicine
College of Medicine
Texas A&M University;
President
Geriatric Consultants of Central Texas
Brownwood, TX 76804

With 5 illustrations.

Library of Congress Cataloging-in-Publication Data
Bloom, Michael V.
    Brief mental health interventions for the family physician
    Michael V. Bloom, David A. Smith.
        p. ; cm.
    Includes bibliographical references and index.
        ISBN 0-387-95235-7 (softcover : alk. paper)
        1. Brief psychotherapy—Handbooks, manuals, etc.   2. Family medicine—Handbooks,
        manuals, etc.
        [DNLM: 1. Psychotherapy, Brief.   2. Family Practice. WM 420.5.P5 B6558h 2001]
        I. Smith, David A., M.D., C.M.D.   II. Title.
    RC480.55 .B565 2001
    616.89'14—dc21   00-067914

Printed on acid-free paper.

Production managed by Terry Kornak; manufacturing supervised by Joe Quatela.
Typeset by Impressions Book and Journal Services, Inc., Madison, WI.
Printed and bound by R.R. Donnelley and Sons, Harrisonburg, VA.
Printed in the United States of America.

9 8 7 6 5 4 3 2 1

ISBN 0-387-95235-7   SPIN 10791734

Springer-Verlag   New York Berlin Heidelberg
A member of BertelsmannSpringer Science+Business Media GmbH

Foreword

Mike Bloom, Ph.D., has been an excellent teacher of family physicians for many years. He has spent those years honing a model of brief intervention suitable for primary care settings and within the therapeutic grasp of most family physicians. Dave Smith, M.D., a family physician, has been a medical school faculty member for 20 years. He has always had a large private practice as well. Throughout his career he has treated mental health problems with the same initiative as he would a myocardial infarction. His brief intervention skills have served as a model for many medical students.

Underneath the knowledge, skills, and attitudes explained in this book is the authors' understanding, indeed their (our) assumption, that the clinicians using these brief interventions will do so out of compassion and respect for the patients and families they serve. Some of the more challenging problems and associated interventions in this text require stretching the doctor—patient—family relationship. This is done in good faith to arrive at new options for healing and adapting to illness, injury, aging, or starting school. A handbook is not intended to be an exhaustive exploration of each topic held within its cover. It is intended to be a quick review, an outline, a refresher of sensible paths toward the resolution of common clinical problems. These goals are achieved in an easy-to-read style with well focused references for those who want to explore further.

In the first chapter Bloom and Smith review the basic components of brief therapy: reframing, resequencing, restructuring. Next comes a review of four steps of a brief therapy interview: (1) exploring the problem; (2) exploring attempted solutions; (3) exploring visions of improvement or goals of the therapy; and (4) delivering the intervention. The following chapters start with an outline and include a case example or vignette plus a tightly written discussion of brief therapy strategies for each disorder. When appropriate, the indications for consultation or referral are presented along with considerations for pharmacotherapy. Because this book describes brief therapy, the reviews of medications are limited although sufficient to guide the reader away from common pitfalls.

Bloom and Smith cover a wide variety of common topics in a concise fashion. After a summary of the brief treatment concept the authors present their perspective on screening in the family physician's office. From there the reader is led through a thumbnail sketch of brief treatment for depression, anxiety, panic disorder, posttraumatic stress disorder, and most childhood and adult mental health disorders. The text covers the full range of common issues and makes it clear in the first chapter that these treatment options are best suited to disorders of recent onset or, when more chronic, before the family is solidly organized in a counterproductive pattern. The authors clarify that as a disorder or symptom becomes more chronic the brief interventions remain worth trying but may not represent the most effective option. The book ends with ideas that smooth the road toward advanced directives and end-of-life decision-making.

This brief text is ideal for keeping handy on the office bookshelf or your desk. Readers can enjoy it by reading it carefully from start to finish, or they can jump into a favorite topic and seek new options for common patient problems. These interventions can help our patients, and they can be done respectfully. Moreover, family physicians and other primary care providers are capable of the interactions skillfully outlined herein.

Macaran A. Baird, M.D., M.S.
Senior Associate Consultant
Department of Family Medicine
Mayo Clinic and Mayo Foundation;
Professor of Family Medicine
Mayo Medical School
Rochester, Minnesota

Preface

The official definition of family practice from the American Academy of Family Practice is that it is a medical specialty that provides continuing and comprehensive health care for the individual and family. It is the specialty in breadth that integrates the biologic, clinical, and behavioral sciences. The scope of family practice encompasses all ages, both genders, each organ system, and every disease entity.

The definition implies that family physicians must be expert in diagnosing and treating the common diseases and disorders of humankind. However, there is no assurance that because a malady is common, it is simple.

The definition also promises that family physicians will provide care through an integrated biopsychosocial model and will treat diseases and promote health in the context of the family. Nowhere in medicine is this a more useful construct than when providing prevention for and treatment of social and mental health problems. These problems are a major part of the activity of the prototypical family practice, and family practitioners deliver a significant portion of this care in the United States (Leon et al., 1995).

Although our activities in this arena overlap with those of social services, psychology, and psychiatry, there are a number of reasons family physicians should be expert and active in the provision of social and mental health care. A family physician, who already has rapport with an individual or family, may be more accessible than other providers and, right or wrong, comes with less stigmatization. The family practitioner can be available for those mental health and social problems that are not serious enough to motivate the patient or family to seek out a specialist. Indeed, minor social and psychiatric problems are so common that were they to present to the formal mental health system that system would be swamped. Yet it is often valuable to "nip things in the bud."

In the process of seeing one's patient's, the family practitioner has the opportunity to be part of their lives, and to recognize changes and identify problems early, before they become entrenched and less apt to be remedied. The family practitioner may even recognize high-risk situations for social or mental health problems and be proactive, instituting preventive measures.

The family practitioner may recognize the potential for parenting problems or a child's grief after a divorce, and so intervene. After the death of a child, the family practitioner may counsel a married couple on the feelings they may naturally have toward each other that might threaten their marriage. At the time of an elder's placement into long-term care the family practitioner may manage his or her medications to prevent polypharmacy and create a milieu and activities care plan to promote a positive adjustment. The family practitioner might even catalyze community mental health activities as a form of good citizenship, interacting with schools to identify children involved in risk-taking behavior or those isolated from their families and peers (the common thread in most recent school violence incidents). Finally, a subtle but extremely important reason for family practitioners to be involved in the prevention and care of social and mental health problems is that the dichotomy of mind and body that pervades our Western culture and infuses the culture of medicine is false.

Psychiatry is becoming rapidly transformed into neuroendocrinology, with the recognition of the genetic, anatomic, hormonal, and neurochemical bases for many mental illnesses. The interrelationship of "mental illness" and "physical illness" is becoming so strong as to blur the boundaries. For example, myocardial infarction occurs more often in those chronically depressed, and death among those who develop depression after myocardial infarction is significantly higher than among those who do not. Polymorphonuclear leukocytes in grief-stricken surviving spouses of long marriages show impaired chemotaxis in vitro. Children are at greater risk of accidental injury for a period of time after relocation of the family home. The evidence that mind and body are one and that the dichotomy of physical and social or mental illness is an antiquated construct are myriad. The family practitioner with a firm foundation in the biopsychosocial model is well positioned to discard old thinking and move into an enlightened future.

Unfortunately, there remain many barriers to fulfilling the potential for family practitioners to deliver care in the social/mental health arena. Some of us still are nihilistic, believing that the social problems of our society are so large as to be unapproachable or that they have no impact. Others, for one reason or another, have not accepted the responsibility of this aspect of family practice. Medical school undergraduate curricula and to a varying degree family practice residency training often fail to emphasize these aspects of health and disease in proportion to their true significance.

Managed care, third-party insurance, and even the government have not provided parity for remuneration of services for social and mental health care compared to services clearly defined as somatic care and far less than for procedural medicine. This may be out of fear of opening Pandora's box and becoming fiscally responsible for all sorts of "touchy-feely" services or never-ending "couch therapy" that almost anyone with a little stress or a little situational sadness might want and for which they might qualify.

Campbell et al. (2000), however, reported that primary care physicians who diagnosed mental health problems in a managed care environment significantly more often than their colleagues were about 9% more economical providers for the organization. This validates the authors' beliefs that much unnecessary medical and social expense is incurred because of nonrecognition and nontreatment of these problems. We suspect that unnecessary laboratory and radiographic testing and symptomatic therapy for somatic complaints associated with anxiety, depressive disorders, dependence, or loneliness—instead of identification and appropriate treatment —may head the list of wasteful, expensive consequences of our current situation.

The increasing pressures of time for the family practitioner are an especially powerful barrier to the provision of excellent social and mental health services in primary care. Managed care and low remuneration per unit of cognitive service tendered by Medicare and Medicaid are potent disincentives for the family practitioner to spend the time perceived to be required for the job.

Finally, perhaps the largest obstacle for family physicians addressing mental health problems is that most of the literature describing treatment is written by mental health specialists. Although this information can be valuable (and in fact informed us significantly for this book), it is often a poor fit for the family practice setting. These treatment protocols must often be altered significantly before they accommodate the family practice content.

In these regards, our book may be of some relief. We offer interventions for prevention, identification, and treatment of social and mental health problems in efficient, provider/time-sensitive increments designed to fit the typical practice patterns of our readers. We are aware of the trepidation we each experience when we catch a glimpse of a potential problem of this sort near the end of a 15-minute office visit for episodic health care while a full waiting room buzzes in discontent. We have experienced the temptation to "let this sleepy dog lie" out of fear that we will be committed to service time we do not have.

Every evaluation and treatment protocol offered in this book has been used repeatedly in academic and nonacademic family practice settings. Furthermore, the protocols have all been taught and learned by family practice residents. We have constantly adjusted and improved them based on feedback received from patients, residents, and former residents now in practice, as well as based on our own experience.

We have made every effort to design the book to be an easy, efficient handbook. Although the chapters can be read consecutively, it is not required and might not be the most effective way to absorb the material. We do recommend reading Chapters 1 and 2 first, as they lay down the basic concepts for the brief therapy interventions used throughout the book. It is then most useful to read the appropriate chapter in response to a patient who presents with just such a problem. The chapters are designed to be read in 5 to 10 minutes. Once a chapter has been read, the outline preceding the text in each chapter can be used as a memory aid and guide. Residents have used some of these outlines in the patient's room to guide the interview.

Readers are invited to send comments to the following e-mail address: mvbloom@usd.edu

References

Campbell TL, Franks P, Fiscella K, McDaniel SH, Zwangziger J (2000) Do physicians who diagnose more mental health disorders generate lower health care costs? J Fam Pract 49:305–310.

Leon A, Olfson M, Broadhead WE (1995) Prevalence of mental disorders in primary care. Arch Fam Med 4:857–861.

Michael V. Bloom, Ph.D.
David A. Smith, M.D., C.M.D.

Acknowledgments

Along with profound technologic changes in medicine, perhaps the most significant other change during the last 75 years is that good medicine now requires teamwork. This book is no exception. In fact the genesis of this book did not come from the authors but from a family practice resident. While seeing a patient in the clinic for insomnia, the resident consulted one of the authors. Within 5 to 10 minutes they had gone over the patient's problem and came up with a treatment plan that the resident proceeded to present to the patient. As the resident was leaving the faculty member's office he casually remarked that the faculty member might write down some of his treatment protocols so the residents could have quick access to them. Whereas the resident might have seen this as a causal remark, the faculty member took the suggestion seriously, and hence the writing of this book. As chapters were produced they were made available to residents, who then gave feedback that provided important guidance for subsequent revisions of the chapters.

A number of physicians, both family physicians and psychiatrists, also read chapters of the book and provided valuable critiques. They include, in alphabetical order, Berne Bahnson, M.D., Michael Glenn, M.D., David Keith, M.D., Richard McClaflin, M.D., Fredric Thanel, M.D., Barbara Yawn, M.D., and Dr. Wesley Nord, who read and critiqued nearly all the chapters.

Esther Gumpert, consulting editor for Springer-Verlag, provided not only editorial support but also overall guidance for the book for more than a year of its development. Terry Kornak, Supervising Production Editor, and her staff did an outstanding job of guiding the book through its production phase. Jane Nyhhaug prepared the manuscripts and provided editorial feedback from start to finish.

Renowned psychologist Erik Erikson in his book *Childhood and Society* (1963) said: "The fashionable insistence on dramatizing the dependence of children on adults often blinds us to the dependence of the older generation on the younger one. Mature man needs to be needed, and maturity needs guidance as well as encouragement from what has been produced and must be taken care of. Generativity, then, is primarily the concern in establishing and guiding the next generation." It has been our calling and privilege to participate in the education of the next generation of doctors. This book is primarily the product of the exchange between patient, doctor in training, and faculty. We hope this interaction has enriched the lives of our patients and the clinical performance of our medical students and family practice residents. We know it has contributed greatly to the development of the two authors as people and doctors. We therefore dedicate this book to our medical students and resident physicians.

Reference

Erikson E (1963) Childhood and Society, 2nd ed., New York: Norton.

Michael V. Bloom, Ph.D.
David A. Smith, M.D., C.M.D.

Contents

1

Approach to Brief Treatment in Family Practice

HISTORY OF THE PROBLEM

1. For brief treatment, open-ended questions regarding the problem, including establishing the patients' and families' view of the problem, are asked.
2. Sequences of events surrounding the problem, including interaction with significant others are determined, as is a description of the problem in the context of a typical day.
3. Attempted solutions by the patient and others trying to help are enumerated.
4. When is the problem even slightly better?

GOAL SETTING

1. Ask—What would be the first sign that a small improvement had occurred? (For example, the miracle question: If you woke up in the morning and your problem was better, how would you know it?)
2. Analyze—What needs did the activities surrounding the problem satisfy (life stages; for example, adjusting to: preschool, a new relationship, separation, retirement, etc.)?
3. Analyze—What has changed to make this a problem now?

TREATMENT

1. Reframing: viewing the problem differently, leading to different behavior.
2. Altering sequences surrounding the problem.
3. Motivating the patient and significant others to make useful changes.

PROTOCOLS FOR COMMON PROBLEMS

1. Self-observational task.
   a. Indications—Patient defines the problem as outside his or her control (e.g., panic disorder, bulimia).

1

      b. Plan—Patient is told to keep a detailed diary of symptoms, thoughts, and interactions with others, from preceding symptoms through resolution of the symptoms.

2. Solution-focused task.

      a. Indications—Patients are motivated to try something new but could become resistant to change. This intervention helps avoid resistance to change.

      b. Plan—Disallow discussion of blame for the problem. Obtain a detailed description of when the problem is slightly better. Develop a plan with the patient and if possible with a significant other to recreate the times of improvement more frequently even if it is only slight improvement.

3. "As if" task.

      a. Indications—Interrupt repeating behavior patterns and habits that lead to needs being met in problematic ways (e.g., frequent relapse from chronic pain treatments).

      b. Plan—Request that the family and patient "act" as though they do not have the problem for a negotiated period (e.g., 1 hour); or to prevent relapse, act as though the problem has returned for a period (e.g., 1 hour) to practice their response.

4. Restraining directives.

      a. Indications—highly resistant patients.

      b. Prescribe that the patient has the symptoms or resists treatment. Give the patient a respectable but slightly uncomfortable explanation for this plan.

It is well known that psychosocial problems in family practice are common. In the past, however, many family physicians have been frustrated by the difficulty of fitting effective treatments into the family practice setting. Treatments commonly used by therapists and psychiatrists, although highly effective, are often not practical for the family physician. This chapter lays the foundation for an overall approach to the patient with psychosocial problems. The family physician's use of brief therapy, psychoactive medication, and referral are discussed. More specific discussion of treatments for specific problems follows in other chapters.

Since the early 1990s there has been a growing degree of activity to develop brief therapeutic interventions that fit into the family practice setting. These interventions are particularly useful for the most common problems seen by the family physician, such as adjustment disorders, depression, anxiety, somatoform disorders, and children's behavioral problems. These therapeutic practices do not solve all the problems patients bring to the physician, and referral and consultation are necessary for some; but they do solve many of the most common problems. Thus the family physician can address most of the common psychosocial problems just as they do for other areas of medicine. Furthermore, when the physician makes a counseling attempt, even if it is not fully successful the patient is then more open to a referral.

The improved effectiveness of brief therapy has been made possible by a shift in the way therapists approach treatment strategies. During the first half of this century psychotherapy was based on the concept that if one could come to understand how the problems developed this understanding would lead to health-promoting change. Research proved this insight-oriented approach was not effective for many people. At the same time a different view of problem-solving was developed that was based on studying how people change, spending little energy focusing on how their problems develop. Most of the therapies recently found to be most effective in helping people change are based on three processes: reframing, resequencing, and restructuring.

Some approaches to therapy attempt to change all three, but it has been found that changing even one of the three often leads to significant therapeutic benefit. One approach, *reframing*, helps people change the way they think about their problem. For example, many people with anxiety disorders come to their doctor believing that the best way to deal with their fears is to avoid them in any way possible. If they come to understand that the more useful approach to the problem is gradually approaching their fear in a step-wise fashion the problem is likely to remit.

Resequencing helps people change by altering the sequence of events surrounding the problem in a strategic way that leads to a different outcome. For example, some parents after a child disobeys confront the situation by repeatedly attempting to explain to the child why he or she should behave as requested. The more they explain, the more stubborn the child becomes. An alternative is for the parents to ignore the child's poor behavior totally but pay increasing attention when the child is behaving appropriately. This altered sequence of events often leads to improvement.

Restructuring is aimed at changing the structure within a family. The most common example is the child with behavioral problems whose parents are attempting to be a friend rather than an authority figure. Changing the structure from a peer relationship to parent as authority figure is often helpful.

In summary, altering the way people think about their problem, the sequence of events surrounding the problems, and altering the family structure often lead to helpful change. Although achieving these goals at first blush may sound simple, the experienced clinician knows otherwise. People tend to avoid change even when they know it might be useful. Homeostasis, that is stability, is a powerful force. Some even define psychotherapy as nothing more than overcoming resistance to change. The process of brief therapy, as discussed here, is based on using approaches that avoid resistance as much as possible, or if it is not possible to avoid it, use resistance as a strategic motivator for change.

There are certain approaches doctors sometimes take that handicap their ability to promote change. One handicapping belief is that people who have problems are motivated to change and come to the physician for help to make that change. In fact, most who come to the physician's office are in some sort of discomfort, and they simply want the discomfort to stop. Far from wanting to change, they want the physician to cure them so they no longer have the discomfort, be it physical or psychological. Therefore the physician's role is frequently to motivate the patient to change.

Another handicap is the belief that you must know the diagnosis and etiology of a problem to treat it. Physicians commonly treat disorders without knowing the exact etiology. In fact, overenthusiastic pursuit of a definitive diagnosis often causes more problems than it solves. For example, physicians who believe they must absolutely know the cause of chronic pain often pursue diagnostic studies with no definitive results, and the problem worsens. When the dangerous etiologies have been ruled out, it is often better simply to pursue treatment even if a definitive diagnosis is elusive.

Another belief that can handicap change is the belief that people must feel better to be motivated to change. In fact, quite the opposite is true. People are motivated to change because they are in discomfort; when they feel better they are more complacent and are willing to leave things as they are. Often the belief that people must feel better quickly moves the physician to use medications that cover up a problem temporarily without developing a lasting resolution.

Another handicap is the belief that patients know and directly communicate their problem. Often the patient knows the pain but not the problem. It takes a good history to define the true nature of the problem. For example, a patient complains of depression without apparent cause. A description of the problem soon reveals that the relationship with the spouse has become increasingly distant and hollow over the last year, and the patient is in fact grieving the loss of this relationship. When distressed, patients often focus on trying to assign blame for their problems rather than on solutions. They focus on historical explanations; and because one cannot change the past, this practice promotes the idea that making meaningful change is impossible. It is therefore useful to avoid issues related to blame or historical explanations.

Another way to fail is to focus on a problem different from that of the patient. A typical example is the physician who confronts a patient with a somatoform disorder, stating that it is a psychological problem not a physical one. It is much more helpful to use the patients' view of their pathology as an explanation to facilitate useful change. For example, "your pain is quite distressing, and from the sounds of things it is really ruining your life style. There are some things we can do to help you regain control over your life and not let the pain ruin it." This explanation avoids the question of whether the pain is physiologic; rather, it focuses on the functional status as something that is treatable using behavioral techniques.

Another common mistake is to neglect to determine what solutions have already been attempted to resolve the problem. The physician then suggests repeating a solution that has already failed. If patients are to be motivated to make a change they must believe that there is something different about this solution from one that failed in the past.

Finally, it is important not to get ahead of or to work harder than the patient or family. For example, doctors enthusiastically make recommendations for life style change, such as exercise programs, when the patient is not yet convinced or ready to even attempt such activity. This is liable to lead to a "yes—but" attitude, which makes motivating the patient to accept change even more difficult. The physician in this case must slow down and continue to search for motivating goals or acceptable activities.

Brief Therapy Process

Although the examination procedure the family physician follows for a brief therapy interview is similar to that followed for a more general examination, there are some differences that help guide the process efficiently to the three change processes previously discussed: reframing, resequencing, restructuring. It is useful to organize the interview into four steps: (1) exploring the problem; (2) exploring attempted solutions; (3) exploring visions of improvement (goals); and (4) delivering the intervention. The intervention should include an explanation of the problem that can motivate the patient to undertake specific activities, which in turn leads to resolution of the problem.

As with all medical interviews, the brief therapy interview begins by exploring the problem. Initially, as with any other history-taking, the physician begins with open-ended questions aimed at establishing the patient's and family's views of the problem. It is important to place the problem in a broader perspective than simply asking for specific symptoms. If a patient says "I'm here because I'm depressed" the physician might ask "How is your day different when you are depressed from when you are not depressed? How does your family see you as being different?" It is then important to understand the sequence of events that surround the problem, including specific actions and dialogue that occur because the person has the problem. For example: "What is different about how you spend your day because you are depressed from how you would spend your day if you weren't depressed? How do people treat you differently because you are depressed, particularly your family and significant others?" Finally, to understand the problem it is helpful to identify times at which the problem is even slightly better. "When you notice when your mood lifts even a little What is going on in your thinking and in your environment when things are even slightly improved?"

After a detailed understanding of the problem is complete, the next step is to obtain a history of attempted solutions from the patient and the significant others. There are two good reasons for understanding attempted solutions. First, such attempts have failed and are now part of the problem. That is, they are part of the sequence of events that maintains the status quo.

Even if they make sense, because they have not yet succeeded in making things better they must be altered in some way to allow a different result to occur. "How have you tried to help yourself out of your depression? How have others tried to help you?"

Goals of treatment should be the next topic. A good way to ask about goals is to ask the patient and family to imagine what would be the first sign that a small improvement had occurred. Another way to ask is the miracle question: "If you woke up in the morning and miraculously your problem was better, how would you know it was better?" Again, dialogue and action sequences should be part of the description, as this is the raw material of therapy that can be altered to create change.

Once the physician understands the goals of treatment, it is time to turn to treatment planning. It is important for goals to be measurable and realistic. For example, "I want to be happy" is not measurable. The doctor should respond to this statement with: "What will be different about your day in how you think and how you interact and do things differently when you are happy?" This is measurable.

In addition to the information already acquired, it is useful for the physician to analyze the whole of the information, thinking about what needs are being met by the problem. This is best conceptualized in terms of life context. For example, if a teenager is acting badly and getting into trouble, one might consider the possibility that the goal of this activity is rebelliousness toward parents and thus gaining a sense of independence. For the teenager to give up the problem behavior, other behaviors that can satisfy the youngster's need to have a sense of more independence from the parents are needed. Otherwise there may be significant resistance to any change, and such change cannot last long term. This is especially important when addictions are involved. What needs has the addiction filled, and what other means of meeting those needs might be considered in the treatment plan?

Another important factor to be analyzed before a treatment plan is developed is why the problem is being brought to the doctor at this particular time. For example, if someone complains that he or she has been depressed for 15 years but just presented for help, something has changed to give this problem a higher priority than in the past.

Assessing the Problem and Treatment Planning

Assessment for a brief therapy intervention requires more complexity than a Diagnostic and Statistical Manual of Mental Disorders (DSM- IV) category. It is useful to begin by analyzing the following issues: (1) In the patient's view: What is the problem on which he or she is motivated to work? What must change for the patient to perceive the problem as resolving? (2) What need(s) is the present pattern of behavior satisfying? What can the physician foresee as possible options for having this need(s) addressed in a less problematic way? Why is the patient likely to resist change? What is likely to motivate the patient to be willing to make changes that are initially uncomfortable? (3) What is easiest to change about how the patient regards the problem or acts on it that is likely to lead to resolution? (4) How are significant others contributing to the status quo?

To be effective the plan usually must include a specific directive or assigned task based on the above analysis of the problem with the goal of the patient and often the significant other changing the way they usually do things. The directive should include a specific set of actions that alter the sequence of events or the thinking process surrounding the events. Usually the directive is given in a way that motivates the patient to follow the specific instructions. Sometimes in highly resistant patients a directive is given in such a way that it increases the patient's likelihood of rebelling against it. In this case, the goal is to motivate the patient to change by rebelling. It is usually best to start by requesting small changes to assess how much resistance there is. Following this step, based on feedback received, the expectation for change is increased until the problem is resolved.

For patients uncomfortable because of their problem, who are motivated to change, and who demonstrate little resistance, a straightforward explanation is often effective. It includes a new explanation acceptable to the patient and a plan that follows from the explanation. For example, a physician sees a 6-year-old child a number of times for various somatic complaints the doctor recognizes are related to missing school. The parents even mention this possibility to the child but dismiss it initially because the child repeatedly says there is nothing wrong at school. After the examination, the doctor tells the parents that the child may be avoiding leaving home or daycare, where things are familiar, not wanting to face the novelty of a new school. The parents must teach the child that feeling sick is not a reason to avoid school. The parents follow through and soon the child's symptoms diminish.

Family physicians commonly treat children with separation anxiety in this way. A new explanation for a problem and a specific directive to alter the problematic sequence often works and is usually the first-line treatment approach to this and other problems seen in family practice. When the patient does not respond to this approach, alternative interventions may produce better results. The four alternative treatment interventions we describe are relatively easy to integrate into family practice. We present them in order of increasing complexity: (1) the self-observational task; (2) solution-focused treatment (i.e., doing more of what works); (3) the "as if" behavioral approach; and (4) restraining directives.

Self-Observational Task

The self-observational task can be used for a host of problems, but it works particularly well when patients define the problem as outside their control. This task can help patients experience ways problems can be brought under their control. Examples of problems that often respond to self-observational tasks are panic disorders, bulimic disorder, certain depressive disorders, some impulse control disorders, and circumstances when parents believe they cannot control their children.

The physician introduces this solution by requesting that the patient and family member, if present, initially not try to change anything but to gather more information. The patient and sometimes the significant others are asked to keep a detailed diary of the symptoms. This diary should include the day and time the symptoms occur and the sequence of events leading up and following the commencement of symptoms, including the thoughts and dialogue with others during that interval. They should include anything that led to alleviation or worsening of the symptoms. Finally, they should describe how the symptoms resolved. The patient and family member are requested to record this information as soon as possible after the symptoms have begun or at least immediately after their resolution to ensure accuracy.

Another variation on this protocol is for patients who tend to dwell on their symptoms. It involves asking them to keep a diary of the times their symptoms seemed to be even slightly diminished. This is particularly useful for depressed patients or patients with generalized anxiety. Other aspects of the diary are the same.

To motivate the patient and family to perform the task, the doctor explains that the problem is complicated and a more detailed understanding would be helpful before any attempts to change are undertaken. For patients with panic disorder, for example, it helps explain that the first step in helping them gain control over the problem is to have a detailed account of the problem.

The outcome of this intervention is often significant attenuation of the symptom soon after they start implementing this plan, likely because the self-observational task gives them a feeling of being more in control almost immediately. Many symptoms, such as bulimia and panic disorder, occur when a patient feels out of control, so this method prompts almost immediate improvement. It is usually not helpful to explain this to the patient. The explanation that "we are trying to gather more information" is usually sufficient for the patient.

Follow-up about 1 week later is recommended. If the patient has improved sufficiently, he or she can be told that simply learning more about the problem is helping them gain better control over it; therefore more of the same is in order. Another option for increasing self-control is for the patient to attempt to bring on the symptom at a prescribed time and then use a relaxation exercise to control it. This also leads to a greater sense of control. The patient should keep a diary in the same way, which leads to an increase in self-control, as the very act of attempting to bring on the symptoms puts one in charge of them.

Family members can be asked to observe this process and keep their own diary as a way to understand the process better. Having the family members observe without getting involved in providing reassurance to the patient helps alter the sequence of events in a direction that increases the patient's sense of being more in control. If the self-observational task works, follow-up visits can consist mainly of requesting that the patient do more of the same until believing he or she has good control over the problem. If the problem persists, another approach can be tried.

Solution-Focused Approach

A solution-focused approach is another type of directive that can be used for a wide variety of problems. It is based on the observation that many people are less resistant to change when change is viewed as nothing more than an extension of what they are already doing. Because a great deal of resistance to change comes from feeling at fault (guilty) for the problems or from fear of the unknown, doing more of what works avoids this resistance. A solution-focused approach is especially useful as an initial approach for patients who have significant potential for resistance to change. For example, family members may be blaming each other for the problem and therefore believe that agreeing to change means admitting that the problem is their fault.

Because the solution-focused approach is based on the concept of doing more of what is already working, it is important to gather a detailed description of the circumstances under which the problem is alleviated even slightly. For example, the patient might be asked, "Although you are depressed, even those who are depressed have times during their day or week when they feel a little better. I'd be interested in a description of when you feel even a little better." The description should include at least one specific time when the patient felt better. It should include the specific dialogue and actions that preceded the better time and what followed afterward. The doctor should understand what the patient believes made this event an exception to the rule, however small.

When assessing problems physicians should ask themselves: "What is different about the times when things go better for the patient? Are their needs being addressed differently during these times? Are negative interactions being avoided?" The purpose of evaluating these issues is not to provide insight to the patient but to recommend activities strategically to the patient and significant others that can expand these positive experiences and increase their frequency. In fact, usually it is best to not offer an explanation for solution-focused directives beyond, "That is what has worked in the past for you, let's figure out a way to do more of it."

For example, a well educated mother of a 4-year-old boy at the end of a preschool physical examination reports that her son throws horrible tantrums before he goes to bed at night. They have become worse lately and in fact have become frightening to both parents because he screams that he would rather die than go to bed. This usually leads to the parents sitting down with the boy and asking him what is wrong. These discussions can last an hour. In the morning they report he is always fine until the next night. When asked if there was ever a time when things seemed to go better, the mother reports a night she and her husband were going out at the child's bedtime. The child threw a similar tantrum when they were leaving. Because they had to meet another couple, they told the child that they had to go and left immediately. The babysitter reported that after they left the child stopped crying and went to bed without trouble. The mother suggested that perhaps it was their fault the child was troubled. The doctor stated that fault was not the issue but that they had learned on this one occasion a way that seemed to work: Simply do not respond to his tantrum; and leave the room. They were warned that his behavior could get worse for a few nights. A week later the mother called back to report that the child had had only had one bad night and since then had been going to bed quite easily. The doctor in this case could have spent a lot of time on the child's separation fears, focusing on the parent's need to be overprotective or the child's need to manipulate for attention. Instead, by focusing on what had worked to improve the problem and expanding it to a regular routine, the child's behavior improved.

"As If" Interventions

The "as if" interventions are slightly more complicated to introduce but are effective for a wide variety of habit disorders and relapse prevention for a host of problems. For example, psychosomatic disorders commonly are alleviated briefly no matter what the treatment, but the patient relapses because of a large secondary gain component. The "as if" directive can be used to prevent relapse once a behavior has improved, and needs are now being met in a new way. It can also be useful in circumstances when the individual's resistance to change is related to a fear of trying something new. It might be a way for a couple to experiment with ways to alter a sequence of events in a problematic relationship, such as a co-dependent or jealous relationship. It is often helpful to start the plan with a challenge such as, "I'm not sure you are ready for this change" or "It might be helpful to see what a change might be like before committing to it" or "Let's experiment with some changes to see if they work for you."

The "as if" behavior can be presented in two ways. The identified patient and family can be asked to act as if they were normal; that is, they act as though they do not have the problem for a negotiated period of time. For example: "Act as if you don't have pain for one-half hour three times a day. The family should act as though you don't have the pain as well." The second way to request "as if" behavior is primarily to prevent relapse once a positive behavior has been attained. In this case the patient and family are asked to act as if the patient does have the problem for a specified period of time. For example, patients might be asked to act as though they do have the pain for 2 hours a day so the family can practice distracting techniques for times when the real problem recurs.

There are a number of approaches that can be used for motivating families to use the "as if" process. One can challenge the family's readiness for facing a difficult behavioral problem. When requesting that the family practice normal behavior for a brief time, another approach is to suggest doing this to explore what it would be like to be normal. For example, a couple who continually battle over jealousy might be asked to act for 2 hours two evenings a week as though they are not jealous of each other to explore what their relationship would be like if they did not have this problem. Another approach is to appeal to a family's and patient's curiosity. For example, the doctor suggests that they practice normal behavior for a specified time to experiment with alternatives to approaching the problem. This behavioral change might be combined with a self-observational task by requesting that they write down the results of these "as if" periods.

The outcome of using "as if" directives is often that patients and significant others try new behavioral interactions they otherwise would not, leading to a lessening in their rigidity and resistance to change. For example, the family who gives each other attention only when someone is sick learns to give attention when the patient is healthy, leading to decreased somatoform behavior. The child who throws tantrums for attention from a parent afraid to ignore this behavior for fear of being rejected by the child learns to get attention in a new way. A family afraid to not rescue a family member from an anxiety attack learns that this member can tolerate some anxiety at least for a short time, which can grow into longer periods. New behaviors that have been resisted because of fear are tried in a safer environment under the "as if" directives.

Restraining Directives

Restraining directives are used for noncompliant patients or those highly resistant to the changes necessary to resolve their problem. The technique is often used when other therapy attempts have failed because the patient did not perform the requested tasks. It is especially useful when rebelliousness, at least in part, motivates the noncompliance. "Yes—but" patients are particularly good candidates for this approach. This type of intervention gives the physician a way to help noncompliant, rebellious patients.

Rebelliousness in fact serves as motivation to make changes. Although highly useful, this type of intervention is sometimes more difficult to deliver because it requires the communication of two seemingly contradictory messages. The direct communication is: "I care for your well-being, but change may be too difficult for you; so don't change." The indirect message is: "I believe you really want to change." For this reason some family doctors elicit the help of a therapist experienced in these interventions. For those who have the time and inclination to gain the experience, it is a useful and powerful aid for treating a difficult group of patients.

Use of a restraining directive is most often chosen after a direct request for change has been resisted. A useful way to introduce a restraining directive is for the doctor to explain that it was a mistake to ask the patient or family to perform the task. Wording such as, "It was too much to ask you to make such a change" is commonly helpful. It is often useful to spell out the needs the problematic behavior may be fulfilling for the patient or family and why there is a disincentive to change or make change. "Because of your problems you are needy now, and if you do more for yourself others will do less." The therapist then suggests that the patient not change, or not change for a while, or at least change slowly.

For example, a 60-year-old man, D.R., suffers a serious myocardial infarction. His wife, who had been an excellent caretaker, died several months before his heart attack. Despite significant damage to his heart he makes a good initial recovery. When it comes time for rehabilitation, however, he becomes dependent on nursing staff and family and makes excuses daily about why he cannot participate in rehabilitation activities. The nursing staff becomes increasingly frustrated by such behaviors as calling them to hand him a glass of water or to push the television remote buttons. Some family members, feeling sorry for him, perform these activities for him regularly.

When direct encouragement and reassurance fail to diminish this overly dependent, sick behavior, a restraining directive is attempted. The patient is told, "Pushing you to become more active might have been a mistake, even if you are physically capable. The health care team mistakenly believed you wanted to get stronger as fast as possible, but the team is now divided on how they should proceed. Some believe that you have suffered so much over the past several months you deserve to be taken care of much more, even if it means you may not recover as well. Others believe you really do not like being dependent and want to work as hard as possible to become independent. As your doctor, I'm not sure who is correct, but I will tell the staff to not expect much change." The doctor then gives the restraining directive, "Maybe for now, because you have suffered so much, it is best for you to accept all the caretaking you can get and not push yourself to get better too fast. The staff will just have to accept a less than optimal recovery." This intervention was given with family present. The patient continued to rebel against the staff, but now the rebellion took the form of more independent behavior and good rehabilitation performance.

When improvement follows a restraining directive it is important to give the patient full credit for improvement to the point of expressing surprise that it occurred, allowing the patient to feel victory in the success. Furthermore, if a restraining technique has been successful, it is important to continue what is working. It is therefore not a time to start being encouraging.

The doctor can give positive feedback to patients for their improvement but at the same time continue to restrain them from further progress. For example, in the above case, after the rehabilitation progress the physician said, "I am impressed by your work in rehabilitation, but am concerned about your getting better too fast. This might lead others to expect too much of you and so not provide enough caretaking, which you deserve after having gone through so much." This technique continued to motivate the patient.

COMMENT: The four above-mentioned techniques have been useful for altering the way patients view their problems and the sequence of events surrounding them. Indeed, any creative way to help patients change while lowering resistance can and should be used.

Use of Medications

Medications for psychiatric problems have been found to be highly effective in many circumstances and are the sine qua non of treatment for others. They are time-efficient for the physician, and patients often prefer them over alternatives such as brief therapy because they act quickly and require little in the way of life style change. Therefore they are much easier for them.

Unfortunately, because of their effectiveness and appeal there has sometimes been overreliance on medication. Take for instance the following commentary from the *Journal of Nervous and Mental Disease* entitled "What should doctors do in the face of negative evidence?" The editor wrote: "Fisher and Fisher call attention to an ostensible contradiction which raises fundamental questions about knowledge and action in medical practice. Although every one of the 13 published double-blind placebo-controlled clinical trials with antidepressants fails to demonstrate an advantage for active drug over placebo in treating adolescents, physicians wrote 4 to 6 million such prescriptions in 1992 for children 18 and under" (Eisenberg, 1996).

The commentary went on to say that physicians often prescribe medication because they want to do something even when drugs are not proven effective. This is no doubt true and understandable, especially when patients are seeking medications. However, we also note that patients often do not continue antidepressant medicines past a year even on the recommendation of their physician. This can lead to relapse, with a cycle of medication, discontinuing medication, relapse, and so on.

We take a conservative approach to medication. That is, we suggest medication only when there is scientific support in terms of double-blind controlled studies (i.e., evidence-based approach). In the common situation where medication and a brief therapy approach are about equally effective, such as with certain anxiety disorders and depressive disorders, we recommend engaging patients in an informed decision-making process, letting them know the advantages of each of the approaches and then deciding with them which is most suitable in their circumstance. We agree with the commentary in the *Journal of Nervous and Mental Disorders* that physicians want to do something for their patients. It is our view that there are often effective alternatives to medications that family physicians are quite capable of undertaking and that patients often prefer once the benefits and risks of alternatives are understood. In some circumstances medications are the treatment of choice, and in others a brief psychological intervention is preferred. Some clinicians speculate that even when efficacy is equivalent for these two treatment alternatives brief psychological interventions are better than medication strategies, as patients are more likely to learn self-help skills and to make attitudinal and life style changes that prevent relapse or help them cope with illness more effectively in the case of relapse. Finally, in some clinical situations the medication strategy and psychological intervention are complementary.

The following review of medication usage is meant only to introduce a basic approach to the use of psychotropic medications for various problems. A more complete discussion appears in chapters on specific problems and diagnoses.

The clearest indications for psychotropic medications are the most severely debilitating disorders, for example, antipsychotic medication for the treatment of schizophrenia. These psychotropic agents have revolutionized the treatment of psychosis, relieved much suffering of patients and families, and helped reduce the census of state hospitals throughout the United States. The effects of the early antipsychotic, neuroleptic drugs on the positive symptoms of schizophrenia (e.g., loose associations, hallucinations, delusions) were essential for treating this condition. Unfortunately, the therapeutic effect was virtually coupled to potential side effects, most importantly extrapyramidal and tardive movement disorders. New-generation antipsychotics, also called atypical or novel antipsychotics, carry less risk of these problems and show benefit for the negative symptoms of schizophrenia, including the amotivational state, apathy, and social withdrawal.

Medications for the treatment of bipolar disorders have also proved beneficial. Lithium and antiepileptics such as valproic acid play a significant role in the treatment of bipolar illness. Many patients with bipolar disorder can lead nearly ordinary lives while taking these drugs prophylactically. Although there are associated side effects, most patients tolerate them well, except when interested in pregnancy.

Studies of medications for depressive disorders in adults show a clear advantage of antidepressants over placebos. The general classes of antidepressants—monoamine oxidase inhibitors (MAOIs), tricyclic antidepressants (TCAs), selective serotonin reuptake inhibitors (SSRIs)—are equally effective. Therefore most decisions as to which medication to use are based on the side effect profiles and matching to patient susceptibilities. In general, it is wise that family physicians become familiar with two agents in each class, though some who practice a great deal of office psychiatry may also wish to learn about a broader armamentarium. Most family physicians do not use MAOIs enough to become comfortable with them, particularly because of the associated dietary restrictions and potential drug interactions.

Tricyclic antidepressants are generally less expensive than SSRIs and are useful for treatment of insomnia. Several pharmacoeconomic studies, however, have shown that the cost of office visits, hospitalizations, and the burden of side effects of TCAs make their prescription more expensive than SSRI alternatives. They are useful for anxiety disorders and treatment of chronic pain. They do have numerous side effects, which many patients find intolerable, such as sedation and anticholinergic effects. They are highly lethal in overdose amounts, making them dangerous for the depressed, suicidal patient. The TCAs have a low therapeutic/toxic ratio with no antidote, and they are not dialyzable. Potential cardiac side effects also must be factored in, which has decreased the popularity of these once widely prescribed antidepressants. They remain a viable treatment choice for certain patients, however, especially when the physician undertakes to treat depression along with some other problems responsive to TCAs and in the occasionally recalcitrant depressive patient requiring combination therapy.

The SSRIs are usually much better tolerated, though they are more expensive. Side effects may include gastrointestinal disturbance, sexual dysfunction (except citalopram), and increased anxiety/insomnia (less likely with paroxetine).

Brief psychological therapy has been shown to be about as effective as medications for depressed patients. Whereas medication strategies usually begin to take effect within 2–6 weeks, brief therapy often takes 2 months before significant benefits are realized. A more complete discussion of medications and brief psychological therapy for depression is undertaken in the chapter on that subject.

Several classes of medication have shown a therapeutic effect for treatment of anxiety disorders. Anxiolytics such as benzodiazepines are helpful for anxiety disorders in the short term, but their long-term benefit is questionable and they tend to reduce the patient's motivation to work on the cause of the anxiety. Inducing drug dependence or addiction is a concern with this class. The benzodiazepines may impair cognition, especially in the elderly and in those with an already impaired central nervous system. Automobile and home accidents are increased in those receiving benzodiazepines. Subtle changes in socialization and motivation may also occur and are difficult to recognize as a side effect, even though they cause significant change in the quality of life and interfere with therapeutic benefit. Benzodiazepines are best used for acute anxiety to help a person return to usual activities.

For more specific types of anxiety, such as panic disorders or the phobias, SSRIs have been of some benefit. To avoid initial exaggeration of existing anxiety these drugs should be started at low dosage and be increased slowly to desensitize certain serotonin pathways involved in anxiogenesis. β-Blockers have been used to control adrenergic physical symptoms (e.g., tachycardia, tremor, panic disorder). Obsessive-compulsive disorder may respond to antidepressants or buspirone.

Long-term treatment of generalized anxiety disorder may be undertaken with buspirone. This nonsedating, nonbenzodiazepine anxiolytic has few side effects beyond gastrointestinal disturbance. Drug reactions are rare, and buspirone is nonaddictive. Some controversy exists regarding effectiveness.

In general, there are good psychological treatments for anxiety disorders that have been shown to be at least as effective as medications with less potential for side effects and more potential for lasting personal growth and change to prevent or self-treat relapse. Therefore brief psychological interventions probably represent the first-line treatment for anxiety disorders. More complete discussions can be found in the chapters on this subject.

Treating insomnia with sedative/hypnotic agents for a short duration (not exceeding 2 weeks) can be effective, easy, and inexpensive. Long-term treatment of insomnia with pharmacoactive agents should be avoided unless the myriad causes of reversible insomnia have been investigated and ruled out. Over-the-counter medications, which usually contain antihistamines, are somewhat effective but quickly lose their positive effect if used longer than 2 weeks. These agents also carry a significant risk for anticholinergic side effects especially in the elderly. Delirium, dry mouth, constipation, fecal impaction, and urinary retention are possible. Because of their safety and efficacy, low cost hypnotics such as the benzodiazepines are the most common treatment choice. They too induce tachyphylaxis and do not affect sleep in a positive way beyond 2 weeks. The chronic user who stops, however, experiences insomnia as a withdrawal phenomenon. This falsely corroborates patients' belief that they still need the drug to sleep. Because of addiction potential, benzodiazepines should rarely be used in patients with a history of substance abuse. Once used, they should be tapered slowly after a week or two to prevent rebound insomnia. Short-acting hypnotics might be better choices when sleep onset is the primary problem. Longer-acting drugs seem more reasonable if terminal insomnia is present, although "hangover" next-day sedation can be a problem with these agents. In addition to the problem of rebound insomnia, alterations in the sleep cycle may lead to less "natural" and less efficient sleep with benzodiazepines. Newer γ-aminobutyric acid (GABA) selective sedative drugs have recently become available and have significant advantages over the older benzodiazepines. The highly sedating antidepressants are frequently best for long-term treatment of insomnia when other means fail.

For most patients a sleep hygiene program such as the one described in the chapter on insomnia works sufficiently well to avoid the use of prescription drugs.

When to Refer

The decision on when to refer need not be complex in most situations. For the most part a brief intervention used by a family physician works so long as the problem is of short duration. When the problem has developed during the last few months, patients generally return to their usual level of function with brief therapy. This is true even when the problem is serious, such as major depression, so long as it is not a long-standing problem. Depression can take 4 months or more to resolve, but behavioral change should be noted after two or three appointments. If the problems are unresponsive to treatment within a couple months the doctor should consider referral. The consulting therapist, psychologist, or psychiatrist will also have a better chance for successful treatment if the problem is not yet chronic.

Long-term problems are much more difficult to treat; they require longer therapy and therefore usually are best referred. Family physician experience and patient preference, of course, must also be considered.

References

Cade B, Hudson-O'Hanlon W (1993) A Brief Guide to Brief Therapy. New York: Norton.

Campbell TL, Doherty WJ, Mooney A (1992) Reaching out to the family in crisis. Patient Care 125–136.

Eisenberg L (1996) Commentary: What Should Doctors Do in the Face of Negative Evidence? J Nervous and Mental Desease 184:103

Eshet I., Margalit A, Almagor G (1993) "SFAT-AM"—treatment approach in 10–15 minute encounters. Fam Pract 10:178–187.

Eshet I, Margalit A, Shalom J, Almagor G (1993) "SFAT-AM" during the Gulf War in Israel. Fam Syst Med 11(3):25–31.

Robinson J, Roter D (1999) Counseling by primary care physician of patients who disclose psychosocial problems. J Fam Pract 48:698–705.

Schuyler D (2000) Prescribing brief psychotherapy. Prim Care Companion J Clin Psychiatry 2(1):13–15.

2

Brief Approach to Mental Health Screening

Although most family physicians acknowledge the importance of screening for mental health problems, in fact few have a systematic way to pursue this goal. Despite the fact there are well studied, effective screening tools such as Prime-MD, screening is seldom undertaken. There are rational reasons why family physicians do not use such instruments. Prime-MD is a good example. It comprises 16 questions, which is time-consuming; and it is difficult to fit into a typical health care maintenance visit in a busy family physician's practice.

For a family physician to adopt a structured screening process it must realistically fit into the health care maintenance visit. It must be cost-effective, which means time-effective. It must be easy to learn. It must be patient-friendly; that is, the doctor must be comfortable introducing the subjects to their patients. It must be sensitive, particularly to the most common problems encountered in family practice. It must have enough specificity that the problem areas identified are serious enough to justify the time required to address them. It is well known that adjustment disorders with depression and anxiety are common among the patients who see family physicians, but many of these disorders are best not diagnosed by the physician as most of them are resolved quite well by the patients themselves. This leads to a sense of competence and self-dependence, which is important for long-term mental health adjustments, not to mention the cost savings. It is analogous to teaching patients that they can take care of their own viral infections unless they reach a pathologic threshold, the signs and symptoms of which the average patient can learn quite competently.

To make a screening process realistic for the family physician, we have developed a three-item mental health screening questionnaire. Its goal is to identify patients with any of the four most common psychosocial problems that present to the family doctor: adjustment disorders, anxiety disorders, depressive disorders, substance abuse disorders. Along with these three questions we developed a flow sheet we have found to be highly efficient in terms of time yet improves the specificity of identifying those problems that benefit from physician intervention.

Screening Questions

The three questions are as follows. "Have there been any major changes in your life or your family's life in the past year?" "When was your last drink or beer?" For adults: "How are your sleeping?" For the elderly and teenagers: "Have you stopped attending your regular activities?"

Rationale for the Questions

The rationale for choosing these questions is as follows. "Have there been any major changes in your life or your family's life in the past year?" is based on the research of Holmes and Rahe (1967). They found that individuals who had suffered a significant loss or other stresses were most likely to develop a form of psychiatric or somatic pathology during the following year. Subsequent research demonstrated that it was primarily a subset of those with significant stress who developed pathology; that is, those who became socially withdrawn and stopped their usual activities were most prone to develop serious problems. We therefore suggest the following line of questioning (Fig 2.1). If the answer to "Have there been any major changes in you or your family's life over the past year?" is negative or only minor changes are described, no related questioning is needed. If the answer is yes, the next question should be, "How are you coping?" If they are coping well, again this line of questioning can end. If, however, they describe not only serious loss but poor coping skills leading to social withdrawal and inactivity, a specific recommendation should be made to maintain the social support system and maintain at least their usual level of previous activity. Finally, one should recommend that if the patient remains significantly withdrawn from their usual social support and activity for a month they should make a follow-up visit.

"When was your last drink or beer?" comes from research on alcohol screening that shows that asking about the frequency and number of drinks in a specific, matter-of-fact way is the best way to uncover possible substance abuse. If the answer to this question is more than 1 week ago, the substance abuse questions can end (Fig. 2.2). If it is less than a week, ask "How many drinks or beers did you have last Friday night?" If the patient had three or fewer drinks on both occasions, this line of questioning can end. If the patient describes more than three drinks on either occasion, the four-part Cage questionnaire (modified based on new research) should be asked as described in Figure 2.2. If the answer to the four Cage questions is negative, the substance abuse questions can end. If one or more is positive, a period of abstinence, such as a 60-day alcohol-free period is recommended, and a further evaluation and a follow-up appointment should be scheduled. If it is clear from the Cage questionnaire that the person has a serious drinking problem, referral to a substance abuse counselor or therapist can be made at that time.

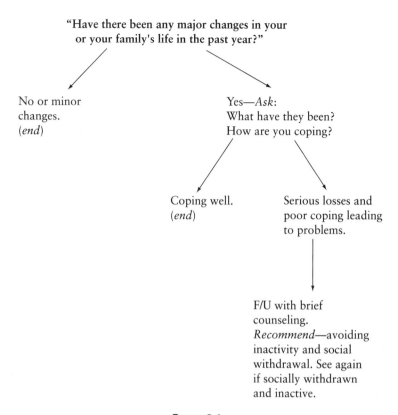

FIGURE 2.1.

"How are you sleeping?" is highly sensitive for a host of disorders, including adjustment disorders, depression, anxiety, mania, and schizophrenia. Among the common disorders for which we are screening, people who have difficulty falling asleep are most likely to have adjustment disorders, anxiety, or both. Those who have depression are likely to have terminal insomnia (i.e., early morning awakening or hypersomnolence in some cases). Some have a primary sleep disorder.

Everyone has occasional sleep problems; it is the regular pattern of insomnia that demonstrates pathology. Therefore in response to "How are you sleeping?" if the patient has only occasional difficulties this line of questioning can end (Fig. 2.3). Those who have regular difficulty achieving somnolence should be asked, "Have you been a nervous person lately?" This has been found on other screening questionnaires to be the most sensitive question for identifying stress and anxiety disorders. If the answer to this question is no, the patient most likely has a primary sleep disorder that will respond to a brief educational description of a sleep hygiene program (see Chapter 11) with a recommendation for follow-up if serious problems con-

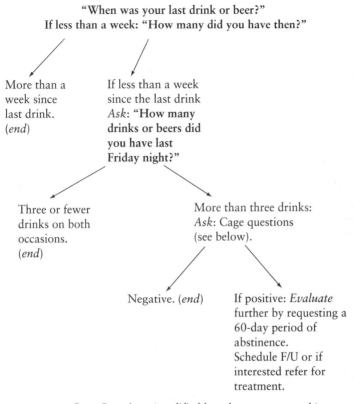

"When was your last drink or beer?"
If less than a week: "How many did you have then?"

More than a
week since
last drink.
(*end*)

If less than a week
since the last drink
Ask: "**How many
drinks or beers did
you have last
Friday night?**"

Three or fewer
drinks on both
occasions.
(*end*)

More than three drinks:
Ask: Cage questions
(see below).

Negative. (*end*)

If positive: *Evaluate*
further by requesting a
60-day period of
abstinence.
Schedule F/U or if
interested refer for
treatment.

Cage Questions (modified based on new research)

1. Have you thought you should cut down?
2. Has anyone complained about your drinking?
3. Have you felt guilty or upset about your drinking?
4. Was there a single day you had five or more?

FIGURE 2.2.

tinue. If they report yes to "Have you been a nervous person lately?" a follow-up appointment should be arranged for further evaluation and treatment of stress or anxiety disorders. Anxiety and sleep problems are common in women who are involved in an abusive relationship. The most sensitive question to date found to expose abuse is the question, "Have you been kicked, punched, or hit by anyone in the past year?"

If the patient's problem with sleeping is early morning awakening, the follow-up question should be "Have you been feeling downhearted or blue lately?" A well studied screening questionnaire showed that this question was highly sensitive and specific for identifying depression. If the answer to this question is no, the patient most likely has a primary sleep disorder. Education about a sleep hygiene program and as-needed follow-up is prob-

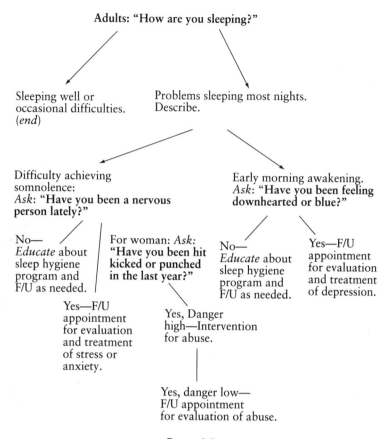

Adults: "How are you sleeping?"

Sleeping well or
occasional difficulties.
(*end*)

Problems sleeping most nights.
Describe.

Difficulty achieving
somnolence:
Ask: **"Have you been a nervous
person lately?"**

Early morning awakening.
Ask: **"Have you been feeling
downhearted or blue?"**

No—
Educate about
sleep hygiene
program and
F/U as needed.

For woman: *Ask:*
**"Have you been hit
kicked or punched
in the last year?"**

No—
Educate about
sleep hygiene
program and
F/U as needed.

Yes—F/U
appointment
for evaluation
and treatment
of depression.

Yes—F/U
appointment
for evaluation
and treatment
of stress or
anxiety.

Yes, Danger
high—Intervention
for abuse.

Yes, danger low—
F/U appointment
for evaluation of abuse.

FIGURE 2.3.

ably sufficient. If the answer is yes, they should be asked if they are having
suicidal thoughts. If they are, the crisis intervention protocol should be commenced (see Chapter 15). If there is no suicidal ideation, a follow-up appointment should be arranged for evaluation and treatment of depression.

Erratic sleep patterns are not unusual for adolescents. Likewise, changes
in sleep are common in the geriatric patient. Some even mistake normal
changes of aging, such as lighter, more interrupted sleep, as abnormal. Questions regarding sleep in these two age groups lack enough specificity to be
useful screening questions. Therefore for both the teenager and the geriatric
patient the question is, "Have you stopped attending your regular activities?" When elderly patients become depressed or anxious, the most common
pattern is that they stop their usual activities and become withdrawn.

For troubled teenagers the most common finding is withdrawal from their
usual activities and social interactions. Another marked change that is common when a teenager drops out of usual activities is a significant increase in

substance usage. Therefore noting changes in activities can be used as a prompt to investigate substance abuse as well.

If the answer to the question about changes in their daily activities or socialization is that there is little change, this line of questioning can end (Fig. 2.4). The doctor can be reassured that the chances of a high level of anxiety or depression in either age group is low. If there is a significant change in social withdrawal or their activity level, the patient should be asked, "What is a typical day for you now?" If there is still some level of daily activity and socialization, educate the patient on the need to increase

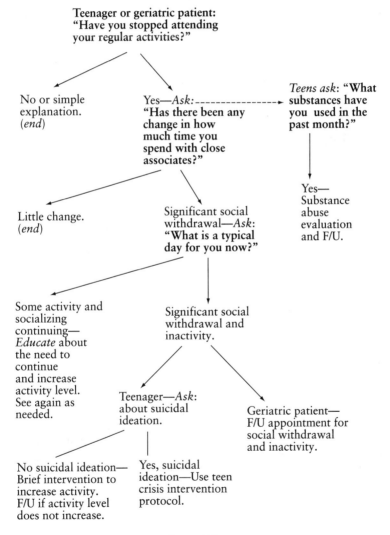

FIGURE 2.4.

their level to normal for them as soon as possible and see them again if this does not occur within a month.

For the elderly patient, if the response to the question "What is a typical day like for you now?" indicates there is significant social withdrawal and inactivity, a follow-up appointment should be made to develop a specific plan to increase this level. The appointment usually requires inclusion of significant others.

If the typical-day description demonstrates a marked decrease in teenagers' usual level of socialization and activity, they should be asked if they have used any substances during the past week. They should also be asked if they have had any suicidal thoughts. If they have not had suicidal ideation or used substances, a brief intervention should be made to increase activity and socialization, and they should be seen again as needed if activity does not increase in a month. If their answer to suicidal ideation is yes, a crisis intervention protocol and evaluation for suicide risk should be instituted (see Chapter 16). If substances have been used, an evaluation for substance abuse should be initiated (see Chapter 21).

Conclusion

For most patients only a minute or two is required to ask the screening questions. Based on the prevalence rates of patients who present to family physicians with psychosocial disorders, about 10% of the patients require a few minutes more to complete the screening evaluation and provide a brief intervention. About 3% of patients are likely to require follow-up or referral. This screening process of asking only three questions and taking only a minute or so may not be quite as effective as a number of other screening processes such as the Prime-MD, but it is much more likely to be used. As one basketball coach who could have been talking to family physicians about screening said, "You miss 100% of the shots you don't take."

References

Beresford T, Blow FC, Hill E, Singer K, Lucey MR (1990) Comparison of CAGE questionnaire and computer-assisted laboratory profiles in screening for covert alcoholism. Lancet 336:482–485.

Berwick D, Murphy JM, Goldman P, Ware J, Barsky A, Weinstein M (1991) Performance of a five-item mental health screening test. Med Care 296:169–176.

Brown RL, Leonard T, Saunders LA, Papasouliotis O (1997) A two-item screening test for alcohol and other drug problems. J Fam Pract 44:151–160.

Fleming MF (1993) Screening and brief intervention for alcohol disorders. J Fam Pract 37:231–234.

Holmes TH, Rahe RH (1967) The social readjustment rating scale. J Psychosom 11:213–218.

Isaacson J, Butler R, Zacharek M, Tzelepis A (1994) Screening with the alcohol use disorders identification test (AUDIT) in an inner-city population. J Gen Intern Med 9:550–553.

Kitchens JM (1994) Does this patient have an alcohol problem? JAMA 272:1782–1787.

Spitzer R, Kroenke K, Williams J (1999) Validation and utility of a self-report version of PRIME-MD. JAMA 282:1737–1744.

Spitzer R, Williams J, Kroenke K, et al (1994) Utility of a new procedure for diagnosing mental disorders in primary care. JAMA 272:1749–1756.

Taj N, Devera-Sales A, Vinson DC (1998) Screening for problems drinking: does a single question work? J Fam Pract 46:328–335.

3

Depression

ASSESSMENT
1. Description of patient's experience of dysphoria and depressive symptoms.
2. Evaluation of symptoms including vegetative symptoms.
3. Detailed description of a typical day including how their depressive mood affects their day as they go through it and the reactions of significant others to their depression.
4. Description of attempts by others to help.
5. Description of their own attempts to make things better.
6. Discussion of any losses or disappointments in their lives over the last year.
7. Description of any guilt feelings they are having and attempts to ameliorate them.
8. Description of any feelings of helplessness and hopelessness; and if positive, ask about suicidal ideation. If present, perform suicidal evaluation (see Chapter 15).

TREATMENT
1. If grieving, avoid long-term social isolation and inactivity. If guilt is a problem, a plan for resolution should be developed.
2. If depression is diagnosed, the advantages and disadvantages of pharmacotherapy or brief therapy treatment should be discussed with the patient (Table 3.1).

BRIEF THERAPY
1. Confronting the pattern of withdrawal and isolation includes a specific plan to become involved in one or two new activities per week, which can be recreational or vocational. If this step is too large, at least have small steps that lead in this direction. A specific plan on how they can begin a new activity should be developed. Exercise activity also has added benefit. It is most helpful if the chosen ac-

tivity helps the patient feel empowered, rather than helpless. It is usually important to elicit the help of significant others to engage the person in the activities. Family members should see the patient not as sick and helpless but as capable of change.

TABLE 3.1. Advantages/Disadvantages of Pharmacotherapy and Brief Therapy

Parameter	Antidepressant medications	Brief therapy
Efficacy	Usually 2–4 weeks, equal to brief therapy	Usually 2–4 months; equal to medications
Side effects	Troublesome to many; most common are nausea, anxiety, headache, reduced libido, and delayed sexual climax	Stressful change
Ease of administration	Easy	Changes of life style; takes time and effort
Cost	From $10/month to $120/month; average about $60/month	6–10 Appointments
Course of treatment	9 Months to lifetime	4–6 Months

2. A daily log can be kept of feelings so patients write down when they feel a little better during the day or a little worse. This log should include the activities and interactions going on at the time.
3. Patients can develop an inventory of strengths and weaknesses. They should identify at least an equal number of strengths and as they do weaknesses. If they are unable to accomplish this on their own, they can solicit the views of others, which improves social interaction. They should bring this written list to the next appointment.
4. If excessive guilt is a problem, a specific plan should address guilt resolution.

MEDICATION

If medication is the approach chosen for the withdrawn, inactive patient, choose an activating medicine, such as fluoxetine or bupropion. If the patient has up-and-down mood swings, bupropion can be considered. If a more sedating antidepressant is needed because of an anxious depression, mirtazapine or nefazodone might be considered or nortriptyline if cost is a significant issue. Maintain the patient on the medicine for at least 9 months. If relapse occurs, reconsider brief therapy or long-term maintenance medication.

Sadness and grief are normal reactions to disappointments and significant losses. Ethologists have noted that grief and sadness are important survival mechanisms. The grief reaction has probably evolved as a powerful negative force for abandoning one's group affiliates, thereby strongly encouraging maintenance of an extended family and tribe necessary for survival. Sadness and disappointment are nature's way of saying you need to change to have your needs met. The initial symptoms of major depressive episodes are often indistinguishable from those of bereavement. They each include a mood that is downcast and sad, anhedonia (lack of pleasure), alteration in appetite, sleep disorder, fatigue and lethargy, alterations in psychomotor activity, guilt, difficulties with concentration, and sometimes difficulty seeing any meaning or value to life. Even guilt has survival value for the human species, as it can be a strong motivator for prosocial behavior and sacrifice for the good of the group. Pathologic depression, however, occurs when these important survival mechanisms somehow go awry or no longer function beneficially in the present environment.

Much of the time the disappointment or loss that initiates a grief reaction is obvious. Sometimes, however, the loss is more subtle, even to the point of the person not being aware of the loss. The most common example is a marriage that has grown increasingly distant over time without overt conflict. The spouse in this situation may feel a sense of loneliness slowly overcoming them; but with the partner denying any change in the marriage, he or she may see the focus of the problem entirely within himself or herself and define the reaction as a depressive mood without a cause. Sometimes the situation is viewed as culturally inappropriate to experience as a loss, such as a child going off to college or getting married, which should be happy experiences. Most major life changes have the potential to induce depression. People who are perfectionists are prone to be disappointed in themselves and therefore often become highly guilt-ridden and prone to symptoms of depression. When a loss or disappointment has occurred and coping mechanisms fail to reestablish a sense of equilibrium, individuals may feel their lives are out of their control and so feel helpless.

Another factor contributing to depressive symptomatology is the response of others to normal sadness and disappointments. It is no fun to be around people when they are sad; therefore the initial response may be to attempt to cheer them up or give them reassurance. Others may provide care-taking and relief from responsibility for the individual until they get back on their feet. If the sadness does not diminish, however, some significant others become irritated and distance themselves. In this situation those who are suffering find themselves becoming more withdrawn and may, as a way to protect themselves from rejection, become further isolated.

Some significant others increase their caretaking in response to increased sadness. This communicates a message to sad persons that they are helpless and sick. It occurs often with the elderly, physically disabled, or highly dependent. If either pattern of behavior goes on too long, the person eventually becomes so stuck in their rut that they develop a sense of helplessness and hopelessness about finding a way out of it, which further exacerbates the symptoms of depression. This is not to say that family members being helpful is harmful; but when someone develops a sense of helplessness it can interfere with recovery. In this case the significant others must learn a new approach to what is helpful, as we discuss in the treatment section, below.

Studies have demonstrated neurophysiologic correlates to grief and depression. Disregulation of serotonin- and norepinephrine-sensitive neurons in the prefrontal and limbic regions is a well known factor in depression and grief. Dopamine and other neurotransmitter sites may also be found to be important. There appears to be disregulation of the corticosteroids as well, and in some people the immune system appears inhibited.

Environmental, neurophysiologic, endocrine, genetic, and other factors are likely involved in depression. Trying to establish specific etiologies is difficult if not impossible for any complex system with feedback loops. Fortunately, this has not been found to be necessary in the treatment of depression.

Assessment

Although many patients nowadays present to the physician with complaints of depression, the ticket of admission to the physician's office has usually been a somatic complaint. Therefore patients who have depressive disorders commonly present with some physical symptoms, such as pain, fatigue, or a sleep disorder. When a physician suspects a mood disorder, asking patients how they are sleeping is an excellent screen (see Chapter 2). A good follow-up question for those with sleep disturbance is to ask if they have felt down-hearted or blue lately. If so, in addition to exploring the patient's description of the problem, it is important to obtain a history of how the symptoms are affecting daily activities. It is also important to understand how the significant others are trying to help and what attempted solutions they have already tried. Usually others have tried to give reassurance, cheering the patients, or admonishing them to get over it and get on with their lives.

For some people these approaches work, but for patients who develop more serious symptoms these measures obviously were not helpful or even made matters worse. Important information to gather includes any losses or major changes in one's life during the past year and how the patient has coped. Guilt feelings in response to these losses or changes should be explored. Specific symptoms of depression to be sought include a sleep disturbance, appetite and weight changes, attention and concentration problems, low energy level, and fatigue. If there has been a sense of helplessness and hopelessness, patients should be asked if they are experiencing suicidal ideation. If so, a suicide evaluation should be commenced (see Chapter 15).

Treatment

If the evaluation is more suggestive of grief than depression, a plan can be offered to prevent deepening into pathologic grief. Such a program should include the patients returning to usual activities within 3 weeks of the precipitating event even if they do not feel ready. Social withdrawal and isolation should be limited. Guilt should not be avoided but dealt with directly in ways that have been helpful in the patient's past. If the patient does not respond with increased activity and socialization in a few weeks, pathologic grief should be reconsidered. This does not mean that continued grief is no longer expected. Dysphoria and other grief symptoms can take up to a year to resolve after a major loss, but a return to activity and socialization is needed much earlier. Pathologic grief and depression are indistinguishable except for an obvious loss in the case of grief. Treatment can be similar for both except that passage of time is more helpful for alleviating grief than depression.

If the evaluation reveals depression, the first decision regarding treatment is whether to institute pharmacotherapy or a brief therapy approach. This can be a difficult decision, as the two are about equally efficacious and there are advantages and disadvantages to both.

Advantages of pharmacotherapy include a short period, usually 2–4 weeks, to achieve clinically significant results and ease of administration. Newly developed drugs are usually well tolerated by patients, although there are side effects. Moreover, successful treatment requires minimal effort on the patient's part in terms of both attendance at therapy and life style changes.

Disadvantages of pharmacotherapy include some patients' intolerance to the side effects, so there is a high rate of patient dropout. There is also a significant rate of relapse unless the patient is maintained on medicine long term.

Advantages of the brief therapy approach are that the patients often achieve life style changes valuable for their long-term mental health. Patients are also less dependent on the doctor for cure at the conclusion of therapy and believe they have developed skills that can help them address future stress. They are often proud of their accomplishment and the changes they have made, which adds self-esteem.

Disadvantages of brief therapy are that the process usually requires more time and energy on the part of both caregiver and patient. The short-term costs are sometimes significantly higher, although in the long run they may not be. It usually takes 3–4 months for the patient to achieve clinically significant results in terms of reducing major depressive symptoms equal to the results obtained with medicine in 2–4 weeks. Finally, patients must accept that they need to make changes in their lives and be willing to accept brief therapy as help in making those changes.

In the past it was suggested that for those who had more vegetative signs medicine was superior, and for those who had more psychological symptoms brief therapy was superior. Outcome studies have not supported this belief. Outcomes beyond 4 months appear to be similar for all but the most severely depressed patients. There also has been some suggestion that using both pharmacotherapy and psychotherapy is superior to either alone, but studies have shown an advantage in only about 10–25% of patients (Keller, 2000). Combined therapy, then, should be reserved as a second-line approach for those who do not respond to one or the other alone.

Given these results it appears that the most patient-centered approach would be to use what has been called the transparency model of decision-making (Brody, 1993), that is, essentially thinking out loud with the patient about the advantages and disadvantages of each approach and then deciding with the patient which one to commence. Clinical experience has shown patients who are self-directed and value independence more often choose brief therapy. Patients who are more dependent, looking to others for guidance and caretaking, tend to want medication.

If brief therapy is the chosen option, it will likely entail three to six sessions. The initial two or three are weekly sessions followed by subsequent sessions at 2- to 4-week intervals. It works best if family members are included. The first session usually lasts 45 minutes to an hour. Subsequent sessions are usually about half that length.

Confronting the pattern of withdrawal and isolation is usually a good starting point. The primary strategy is to direct the patient to become involved in activities that in the past had been meaningful. This should certainly include work and some social activity. Exercise has been found to be a valuable adjunct (likely stimulating the reticular and limbic system, particularly the serotonin–, norepinephrine–, and endorphin-sensitive neurons). Confronting guilt feelings, if excessive, is important as well. Patients must feel that the new activities give them some greater control over their life circumstances. They must move from a helpless outlook to an empowered one.

Becoming involved in at least one new activity is usually valuable. The new activity should be chosen with several factors in mind: It should give patients a new sense of mastery in their life that improves their sense of being in control. If a loss is involved, it should allow the person to have some needs met that had been met by the lost person or object. Some small step in the direction of becoming involved in this new activity should be taken every week. Too large a step should be discouraged, as it often leads to failure and an even greater sense of helplessness. For example, persons who become depressed soon after their retirement might explore what needs were fulfilled by their job. Some new activity directed toward fulfilling the same needs might be explored and some action taken each week in the direction of becoming involved in that activity.

It is often helpful to request significant others' help in involving the patient in the new activity at least at first. A task such as this also helps families move away from treating patients as sick or at fault for their depression; they can now be view as capable of being involved in activities. This moves the family to support empowerment rather than helplessness. For the patient and family who feel a need to communicate about the sadness and depressive material, the discussion can be encapsulated into a brief period of time. For example, the patient should be advised to talk about the sadness for 10 minutes twice a week and then ignore it the rest of the week. Another sometimes helpful task in this regard is to ask patients to keep a daily log in which they write down everything that made them feel even slightly better or made them feel badly during that day. If they tend to write down only things that make them feel badly, at the next appointment the assignment should be to record only the things that made them feel even slightly better. Subsequent sessions should focus on gradually increasing these activities during the week.

Another task that helps to enhance self-esteem and reduce social isolation is to have patients inventory their strengths, including the good things about their personality. They should solicit the views of others and include them in the written list they bring to the doctor.

Excessive guilt can be dealt with in ways that are common for everyone, such as: (1) education about the realistic likelihood that the patient was responsible for the target event (e.g., discussion of an autopsy report after a loved one has died); (2) asking the appropriate person for forgiveness; (3) asking a secular or religious authority for forgiveness; (4) developing a plan for doing penance in a non-self-destructive way; or (5) writing a letter to the lost significant other to close unresolved issues. (If alive, this may or may not be sent.)

In summary, brief therapy should be aimed at slowly increasing activity and social interaction leading to an improved sense of competence, resolving excessive guilt if present, and changing interactional patterns with significant others away from being seen as sick and helpless to being seen as sad but capable.

Medication

If medication is the preferred treatment, the choice of which medicine to use is based on several factors. There is no significant difference in the efficacy of the various classes or individual antidepressants. Any one drug has an approximately 70% chance of being effective in an individual case. Therefore it is the side effect profile matched to the symptoms and susceptibilities of the patient that should guide the physician to the best choice.

Although many drugs are available on the market, the physician would do best to choose a limited number of antidepressants, use them regularly, and become comfortable and familiar with them. Within a class it seems reasonable to choose agents at either end of a spectrum of characteristics (e.g., sedation or activation, appetite-stimulating or appetite-depressing, long or short half-life) to be prepared to cover most clinical situations. For the patient who is withdrawn and inactive with psychomotor retardation, the more activating and less sedating medicines such as fluoxetine (Prozac) and sertraline (Zoloft), bupropion (Wellbutrin, Wellbutrin SR), and venlafaxine (Effexor, Effexor XR) might be most appropriate. For patients who have up-and-down mood swings, bupropion may be the best choice. For those who have high anxiety along with their depression, the physician might best choose a more sedating antidepressant such as: one of the tricyclic antidepressants; or nefazodone (Serzone), paroxetine (Paxil), or mirtazapine (Remeron), though the latter requires monitoring the white blood cell count.

Tricyclic antidepressants (TCAs) were once widely prescribed and effective in the treatment of depression, but they are now less preferred owing to the dangers of overdose, anticholinergic side effects, and risks of cardiotoxicity. In selected cases TCAs may still be the preferred agents, and they are much less expensive than alternative antidepressant choices. They can be useful when treating depression concomitantly with chronic pain syndromes, urge type or mixed urinary incontinence, and gastric hyperacidity.

When prescribing an antidepressant the patient's age and metabolic status must be considered when establishing the initial dosage. In the elderly the axiom "start low, go slow" is important, although the family physician should be comfortable with advancing antidepressant doses at appropriate intervals within the manufacturer's recommended guidelines rather than simply continuing for long periods of time at nontherapeutic or subtherapeutic doses (an extremely common clinical error). Obviously, at any one dose the physician must reevaluate for efficacy and side effects before making an upward titration based on the expected half-life and time to reach the efficacy characteristic of that antidepressant. A period of 2–6 weeks is needed for almost all antidepressants before one can say that a certain dose is not efficacious. From a practical standpoint 6 weeks is just too long for most patients to wait, so many practitioners use the 4-week mark as the logical reappointment interval. Most failures in treatment of depression by family physicians and subsequent referral to psychiatrists simply involve failure of the family physician to continue upward titration of what would eventually be an effective antidepressant dose. Another common error is to treat depression with tranquilizers rather than using an antidepressant.

When a certain antidepressant has proved nonefficacious or has caused side effects requiring its discontinuance, the family physician must choose a second agent. If the drug to be discontinued is a short half-life selective serotonin reuptake inhibitor (SSRI) (all but fluoxetine) or venlafaxine, it is wise to taper the drug before discontinuing totally because of the frequent occurrence of SSRI withdrawal syndrome. It is also wise to allow a 7- or 10-day "washout" period to avoid drug interaction, though for some switches this is not necessary. When changing the drug, the physician may switch to another member of the same class or go to a totally different class of antidepressants. These two strategies, surprisingly, work about equally well.

When switching from one serotonin-activating antidepressant to another, the "washout" period should be carefully observed to avoid the serotonin syndrome. Patients who are switched from one drug to another too rapidly or who undergo combination therapy may develop hyperpyrexia, tremors, seizures, and altered consciousness. The condition may be mistaken for neuroleptic malignant syndrome, but it differs in that the patient is more tremulous than rigid. Supportive therapy is all that can be provided. This medical mishap is often fatal.

Once antidepressant medication has been started and has proved efficacious, the physician should expect to treat the patient for at least 6–9 months during the first episode. Relapse is common, and stopping the drug too soon increases the likelihood. Elderly patients suffering their first episode of depression should probably be treated for 12 months, though some clinicians believe that relapse is so common as to warrant lifelong therapy in this age cohort. Nonelderly patients suffering a second episode should also be treated for 1 year. Those suffering a second episode with complications (psychotic features, suicidal ideation) should be treated for life, or brief therapy should be recommended. All those suffering a third episode should be treated for life. Brief therapy is an option in all the above situations when relapse occurs or medication fails.

Elderly patients who "take to bed" and stop eating as a symptom of their depression (a passive suicidal intent) require urgent treatment. If initial therapy with ordinary antidepressants is not quickly efficacious, brief therapy should be considered.

Patients who have suffered depression without treatment for more than 6 months often are extremely difficult to treat, and referral might be considered. The severity of symptoms is not as important in the decision to refer as is the longevity of the symptoms, although they are interrelated.

Case Report

D.R. was a 58-year-old caucasian woman who presented with vague gastrointestinal (GI) complaints. In the process of history-taking her physician asked, "Have there been any major changes in your life or your family's life in the past year?" D.R. answered that she had retired from retail sales and that 14 months ago her husband had passed away. The physician proceeded with the physical examination but persisted with this line of questioning and learned that the patient's husband had died of a myocardial infarction while having an extramarital affair. The patient showed no signs of being suicidal. The return appointment was scheduled with the physician's nursing staff who performed a Beck Depression Inventory and scheduled the patient to see the family physician again in just a few days. On the basis of the inventory and her history the physician diagnosed pathologic grief.

At the second visit the physician learned that D.R. had depended heavily on her husband for managing household finances and in many other ways. She was embarrassed and angry about the circumstances of his death but guilty that she had somehow let him down. She was confused by ambiguous feelings of anger, remorse, loneliness, and grief. The patient had become withdrawn from many of her prior activities and had quit her job (although the physician had a sense that she might have been asked to leave). At this appointment the patient was no longer experiencing gastrointestinal symptoms, and she was told her GI workup was negative. Several follow-up sessions were planned.

At each of the sessions the patient vented her feelings about her husband's death. At the third visit, the patient was asked to bring family photo albums, and the physician and patient looked at them as the patient recalled many of the good times they had had together. The physician requested that the patient write a letter to her deceased husband sharing with him symbolically her feelings about abandonment, her anger with the circumstances of his death, and her feelings about missing him. At first the patient seemed reticent to perform this assignment, but with encouragement and an explanation of the purpose of the exercise the physician gained her cooperation.

At a fourth session the patient and physician discussed the aforementioned letter. The patient seemed to gain some closure on these issues as they talked. D.R. was encouraged to begin brisk walks, perhaps enlisting a friend to walk with her on a daily basis. She was asked to undertake an assignment of going to one social event per week. She was also asked to begin a "pleasant events diary" documenting all daily events that produced some pleasure. She was asked to review the previous day or two each time she felt "blue."

At the fifth and sixth sessions the physician continued to reinforce the assignments the patient had been performing fairly compliantly. The patient was asked to increase social involvement a bit more.

At the sixth and final session the physician discussed the possibility that the patient might wish to return to some type of employment. The patient volunteered that her church had been looking for a new secretary; it would be part-time and she thought she might enjoy it without undertaking a full-time schedule that might compete with her retirement plans.

References

Bhatia S, Bhatia S (1997) Major depression: selecting safe and effective treatment. Am Fam Physician 55:1683–1693.

Coyne J (ed) (1986) Essential Papers on Depression. New York: New York University Press.

Brody H (1993) Healer's Power. New Haven: Yale Univ. Pr.

Dietrich A, Eisenberg L (1999) Better management of depression in primary care. J Fam Pract 48:945–946.

Keller MB, McCullough JP, Klein DN, et. al. (2000) Comparison of Nefazodone, the Cognitive Behavioral-Analysis System of Psychotherapy and their Combination for the Treatment of Chronic Depression N Engl J Med 342:1462–70.

Kruszewski S (2000) Approach to depressive disorders. Arch Fam Med 9:19.

Shearer S, Adams G K (1993) Nonpharmacologic aids in the treatment of depression. Am Fam Physician 47:435–440.

Smith D (1995) CNS Side Effects of Drugs in the Elderly Monograph. Providence, RI: Manissess Communications Group.

4

Anxiety

ASSESSMENT

1. Obtain a description of the presenting symptoms of anxiety, including a detailed sequence of events from before the onset through resolution. It should include the environmental context and interpersonal interactions.
2. When is the anxiety most likely to occur in the context of a typical day? Least likely to occur?
3. What stressors are most likely to bring on the fear? Under what circumstances is the fear least likely to occur?
4. What have significant others tried to do to help (e.g., reassurance)?
5. What significant changes have occurred in the patient's life or the family's life over the past year?
6. What would be different if the anxiety feelings were not present, or what change would occur if the problem were even slightly alleviated?

PLAN

1. Reframe the problem.
   a. Phobia—Define the problem as the patient's pattern of learning to avoid the fear, whereas overcoming the problem requires learning to approach the fear gradually in a more controlled way.
   b. Obsessive-compulsive disorder—Define the problem as dealing with fears by repeating rituals that are reassuring and overcontrolling for fear of losing control. The resolution can be described as finding less problematic ways to feel in control.
   c. Generalized anxiety—Define it as patients feeling out of control of their lives. The resolution is learning how to deal with stressors in a way in which they feel more in control.
   d. Panic disorder—See Chapter 5.

2. Initiate treatment by recommending that the patient not change anything at first but perform a self-observational task. The purpose of this is to help the patient and physician understand the problem in greater detail. A detailed diary should be brought to the next appointment. Family members, if possible, should also be given this task; but they are not to discuss with each other what they have written.

3. Progressive relaxation exercises can be taught to patients, or they can be asked to get a tape from the library. They should practice the exercises two or three times a day but not use them in relation to the stressors until they have learned them well.

4. At the next appointment, if the patient has improved as a result of the self-observational tasks, they can simply be asked to continue this process, as gaining an understanding helps both them and the doctor. If they have not improved, a step-by-step process to approach the problem gradually should be developed. Relaxation exercises can then be used to help them feel in control as they approach the anxiety-producing stressor. In the case of obsessive compulsive disorder (OCD), this process might be accomplished by them bringing on the obsessional thoughts as described in their diary at a specified time. It is most helpful that they do this at a time of day when they are most likely to be having these thoughts anyway. They can then use the relaxation exercises to gain a sense of being in better control. In the case of generalized anxiety, one stressor should be chosen that they can then use as a model to apply to other stressors in their life.

5. Family should be given various tasks aimed at distracting the patient from anxiety. An "as if" task can be suggested to practice normality by setting aside 1–2 hours a day to act normal. The main target is to make their lives less focused on the problem of anxiety. If secondary gain is an issue, it is important during these periods of acting normal to make sure patients are having their needs met (e.g., getting enough attention) for nonpathologic behavior.

MEDICATIONS

1. Medication is the second-line treatment. Benzodiazepines can be used short term for specific goals, such as helping them return to feared tasks. They should be started at a dose sufficient to clearly control the anxiety. After 2 weeks, a minimum of a week-long taper should begin to avoid iatrogenic rebound of symptoms.

2. If long-term medication is the treatment chosen, antidepressants with anxiolytic effects are best, such as mirtazapine, nefazedone, or nortriptyline. Medications, if used exclusively, are likely needed long term.

Everyone accepts fear as a normal part of life. Like pain, it can be seen as an instructive device for providing feedback that certain things are to be avoided. The problematic form of fear, *anxiety*, develops when something has occurred that changes the fear into an ever-increasing interference in one's life. The individual afflicted with anxiety may develop a pattern of being afraid of being afraid (e.g., panic disorder; see Chapter 5), and as a result they feel out of control of their lives. They try to alleviate the problem primarily by avoiding feared situations (e.g., phobia) or by surrounding themselves with familiar objects and experiences that reassure them (obsessive-compulsive disorder). Usually significant others try to help by offering reassurance. The individuals and families become more and more focused on the fear and the attempts to avoid it. This ultimately leads to the unfortunate corollary of the fears becoming worse and worse. For people who crave attention, this pattern can also lead to their fears becoming a way to get people to pay more attention to them. (This is usually learned unconsciously.)

Evaluation and Assessment

When the physician requests a description of the presenting complaint the patient often starts with the physical symptoms. Most often they are sympathetic nervous system responses (e.g., racing heart or profuse sweating). After obtaining a description of the problem, it is helpful to request a detailed sequence of events: how, when, and where these symptoms occur throughout the day, including what is on the person's mind before, during, and after. Because the fear of losing control or dying is prominent, it is useful to ask about these feelings specifically. If stresses related to the fear cannot be specifically identified, the focus can be on what would be different if the feelings of anxiety were not present. It is also helpful to obtain a detailed description of when things are even slightly better.

It is also important for the doctor to understand how significant others are involved. For example, how do others help out, what do they do differently as a result of the disorder? Usually the way others help is by offering reassurance and paying close attention to the patient when they are fearful. It may be that by the time the patient presents to the doctor some of the significant others have become frustrated and hostile toward the patient.

The next step is to explore the attempted solution. The most common patterns involve an avoidance pattern, which often includes not just triggers of anxiety but all stresses. For example, if work has been uncomfortable, work is now avoided. Significant others often respond with reassurance and help the patient avoid stressors. Most commonly this makes things worse: If it had made it better, the patient would not be seeking the doctor's help. Furthermore, it focuses attention on the fears and away from the normal issues of life, so the fears are exacerbated.

Goal setting should be explored next. The most common response to this inquiry is for the person to envision having "no fear." It is important to obtain a detailed description of how this would affect one's overall life. If they did not have the fear, how would their lives be different in specific ways; or if the fear was somewhat diminished, what would be the first things that would be different about their lives? If they were to have a wand or wake up tomorrow without the fear, what would they be doing differently and what would their significant others be doing differently? This information helps the doctor develop motivations for change.

Treatment

It is often helpful to define the problem as a natural process that has gone awry. For example, "It is natural for people to avoid fear, and when this doesn't work it is natural to feel overwhelmed by it. However, as with all fears, the best way to overcome it is to learn to approach the fear gradually." A useful first step that sometimes leads to significant improvement is simply to request that both the patient and family members keep a detailed diary about the fear so the doctor can learn more specifically what occurs. Patients are instructed to not alter anything but to record promptly everything they observe, including their thoughts and interactions from before the onset of the symptoms to their resolution. Family members are requested to do the same but not to discuss it with each other. It is helpful to encourage detailed, specific reporting.

This simple self-observation exercise often leads to the person feeling more in control and therefore creates an alteration of the pattern. Rather than avoiding the stressor, the person becomes intrigued and therefore is not afraid of losing control.

Another step is to teach progressive relaxation exercises and have the patients practice them several times a day. They should not apply them to the feared response until they have learned the exercise well. This again helps individuals feel more in command of their body, which confronts their feeling a loss of control.

If the person at the next session is already improved, simply doing more of the same can be suggested. If the person has not significantly improved, the next step would be to develop a hierarchy of feared situations and then approach them in gradual steps from the least to the most feared situation, usually over a period of weeks. Using the relaxation exercises in response to the fear continues to help them feel in better control. A useful first step may be to have them imagine performing the feared activity including feeling the anxiety. The relaxation exercises are then used to gain more control over the symptoms. Relaxation tapes can help. Because they feel more in command, they do not have the same experience of being out of control, and improvement occurs. The next step is to continue to approach the fear gradually in small steps, using the relaxation exercises to maintain control.

If the anxiety is more generalized, the process can still be defined as becoming more comfortable performing daily activities. In this case, focusing on one stressor as a prototype for gaining control of anxiety can help. Once a stressor is chosen, an approach similar to that used above can be employed. For example, making a mistake at work might be a reason for a perfectionist to have generalized anxiety. The person might be expected to make a small mistake deliberately and then do relaxation exercises, which interferes with the usual avoidance mechanism and teaches them they can live with mistakes. Making a mistake on purpose also adds to a greater sense of being in control.

Another helpful approach is to use the information about when things are "even slightly better" to plan ways to recreate similar circumstances more often. For example, if socializing with the family is relaxing, finding more ways to socialize might help.

It is helpful to include the family in the treatment process. This is commonly done in several ways. The family can rehearse with the patient what life will be like when things are back to normal. For example, normal activity can be practiced for 1–2 hours a day by the family with routine activities. During this time the patient and family pretend that the patient does not have a problem. If the patient has any difficulties, the family, for this hour, is to ignore them and go on with their normal routine. Another approach is to have the family use distracting activity, performing normal routines when the person is pretending to have anxiety attacks, so they can learn how to distract them. Another approach is to have the family help patients perform the relaxation exercises more effectively by having them practice them while challenged with reminders of the precipitating fears. All of these approaches have the same purpose: moving the patient and family out of the avoidance pattern that centers their life on the anxiety. Asking the family to perform pleasant activities together for distraction from anxiety also can improve success, as it provides alternative ways for care-taking behaviors to occur without the need for increased symptoms. The goal is for the patient to receive attention for nonpathologic behavior (eliminating secondary gain and learned helplessness and making their lives non-symptom-focused).

Once improvement is recognized by the patient and family, a go-slow approach can help. The patient and family can be told it may be safest to improve slowly, as certain other changes may follow for which they may not be ready. For example, "You may not be comfortable with the increased freedom improvement might offer. You may develop increased expectations for the patient because he [or she] is no longer handicapped, and these changes and challenges are best faced only very slowly." This go-slow approach can help keep the improvement moving forward.

Medication

Medication should be second-line treatment for anxiety. When medications are considered, benzodiazepines are reserved for short-term use only (a few weeks). The risk of using the medicine this way is that patients who receive immediate relief are not motivated to work at the more gradual approach to relieving the anxiety. They quickly develop a psychological dependence on drugs. Benzodiazepines may help prevent the patient from developing a pattern of avoidance. In this case the patient should receive an adequate dose to start but should be required to return to usual activity as a condition of receiving the medication. After 2 weeks a week-long tapering process should be instituted to decrease rebound symptoms.

If long-term medication is the treatment chosen, antidepressants comprise a more effective choice. Because the more activating drugs often cause generalized anxiety, it is usually better to choose one of the more sedating ones, such as mirtazapine, nefazodone, or nortriptyline. If SSRIs are used they should be started at half the usual dose and titrated up slowly to avoid symptoms of generalized anxiety. Some types of anxiety, such as obsessive-compulsive disorder, respond best to this approach.

Long-term treatment of generalized anxiety may be undertaken with buspirone. This nonsedating, nonbenzodiazepine has few side effects beyond gastrointestinal disturbance. Similar to antidepressants, this drug requires approximately 2 weeks to start having an effect.

If used exclusively, medication is likely to be needed long term.

Case Report

J.N. is an 18-year-old high school senior who was initially seen because of a fine tremor in his fingers. His father, a physician, had told him 3 years previously when he discovered it that it was not abnormal and not to be concerned about it. However, he played the fiddle in a bluegrass music group and was concerned that it would cause him to make mistakes. It had become increasingly worse before performances, so a physician placed him on β-blockers. This seemed to help initially but had gradually become less effective. Things recently reached crisis proportions when he, after his 18th birthday, began emergency medical technician (EMT) training. He proceeded well with the training, but while learning to start intravenous infusions (IVs), he had shaken so badly the exercise had to be terminated. On his demand his father had agreed to have him seen by a neurologist, who diagnosed the problem as idiopathic tremor exacerbated by anxiety. He had refused the neurologist's suggestion to see a psychiatrist but had agreed to go back to see the family doctor. He was considering quitting EMT training. The family doctor, after evaluating him, reframed the problem for J.N., telling him that he had performance anxiety, which made his fine tremor worse. He told him the benzodiazepines that he was seeking were not a good drug in situations that required rapid reaction time, such as being an EMT or a musician.

The physician proposed that he learn how to "be in control of his body instead." He was given relaxation exercises to learn and was told to keep a detailed diary of everything that was going on around him and in his mind whenever the tremor appeared so they could learn more about the problem.

At the next appointment J.N. reported he had acquired a tape on self-hypnosis at the library and had played it enough times that he felt he was pretty good at it. His diary revealed fear of mistakes as the primary source of his anxiety. He admitted to perfectionist tendencies. He was given three tasks at this appointment. One was to try to make his tremor worse by sitting once a day and telling himself all the mistakes he was going to make while practicing his fiddle and then using the relaxation exercises to help him gain control over his extremities. Next, while practicing with his band, he was to make a mistake purposefully and come up with some sort of humorous joke or routine to deal with the mistake. This was framed as his need to learn how to deal with imperfections and mistakes rather than fear and avoid them. Finally, he was to obtain some pigs' feet, draw a line on them, and puncture them repeatedly with needles as practice for starting IV lines. He was to use his relaxation cues to establish a relaxed state just prior to the puncture. He was to repeat this at least 100 times a day. The next appointment was set for 2 weeks to give him enough time to work on these tasks.

At the next appointment he expressed delight with the results. In fact, the comedy routine he developed around his mistakes had gotten such a good laugh at practice that he was disappointed when he did not make a mistake in his performance and had no opportunity to use it. He also felt much more confident about his EMT training.

At this final appointment he was told that he could use this overall approach of learning how to approach his fear rather than avoid it for other times in his life when fear was interfering with his abilities. He was then comfortable, returning on an as-needed basis.

References

Bruce T, Saeed S (1999) Social anxiety disorder: a common, underrecognized mental disorder. Am Fam Physician 60:2311–2320, 2322.

Danton W, Altrocchi J, Antonuccio D, Basta R (1994) Nondrug treatment of anxiety. Am Fam Physician, 49:161–166.

Lehman A, Salovey P (1990) An introduction to cognitive-behavior therapy. In Wells RA, Giannetti VJ (eds) Handbook of the Brief Therapies. New York: Plenum.

Michels P (1997) Am Fam Physician: Anxiety Monograph (212th ed). Kansas City, MO: American Academy of Family Physicians.

Nymberg J, VanNoppen B (1994) Obsessive-compulsive disorder: a concealed diagnosis. American Family Physician, 49:1129–1137, 1142–1124.

Smith D (2000) Recognition and treatment of anxiety in long term care. Ann Long TermCare 8(3):88–89.

Stein M (1999) Coming face-to-face with social phobia. Am Fam Physician 60:2244, 2247.

Walley E, Beebe D, Clark L (1994) Management of common anxiety disorders. Am Fam Physician 50:1745–1753, 1757–1748.

5

Panic Disorder

ASSESSMENT

1. Patients with panic disorder most commonly present with neurologic symptoms mediated by the sympathetic system, including chest pain, choking, dizziness, flushes, hyperventilation, nausea, paresthesias, shortness of breath, tachycardia, trembling. Psychological symptoms include fear of dying, fear of losing control, going insane.
2. Medical workup is indicated in some cases. The patient should be told that a negative workup is expected.
3. History should include a detailed description of the sequence of events starting before the onset and then through resolution, the thoughts going through the patient's mind at each step of the occurrence, and how significant others respond to the panic attacks.

PLAN

The central theme of brief therapy is that the psychological trigger is the fear of losing control, essentially fear of being afraid. Once the patient has gained a sense of being in control, the panic attacks subside.

1. Prescribe progressive relaxation exercises. Patient practices them twice daily but does not apply them to the anxiety until good at them.
2. Self-observational task. Explain that understanding the attacks in more detail is helpful. Patient should keep a diary either during the attack or as soon afterward as possible and bring it to the next appointment. The family should do the same but not discuss it.
3. At the next appointment the primary goal is to learn to practice bringing on the symptoms. Use the descriptions in the diary as a trigger to bring on the attacks. Once the attack occurs, use the relaxation exercises they practiced. They should continue the diary. Family should be encouraged to avoid reassurance and should engage in distracting, normalizing activities.

4. At the next appointment the prescribed task can be that when they have a panic attack to first try to make it worse using what they have learned from their diary. Once they have made the attack worse, use the relaxation exercises to help it subside. Often even before this task is presented, the panic attacks have begun to diminish markedly.

MEDICATION FOR TREATMENT OF PANIC DISORDERS

1. Medication is second-line treatment. Benzodiazepines are avoided where possible. At most they should be used for only 2 weeks with a week taper to maintain patients at their usual level of activity.
2. SSRIs have been shown to be effective for panic but can increase a generalized anxiety disorder in the prone patient. Gradually titrating the dosage upward helps. The more-sedating antidepressants (e.g., mirtazapine, nefazodone, nortriptyline) are likely more effective. Tricyclics, if tolerated, are less expensive. Starting at low doses and gradually increasing the dose is highly desirable. If used, patients should expect to be on these medicines long term.

Patients with panic disorder are commonly seen in family practice. It is highly desirable to begin prompt treatment when a patient presents with new-onset panic disorder to prevent the frequent sequelae of agoraphobia and depression. As with most other problems, early treatment makes resolution easier and more successful.

Patients most often present with somatic symptoms that reflect a high level of sympathetic activity and fearfulness. Symptoms may include the following.

Chest pain or discomfort
Choking
Dizziness, unsteady feelings, faintness
Flushes or chills
Hyperventilation
Nausea or abdominal distress
Paresthesias
Shortness of breath or the sensation of smothering
Tachycardia
Trembling or shaking
Depersonalization or derealization
Fear of dying
Fear of doing or saying something uncontrollably
Fear of going insane

When asked what they are feeling during an attack, common responses are that they have a sense of being out of control, of being insane; or they fear they are dying. Often the initial panic experience occurs at stressful times (e.g., prior to a final examination, before participation in an athletic event, during an argument with a friend). The patient, however, sees no reason for being panicked and considers it an out-of-control response. They worry about it occurring again. This worry is most prominent at times of relative inactivity. For example, in the evening a patient is watching a boring television show and begins to wonder if his or her heart rate is faster than normal. At that moment, it likely speeds up and is faster than normal. This frightens the patient and sets off a cascade of events that causes high sympathetic arousal and fear of dying and being "crazy," out of control.

For some people these panic attacks are infrequent, isolated occurrences that have little impact on their lives. For others they recur repeatedly and often with increasing frequency, which causes individuals to become more and more isolated as they orient their life around avoiding the attacks. They become fearful of being fearful.

A medical workup is indicated in some cases, but repeated testing and referral to subspecialists raises the alarm level and can be counterproductive. The differential diagnosis might include other anxiety disorders, drug abuse (especially stimulant drugs), endocrinologic disorders (hyperthyroidism), arrhythmias (or other heart disorders or transient ischemic attacks primarily in older patients), and anticipatory grief (e.g., fear of a spouse's separation). It is a good idea prior to commencing the workup to tell the patient it is unlikely that organic pathology will be found; otherwise the patient may press for more workup, fearing that something may have been missed.

When gathering the history it is helpful to obtain a detailed description of the sequence of events that precedes the episodes and of the panic attacks themselves and how they resolve. This description should include what thoughts are going through the patient's mind at each step of the occurrence and how others interact with the patient before, during, and after the attack.

Treatment

Particularly with new-onset panic disorder, brief therapy is highly effective. The primary advantage of the brief therapy approach is that not only does it have a high level of success (about equal to that of medicines), when patients have completed the therapeutic process they have a greater sense of being in control of their lives and having overcome a serious problem. Pharmacotherapy, on the other hand, leaves the patient feeling dependent on the doctor for cure. Therefore patients using medication are likely to require them for a long time.

The disadvantage of brief therapy is that it requires a time commitment by the physician of at least two or three meetings of a half-hour each and several follow-up visits of at least 15–20 minutes each. It also requires a considerable effort on the part of the patient. Pharmacotherapy, on the other hand, requires little time by the physician and little effort by the patient. A combined approach yields some of the advantages and disadvantages of both approaches, and the efficacy rate is slightly higher than when either approach is used alone. Once they use medication, some patients lose all motivation for brief therapy, as their symptoms resolve without effort. For some, medication prevents them from entering a pattern of withdrawal from activity while they are learning behavioral techniques.

Brief Therapy

The central theme of the brief therapy approach is that the psychological trigger for the fear response is fear of losing control. Once patients gain a sense of being in control of themselves, they do not have the panic attack. For brief therapy, start with a short description of the relation of fear and the sympathetic response (fight and flight response). Explain that the more they learn about their fear response and being in control of their body, the more easily will the symptoms resolve. They are then briefly taught a progressive relaxation exercise (see Chapter 14), or a relaxation tape is prescribed and they are told to practice with it at least twice a day for the next week. They are then given a self-observational task.

They are told initially not to try to alter anything; learning about their attacks is the first step. They should keep a diary of all their panic episodes, including what they were doing and thinking prior to the attack and what action, dialogue with others, and thinking occurred during the attack and afterward. They are to write this down as soon as the episode is over or, even better, as they are experiencing it. Finally, the patient is told that no matter how uncomfortable they are they should not avoid their usual activities—that avoiding them will only make them feel worse. In fact, so long as they stay busy they are less likely to have the panic attacks. It is not unusual that the self-observation exercise itself helps improve panic.

At the next appointment the primary goal is to learn to practice purposefully bringing on the symptoms to learn to be in control of them. After reading the patient's diary of attacks, it should be easy to determine how the episodes usually start. Patients are then told to reproduce this sequence at least two or three times a day, bringing on a panic attack. For example, initiation of symptoms commonly begins when they tell themselves that their chest is beginning to feel funny, that they are breathing fast, that they are losing control. They are told to repeat these thoughts that usually precede an attack until they bring on a panic attack. When they have brought on the attack, they are told to then use the relaxation exercises they have learned to help gain a sense of control and help the panic attack dissipate.

There may be some resistance to this plan, but they can be told that if they can make the panic attacks occur they can ultimately make them go away. They are again encouraged to maintain their usual activities and continue to practice the relaxation exercises twice daily.

It is helpful to have a family member or significant other present at this appointment. Family members, in attempts to help, commonly make two mistakes that exacerbate the problem. First, they provide reassurance that there is nothing to worry about, which only focuses more attention on the anxiety and has the effect of making the person feel crazier because it defines their fear as "sick." The other common attempted solution is to be protective and help the person avoid anxiety. This leads to much attention and care focused on the patient for "sick" behavior, a secondary gain that tends to exacerbate the problem. Instead, they are told to help the person distract themselves from the attacks by proposing to undertake "normal" activities the patient has enjoyed in the past.

Follow-up should again occur in about 1 week. Often at follow-up patients confide that although they attempt to bring on the attacks they cannot. This is explained by the fact that the very process of trying to bring on an attack abrogates the sense of feeling out of control, and therefore the patients cannot bring them on. Even if they can, the panic attacks are not experienced so fearfully. If the patients have been able to bring on a panic attack and then practice relaxation, they are congratulated. If they have not been able to bring on the panic attack, they are told this is okay but that there is a way to make it a bit easier for them. In both cases their specific prescription is that in the future whenever they feel a panic attack coming on they are to attempt to make it worse by telling themselves all the usual things they tell themselves when they are beginning to have a panic attack. This interrupts the usual sequence of events where the patient (and others) attempt to calm themselves by saying there is nothing to worry about, which only leads them to feel worse. They are instructed that once they have attempted to make the panic attack "worse" they should use the relaxation exercise to gain mastery over their sympathetic response. Again the usual response is the patient feels more in control and improves.

Once improvement has occurred, the appointments can begin to be spaced out to every 2 weeks, then every 3 weeks, and so forth. If the person continues to have an occasional panic attack, it should be reframed as not a relapse but as an opportunity for the person to work on continuing to gain more and more control by practicing to make it worse and then using relaxation exercises to make it better. If the patients do not improve within a month or two, a referral is indicated.

Medication

Medications can be effective treatment for panic disorder. They are best used when other attempts at preventing patients from dropping out of usual activities are not effective. Sometimes patients are so resistant to even brief therapy by the family physician that it is the best alternative.

Benzodiazepines are commonly used to treat panic disorder because they are easy, quick, and effective in the short term. The primary drawback is that a large number of patients develop psychological, if not physical, dependence. Psychological dependence develops rapidly in some patients. Even at low doses these drugs have a small but noticeable effect on sensitive tests of mental status such as IQ tests. At higher doses the effect on mental ability is more pronounced. If they are used, they are most effective on a scheduled dosage rather than as needed, so they prevent the surges of panic and anticipatory anxiety. They also help reduce chronic anxiety between attacks. Long-term follow-up of pharmacologic intervention suggests that the relapse rate following termination of treatment is high for benzodiazepines. Therefore psychological dependence often quickly develops, and there is a potential after long-term usage for physiologic addiction.

The SSRIs have been shown to be effective for panic disorder with fewer side effects than tricyclic antidepressants. When SSRIs are used to treat panic initially, they should be started at one-half or less the initial antidepressant starting dosage. This decreases the potential for developing iatrogenic generalized anxiety in these especially susceptible patients. The initial small dose should probably be used for several weeks before titrating upward. During this titration period it may be necessary to use a benzodiazepine temporarily for quick relief of anxiety, though it should be discontinued when the SSRI has reached a higher dosage level. It is important to remember that most SSRIs cause significant sexual dysfunction. Such a prescription may be an especially egregious error in patients who are having relationship problems or who are feeling insecure. Like tricyclic antidepressants, the SSRIs effectively treat and perhaps prevent the development of co-morbid depression, an event that occurs perhaps 40% of the time.

Tricyclic antidepressants are also effective for the treatment of panic disorder. They have the advantage of having a much lower potential for psychological dependence and no known physiologic dependence. They have the benefit of treating concomitant depression when it is apparent as well. When gradually withdrawn after several months of usage, they are associated with a much lower rate of relapse than the benzodiazepines. Usually it is best to start at a rather low dosage and gradually increase it. It is important to remember that some panic disorder patients become so distressed they may attempt suicide to escape from a severe panic attack. Tricyclic antidepressants are "perfect poisons" and so should be used with great caution if the panic disorder is severe and the patient is considered suicide-prone. Suicide may occur with panic disorder even when there is no co-morbid depression.

It has been suggested that medications are useful in conjunction with brief therapy, but this is not necessarily true. In many cases patients who start taking medication are not motivated to work on problems. Hence once medication is started it may be difficult to stop it without a relapse.

Case Report

J.S. was a 23 year old caucasian woman, frail-appearing and short of stature. She was a fourth-grade teacher who had functioned well in her job and her marriage until 2 months before presentation to her family physician. She reported recurring episodes of gripping fear for no apparent reason, with chest tightness, pounding heart, shortness of breath, and a feeling of unreality "as if I'm going to explode." She asked if she were "losing her mind." She denied depression or suicidal thoughts but did have problems with sleep onset. When questioned she reported that the "trigger" for these episodes was often, but not always, leaving the house. She could guarantee that the episode would occur if she drove into the Texas countryside, "where I am away from everything and it is wide open." After a brief physical examination and obtaining a history of no illicit drug use or prescription drugs that might cause anxiety, the physician made a presumptive diagnosis of panic disorder with agoraphobia. He immediately discussed this diagnosis with the patient and educated her on the physiology of the fight/flight reflex, assuring her that she was not going "crazy."

The family physician prescribed that a diary be kept of the panic episodes, specific details, how far she needed to travel before one would occur, how long each lasted, and how severe it was. The patient was asked not to do anything about these attacks as yet, indicating that there was a need to develop baseline data before planning a treatment. The physician did, however, ask the patient to begin relaxation exercises and taught her how to "self-talk," reminding herself that "*it* doesn't stress me, *I* stress me." A visit was planned in 1 week.

At that visit the family physician asked J.S. to undertake bringing on the panic attack right there in the office and then to perform the relaxation exercise and self-talk to "bring herself back down." At first the patient was reticent, but she was reassured that the physician would remain with her during the exercise and she agreed. She was told that by doing this exercise she was gaining control of her body. She surprised herself by being able to perform this task and seemed quite proud. The physician told J.S. that she could repeat this exercise at home as many times as she wished and could use the technique when a panic attack occurred of its own accord. He said that he expected a full report about this in her diary at the next visit. Again the patient was reticent and required that the physician reassure her that this was the proper technique to relieve herself of these attacks. He reminded her of her success here in the office and praised her.

At the third visit the physician began to work on the agoraphobia component of the patient's disorder. J.S. had successfully practiced control of self-generated panic attacks and of two spontaneous attacks. The physician prescribed daily walks one-half block farther from the house each day. At the fifth visit the patient related success with this exercise, and treatment was advanced to include short drives in the car alone but in town. The previously learned techniques were used each time her ventures out of the home precipitated panic. Finally, the patient was asked to venture into the barren countryside with her husband driving and then alone in her car. Again she was to use her techniques for dealing with an attack. A month later the patient returned, indicating that the program had worked beautifully, with each successive panic attack being less severe and more easily controlled until she had had none for a week. She had then experienced a small attack the day before and was frightened that she might be relapsing. The physician told the patient that this was not unusual and asked whether she had been doing the relaxation exercises or practicing causing and relieving the panic attack at home. The patient reported that she had not. She was told that this still be necessary for an indefinite period and she should simply perform these exercises as often as necessary to relieve or even prevent future panic attacks.

Four months later while seeing the patient's daughter for an upper respiratory infection the physician was able to ask J.S. whether she had been troubled by her panic disorder and agoraphobia. She reported that it was seldom a problem and went on to discuss her daughter's illness.

References

Barlow D, Gorman J, Shear M, Woods S (2000) Cognitive-behavioral therapy, imipramine, or their combination their combination for panic disorder: a randomized controlled trial. JAMA 283:2529–2536.
Katernadahl D (1996) Panic attacks and panic disorder. J Fam Pract 43:275–282.
Rosenbaum J, Pollock R, Otto M, Pollack M (1995) Integrated treatment of panic disorder. Bull Menninger Clin 59:A4–A26.
Saeed S, Bruce T (1998) Panic disorder: effective treatment options. Am Fam Physician 57:2405–2412, 2419–2420.
Vanin J, Vanin S (1998) Panic disorder: diagnosis and treatment in primary care. Am Fam Physician 57:2328, 2334.
Zarate R, Agras W (1994) Psychosocial treatment of phobia and panic disorders. Psychiatry, 57:133–141.

6

Posttraumatic Stress Disorder

PREVENTION

Following exposure to a traumatic event, symptoms, including nightmares, flashbacks, emotional lability, poor sleep, impaired appetite, and guilt, usually resolve over the course of 3 months to 2 years. To shorten the initial symptoms, a four-step process can be initiated.

1. Have patients describe the events and help them come to terms with their reality. This may have to be repeated with significant others.
2. Help patients express their feelings and normalize them.
3. Encourage the use of coping mechanisms that in the past have been helpful during highly stressful situations.
4. Encourage a return to normal activity with the expectation that things will continue to improve.

Risk factors for developing chronic posttraumatic stress disorder (PTSD) include people who have a long-standing sense of little control over their lives, a sense of helplessness, poor self-esteem, little support from significant others, and high guilt for the trauma unmediated by realistic assessment. There was also a past history of trauma, and the trauma was extreme.

For those at high risk for developing chronic PTSD, a more specific plan should be developed for return to normal activity and helping them confront excessive guilt feelings. Significant others should be directed to help provide nonjudgmental support and reinforce a return to normal activities.

ASSESSMENT

1. If symptoms do not continue to diminish after 3 months or have not significantly resolved by a year, a more comprehensive treatment program is indicated.
2. Symptoms of chronic PTSD include intrusive recollections, distressing dreams, flashbacks particularly after exposure to cues, dysphoric state, avoidance of cues, amnesia for the event, loss of inter-

est in usual activity, hyperarousal, angry outbursts, difficulty concentrating, and an exaggerated startle response. Substance abuse and depressive symptomatology are also common.
3. If substance abuse is significant, it must be addressed before other treatments can produce benefit.
4. Symptoms should be evaluated in the context of a typical day. When and what makes them better or worse? How do significant others respond? What has been tried already?

PLAN

1. The problem should be reframed for the patient as a sense of helplessness and powerlessness that must be overcome.
2. Treatment can start with a self-observational task directed toward cues and other stressors.
3. Stress reduction techniques, such as progressive relaxation, should be taught and used when confronting the anxiety to help persons feel more in control of their lives. A desensitization process to cues should be implemented, as should a specific plan to return to normal activity.
4. The overall goal is to help the person gain a sense of control.
5. Medication plays a limited role. Benzodiazepines are not helpful long term. Antidepressants with anxiolytic qualities may be helpful if there is significant depressive symptomatology.

Most people subjected to psychological trauma, especially severe trauma, suffer significant psychological pain similar to a grief reaction. This initially includes shock and denial, which soon give way to nightmares, flashbacks, emotional lability, poor sleep, impaired appetite, and guilt/self-recrimination. Most victims of psychological trauma, however, improve rapidly for 2–3 months, then more gradually over the course of 2 years. Studies show that about 4–10% are left with significant sequelae of PTSD after 2 years.

The diagnosis of chronic PTSD indicates the presence of symptoms for at least 3 months following a severe stressor such as rape, assault, severe accident, witnessing a catastrophe, or being involved in a disaster. Patients with chronic PTSD reexperience symptoms such as intrusive recollections, distressing dreams, flashbacks, and distress at exposure to such cues including associated effects: anxiety, dysphoric state, and other physiologic reactions to the exposure to cues. There is often an avoidance pattern of cues specifically or generally, such as amnesia for the event, diminished interest in significant activities and overall withdrawal, restricted affect, and a sense of no future. Patients have increased arousal, for example, a sleep disorder, irritability, angry outbursts, difficulty concentrating, hypervigilance, and an exaggerated startle response.

There are known risk factors that differentiate those who are likely to recover spontaneously from those who are likely to develop chronic PTSD. Therefore the strategy of early treatment by the family physician should be to help the victims through the initial traumatic phase and provide more comprehensive early intervention for those at risk for developing chronic symptoms. This is especially important because there is a high incidence of substance abuse and depression associated with chronic PTSD; and once these symptoms are established, treatment is markedly more difficult than preventive measures.

Psychological First Aid for Exposure to Trauma

Psychological first aid, primarily debriefing, can provide an attenuation of early symptoms. However, long-term studies have not shown a benefit of debriefing to prevent chronic PTSD. Because it requires no more than one or two visits for debriefing, it probably is worth offering to patients to decrease their short-term suffering.

If it is to be useful, debriefing should be offered as soon after the event as possible. If a widespread disaster has occurred, it is often most helpful to do the debriefing with a group of people who have shared the traumatic experience, whereas in the case of response to a rape or assault it may be done on a one-to-one basis or, better, with a significant other present. Usually the process is in four steps. The first stage includes the person describing the event and helping him or her come to terms with the reality of it. The second task is helping them express their feelings and reactions and then normalizing them. They often believe their reactions are crazy, whereas a wide range of reactions is quite normal. A useful way to elicit an emotional response is to empathize openly. For example, "If that was happening to me I'd be frightened and angry." Third, explore coping mechanisms; that is, what in the past has been most helpful when they have had to face tragedy or grief. Finally termination, which should include the expectation that things will improve, developing an optimistic attitude, and perhaps some discussion of what can be learned from the event. There should be a definite plan to resume normal activities within a rather short time (i.e., days or a few weeks at most). Avoiding normal activity can lead to chronic problems. Patients should be told that normal activities distract them from uncomfortable memories. Relaxation exercises can help the patient feel more in control when bothered by anxious memories. Explore any guilt feelings that might hamper improvement. If guilt is a problem, help patients evaluate their guilt feelings realistically while respecting them: "I know you feel you should have done more, but it sounds like you did what could be done."

For those who have good support (i.e., nonjudgmental caring family members or a significant other) and few risk factors (as noted below), this is all that is necessary. Patient and significant others should be told the person needs a chance to discuss the feelings at first. The family should be taught to validate the patient's feelings as normal after trauma. Over a period of weeks the person should be expected to return to more normal activity. The family can be taught the value of distracting activities.

Assessing Risk Factors for Chronic PTSD

Those at high risk for chronic PTSD have a long-standing sense of little control over their lives (a sense of helplessness in the face of stressors), poor self-esteem, little support from significant others, high levels of guilt about the trauma, and a past history of significant trauma. The trauma was likely extreme (e.g., torture, witnessing grotesque death, humiliation, serious injury, extreme terror), or loved ones may have been lost as a result of the traumatic experience. Generally, the more negative factors, the more likely is the patient to develop chronic PTSD.

Because of the fact that once chronic PTSD develops it is much more difficult to treat, for those with high risk factors preventive treatment is desirable. Interventions for those at serious risk include stress reduction techniques (e.g., progressive relaxation, biofeedback, meditation), which can help them feel more in control of themselves when anxiety symptoms occur. A specific plan (including a time frame) for returning to normal activities, including work, can help them gain a sense of mastery. A counseling session with significant others present is directed at helping them provide nonjudgmental support but not reinforce illness behaviors by giving more attention to normal behavior than sick behavior. This is particularly important for dependent patients. For those with excessive guilt feelings, developing a plan for resolution can be helpful (see description of treatment for excessive guilt in Chapter 27). The patient should be asked about suicidal ideation if feeling excessively guilty. If the patient is suicidal or potentially violent, referral is indicated.

Treatment for Chronic PTSD

If symptoms of chronic PTSD have developed, treatment directed at these problems should be instituted as soon as possible because, as previously stated, the longer they become a part of the person's life the more recalcitrant they are to treatment. Although initially disclosure and emotional venting are helpful, as time goes on this becomes less useful and treatment should be directed more at helping patients gain a sense of mastery to return to a more normal life. It is helpful to frame the problems to them as: "You are still letting the trauma [e.g., the rapist] control your life, and it is time for you to kick that person [or event] out of your life so you are in control again."

Helping with control of anxiety and desensitization to cues is often most helpful. For example, if this person is now afraid of relationships with men, an approach to becoming more comfortable with men, particularly a sense of being in greater control, should be seen as the central plan. Using a self-observational task (e.g., keeping a diary) for symptoms of anxiety can help the patient gain a greater sense of mastery and self-control (see Chapter one). If there is avoidance of cues, it is helpful to use a desensitization approach. Involving a significant other to help the patient gradually approach the cue while performing relaxation exercises, rather than avoid it, can be helpful.

For example, a combination desensitization plus self-observational approach might go as follows. You said, "You were raped by a man who followed you out of a bar, grabbed you in the parking lot, and dragged you into his car. Now you have flashbacks and become terrified whenever you go into a parking lot. I'd like you to practice the following program next week."

1. Relaxation exercises twice daily.
2. Once daily imagine yourself at a parking lot for 5 minutes, write down everything going through your head; daily increase this exercise by 1 minute.
3. After 5 days of steps 1 and 2 go to a parking lot with a support person, get out of the car, and stand there for 5 minutes. Write in a diary everything going through your head until you get home. Do this daily for 3 days, increasing your time 2 minutes per day. When you get home practice your relaxation exercises. Your support person must remain silent, *not* giving reassurance.
4. Follow-up appointment: If improving, keep gradually increasing the time in the parking lot and have the support person move gradually farther away in the parking lot. Continue writing in the diary. If there is no progress, explore the secondary gain and attempt to pay more attention when there is progress. For example, go out to dinner with friend or significant other when you have made progress.

If there is more than one cue causing problems, it is best to address one cue at a time. If substance abuse has already become a problem, it usually must be addressed before other treatments can be useful.

Medication

Medications have been disappointing in the treatment of PTSD. Tranquilizers and especially benzodiazepines are to be avoided. In many old movies the physician runs to the bedside and gives a sedative to the hysterical victim of some tragedy. This is not to be emulated, as preventing a victim from "working through" the psychological stresses of tragedy can actually worsen the problem. Prevention of chronic PTSD should be accomplished most of the time without medication. Once chronic PTSD has become established, medications are still ineffective. If agitated depression is a characteristic of the clinical picture, however, antidepressants with anxiolytic qualities may be helpful. Sertraline is the only agent approved for PTSD, but mirtazapine, nefazodone, or nortriptyline might be considered. Sedative hypnotics are to be avoided for treatment of sleep problems associated with PTSD. These drugs affect rapid-eye-movement (REM) sleep unfavorably. Because substance abuse is characteristic of established PTSD, these potentially addictive drugs are often misused.

Case Report

C.T. was a 20-year-old college freshman away from home for the first time. She supplemented her allowance from her parents for living expenses at college by working at the local convenience store. This somewhat unattractive young woman had few friends and low self-esteem. However, she and her roommate had similar backgrounds and social status at the college and had developed a warm friendship. C.T.'s roommate was keeping her company during a late shift at the convenience store when a gunman came in demanding money. C.T. quickly filled a brown bag with the contents of the cash register as she had been instructed and handed it to the gunman. By pure accident a police cruiser drove by at that moment, and the gunman grabbed C.T.'s roommate around the neck and chest dragging her along as he hurried to his automobile to get away. The girl's screams alerted the police to the trouble, or they might have simply driven by. Instead, shooting began and as the gunman dove into his automobile he threw down his hostage but unfortunately ran her down during the getaway, causing her death.

C.T. left school and returned home. She remained in her room all that week, leaving only to attend her roommate's funeral along with her parents. When she did not return to school the following week and continued to be reclusive in the house her mother took her to their long-time family physician.

At this visit C. T. indicated that she was unable to sleep because when she did she dreamed of the robbery. She told her physician that, "I feel like it should have been me; it was my job not hers" and that "I don't know why I deserve to live when she died." She idealized her friend in her descriptions.

The family physician determined that there was no concern about substance abuse or suicidal ideation, but that the patient had severe anxiety and depressive features. She was clearly ruminating about the terrible event, and it was almost never out of her mind. Although behind on his schedule, the family physician spent about 30 minutes alone with C.T. as she carefully retraced the events of that night. The family physician was fairly direct in telling C.T. that the world is a dangerous place and sometimes bad things really do happen to nice people for no other reason than that they are in the wrong place at the wrong time. C.T. indicated that sometimes it seemed as if this could not possibly have really happened and the physician sympathized, but that indeed it had happened and the tragic consequences were permanent. He indicated to C.T. that although she would probably never forget that night and should not forget her lovely friend in time the anguish would decrease and she would not suffer this extreme anxiety and depression forever. He predicted that she would grieve "hard" for another week but then things would begin to brighten. He asked if she would be able to make herself leave the house and shop with her mother at the grocery store during daylight hours. He also asked if she would get out and shoot some baskets on the driveway, as he knew that she had played some high school basketball. He indicated that he wanted to see her again in 1 week and that he would get a report on how she had done with these activities. He asked C.T.'s mother to come in and reiterated to her in C.T.'s presence the prediction that the grieving would an intense for short time and then diminish. He reiterated the assignments that he gave to C.T. and asked the mother to remind her of her promise to the doctor if she didn't carry through with them.

At the next weekly visit, scheduled for a half-hour, C.T. was again debriefed about the incident but not with such a lengthy discussion. The physician found that she had undertaken her assignments, although without pleasure. C.T. reported that she still was ruminating about the tragedy most of the time. The physician indicated that he thought C.T. should return to school as soon as possible, though she need not return to work. He told C.T. that getting back to her normal activities was essential for getting through this time, that it would be tough but he knew she could do it. Together they called the student health department at the college and arranged for a counselor, a Ph.D. candidate in clinical psychology, to have appointments with C.T. to continue her psychological treatment. The family physician left his name and telephone number for the counselor to visit with him prior to the first visit with C.T. and periodically thereafter as needed. After that first call and before C.T. began to see the counselor, the physician telephoned her at her dormitory and told her of the telephone contact and that he had confidence in the counselor with whom she would be working. An agenda was followed to return C.T. to her normal activities gradually and to ventilate her about the tragedy but with gradually decreasing intensity while gradually turning more effort into building self-esteem by focusing on a successful return to activities.

When C.T. returned home at Christmas break she went for her annual female examination (which was normal) with her hometown physician. During that visit the family physician found that although C.T. still was remorseful about the incident she no longer dwelled on it or felt guilty about being the survivor, and she had no sleep problems or bad dreams. She meticulously avoided the convenience store area of her college town but had found another job as a clerk in a boutique. Her college counselor had wisely encouraged her to become involved in some extramural activities, and as a result C.T. had found several new friends and one new best friend.

References

Lundin T (1994) The treatment of acute trauma. Psychiat Clin North Am 17:385–391.

Morrison R (1994) Early identification of chronic posttraumatic stress disorder by nurse clinicians. Orthop Nurs 13(4):22–24.

Raphael B, Meldrum L, McFarlane A (1995) Does debriefing after psychological trauma work? Time for randomised controlled trials. BMJ 310:1479–1480.

Samson A, Benson S, Beck A, Price D, Nimmer, C (1999) Posttraumatic stress disorder in primary care. J Fam Pract 48:222–227.

Solomon SD, Gerrity ET, Muff AM (1992) Efficacy of treatments for posttraumatic stress disorder. JAMA 268:663–638.

7

Somatoform Disorder

ASSESSMENT

For somatoform disorders the physician should maintain the focus of attention on the physical complaints, avoiding making patients feel as though their physical problems are primarily psychological.

1. Obtain a thorough history of the physiologic symptomatology including understanding how exacerbations and attenuations fit in with daily activities. Have patients describe a typical day and how the illness affects their activities, noting any losses in functional status. Understand how significant others respond to the symptoms.
2. Have patients describe how their life would be different if they did not have the physical problem.
3. If possible, obtain a history from the family and other significant people, such as employers and teachers. Make sure previous medical records are on hand before a plan is developed.
4. Assess what needs are being met by the illness behavior. A positive diagnosis of somatoform disorder requires recognition of some need being met by the illness behavior.

PLAN

1. Early during treatment decide what workup must reasonably be done and do as much as possible as early as possible. Let the patient know that both negative and positive findings help guide treatment.
2. Provide patients with an explanation for their symptoms. Usually a descriptive explanation is best, such as "chronic nausea." Avoid a psychological diagnosis unless the patient appears receptive.
3. Develop realistic goals with the patients and significant others. Improvement in functional status should be the primary goal.
4. Develop gradual steps that help the patient achieve improved functional status and activity. Recognize what important needs are being met by the illness behavior and make sure the plan allows these needs to be met. Often this means making sure dependency needs

are taken care of by the patients getting more attention for healthy behavior than sick behavior.
5. A restraining technique might help for highly resistant patients.
6. For patients who acknowledge that stress makes symptoms worse, relaxation exercises or biofeedback can be useful.
7. Distracting activities that are enjoyable and help the patient have their needs met should be prescribed for the family.
8. Doctor's appointments should be time-contingent versus symptom-contingent.

The problems of a somatoform disorder are commonly the result of people having their needs met by exhibiting illness behavior rather than through other activities. These patients are usually unaware that they are acting in this manner and are unaware of any problems beyond their physical ones. In fact, they are usually uncomfortable with the concept of psychological problems, especially the idea that psychological distress could cause physical symptoms. Therefore it is usually important to maintain the focus of the interview and treatment on the presenting physical problem and work only indirectly on the psychological issues. Some of the most common needs being met by physical symptoms are dependence on significant others, avoidance of unsavory activity or work, avoidance of a conflict with a significant other, avoidance of sexual problems, or in the case of a child distracting parents from martial conflict. Caretaking behavior by the doctor is often a reward as well.

Often doctors put forth a great effort to take care of these patients, seeking to care and relieve their symptoms, a goal not shared by the patient. The physician then becomes frustrated because these patients rarely improve for more than a brief time. There is always one more symptom or one more relapse. This sometimes leads to an unproductive cycle where the doctor tries to put the patient off while the patient, feeling neglected, pursues treatment more vigorously with increasingly exaggerated symptoms. If the goal of the doctor changes from symptomatic cure to management, a more productive treatment course can be charted.

Assessment

When the patient presents with a physical complaint that the physician suspects stems from a somatoform disorder, it is important for the physician to maintain the focus of attention on the physical complaint and not turn to psychological issues. The physician should begin by obtaining a thorough history of the physiologic symptomatology. It should include understanding how exacerbations and attenuations fit in with daily activities. This is best understood by having patients describe a typical day and how the illness affects their activities: the more detailed the better. This account provides both a clear understanding of the sequence of events surrounding the illness and the effect of significant others on the problem.

It is important to understand from the patients' perspective what losses in functional status have occurred as a result of the physical problem. It is also helpful to understand how their lives would be different if they did not have the physical problem. This information helps the physician identify the motivators that can be used to help the patient change. It is also helpful to understand what significant others have had to do to alter their life style as a result of the patient's illness. Obtaining this information from both family and patient is helpful. It may also be advantageous to secure information from employers or teachers. The doctor should explore how the patient and family have tried to make things better.

All previous treatments by other physicians should be explored as well. It is most helpful to have the previous medical records on hand before a treatment course is developed. The physician does not want to repeat treatment that has already failed.

The diagnosis of somatoform disorder should not be a diagnosis of exclusion. It is not enough for the physician to conclude that because they have no reasonable explanation for the symptoms the problem must be "in their head." The diagnosis of somatoform disorder must be based on finding that some important need is being met by the illness behavior. This is a positive finding. As stated, receiving caretaking that satisfies dependency needs is the most common need met, but other needs also motivate illness behavior. As long as an explanation cannot be found, be it physiologic, psychological, or both, it must be accepted that the illness remains *undiagnosed*. On the other hand, when the doctor has diagnosed a somatoform illness it is not useful to continue doing more tests or getting more consultants to rule out "zebras." As early as possible the doctor should decide what workup is reasonable and to have it done. When discussing the workup, the doctor should explain to the patient that negative findings are as helpful as positive ones because they also help guide treatment. To continue doing tests that are unreasonable in an attempt to reassure the patient has the opposite effect of reinforcing illness behavior, as it devotes a great deal of attention to the illness and proves to the patient that there is always one more diagnostic procedure.

Plan

Once the doctor has identified the "needs being met by the illness" behavior, he or she can begin to strategize how the patient's needs might be better met by other behavioral patterns that reduce the somatoform symptoms. Patients will likely remain as dependent as ever but can have their needs met through healthy rather than sick behavior. To secure the patient's cooperation, the doctor starts with an acceptable explanation for the symptoms. Because these patients are nearly always upset by a psychological diagnosis, a descriptive one might be best, such as chronic pain disorder, chronic nausea, or chronic numbness. Often there is a physiologic diagnosis that explains some of the symptoms, but patients are much more debilitated by the symptoms than they have to be. For example, the doctor might say, "You have reflux we have not been able to control as well as we would have liked. We'll keep working on developing a treatment program that provides better control, but at the same time we need to work on how these problems are affecting your life." This diagnostic explanation is both likely to be acceptable to the patient and allows the doctor to address behavioral changes that can help alleviate the problem as well.

The first treatment step is to develop realistic goals. It is unlikely that there can be complete resolution of symptoms, so negotiation of goals should be aimed primarily at the functional status. The physician might ask, "If the symptoms were to subside somewhat, what would you do during the day that would be important to you?" Based on the answer, a specific plan can be developed that moves the patient in gradual steps toward achieving that level of functional status and activity. The plan must also satisfy the patient's most important needs, be it attention from others or a more rewarding job. In almost all cases of somatoform disorder, significant others must be part of the planning and treatment process. Usually the patient must receive more attention from significant others when they act healthier than when they behave sicker.

Take the case of Mrs. M, a 74-year-old ex-schoolteacher residing in an assisted living facility. After suffering a fracture from a fall secondary to osteoporosis, she had literally and figuratively not been able to get back on her feet. She had become withdrawn and isolated in her apartment. She called for nursing help frequently and called her family to come over and take care of her so often that all those involved were ready to move her to a nursing home. Mrs. M resisted this move vigorously.

Mrs. M had previously been involved with other people at the assisted living center but even prior to her hip fracture had not felt fulfilled with this life style. Her mental status was still sharp, in contrast to her difficulties with ambulation. A meeting was held with the assisted living staff, her family, and the doctors involved. It was pointed out to Mrs. M that there were people who could use her help desperately: immigrants who were having difficulty learning English. Having been an English teacher, they would greatly benefit from her tutoring them at the cultural center, but she would have to obtain better control over her weakness and ambulation before she could do this. Rather than being withdrawn and staying in bed, she would first have to attend her physical therapy; then she could begin to go to the cultural learning center to tutor. She was told firmly but matter-of-factly that nursing home placement would be unavoidable if she did not reduce her need for her family and nursing staff. Limits on how often they would come to her apartment were specifically laid out. She would need to take her meals in the general dining room.

Within 1 month of instituting this plan, Mrs. M was not complaining of weakness, was out of bed, and was attending the learning center on a regular basis to tutor. Her family continued to visit her at the specified frequency but provided no caretaking, which was left to the nursing staff. The critical element in this treatment program was to not respond to her illness behavior, so her needs for socialization and attention were met by prosocial behaviors. Her new behaviors not only provided her with much needed attention but also improved her self-esteem.

For some patients and families who are highly resistant, a restraining technique may help (see Chapter 1). In such cases the doctor states, "It takes a great deal of courage and strength to be able to accept that one will be afflicted with this physical ailment the rest of one's life. Accepting this as being a forever situation is extraordinarily difficult. You may feel better for the present by keeping your hopes up, by getting more consultations." This communication avoids a direct confrontation that could lead to a power struggle. The physician agrees with the family's desire for more medical workup while framing it under the idea that it is because of the discomfort of accepting the inevitable. The family members feel understood but are given the freedom to change direction when they are ready. Framing this change as strength is encouraging as well. Under this framework most families commonly respond by saying, "I don't need any more consultations, I have already been through that. I am ready to work on my life being better." If the family responds in this way, the doctor should initially be skeptical of their readiness before "giving in" to this acceptance.

For patients who acknowledge that stress makes symptoms worse, some specific stress reducers can help. Relaxation exercises or biofeedback can be useful. These techniques help patients have a sense of control over their bodies. It is also important to recommend to the family that because thinking about illness is stressful distracting activity can benefit the patient. Distracting activities that are enjoyable to everyone involved are best. This again provides alternative reinforcers for nonillness behavior. In some cases the families are so anxious about the patient's health they are constantly looking for feedback on how they are doing. For these families the physician can suggest a specific time for "sick talk." For example, "To help everyone be reassured that they understand whatever problems are present, let us set aside 15 minutes before the evening meal for nothing but "sick talk," but at all other times this should be avoided."

Doctor appointments should be time-contingent rather than symptom-contingent. This models for the family the concept of not giving extra time for being sick. The doctor can reinforce it further by stating that there may be a need for extra appointments when real change has occurred. For example, when there are more normal daily activities, extra time may be required for planning the next step.

When significant improvement has occurred, usually a go-slow approach helps it continue. During follow-up sessions this can be explained by saying, "People are sometimes excited about the positive improvements they make and then go too fast, building up overly positive expectations in themselves and others. Therefore continue to make improvements slowly." Sometimes if the doctor suspects the patient might relapse, predicting the relapse in this vein may also be helpful, stating, "Sometimes down deep when one gets to feeling healthier they worry no one will pay attention to them. Therefore don't allow yourself to get better too fast. You may even make sure you have a bad day once a week." This restraining technique usually reduces the potential for relapse.

When considering this protocol, physicians may initially view the up-front time requirements as too costly to them and their company, especially in a managed care environment. In the long run, however, an investment in time with the patient suffering from a somatoform disorder "pays off" in many ways. Iatrogenesis associated with unneeded diagnostic testing and ill-fated symptomatic treatments creates a malpractice risk for these patients who, when treated in a way that does not improve patient satisfaction, are likely to be discontented. An initial investment in time is likely to lead to decreased patient utilization of medical services especially in high-cost circumstances such as the emergency room or the urgent care clinic. This investment in time also decreases the cost of diagnostic testing. As a result, the physician skilled in the treatment of somatoform disorder early on displays a profile suggesting poor performance in terms of patient return visits but later shows a favorable cost/outcome managed care profile.

Perhaps even more important, the functional status of most patients improves and there is reduced medical utilization. As a result most physicians feel less frustrated by these patients, which can enhance their overall job satisfaction.

References

Johns M (1999) Communicating effectively with a patient who has a somatization disorder. Am Fam Physician 59:2639–2640.
McDaniel SH, Campbell TL, Seaburn DB (1990) Family-Oriented Primary Care: A Manual for Medical Providers. New York: Springer-Verlag.
McDaniel SH, Hepworth J, Doherty WJ (1992) Medical Family Therapy: A Biopsychosocial Approach to Families with Health Problems. New York: Basic Books.
Righter E, Sansone R (1999) Managing somatic preoccupation. Am Fam Physician 59:3113–3119.
Servan-Schreiber D, Kolb NR, Tabas G (2000) Somatizing patients. Part I. Practical diagnosis. Am Fam Physician 61:1073–1078.
Servan-Schreiber D, Tabas G, Kolb NR (2000) Somatizing patients. Part II. Practical management. Am Fam Physician 61:1423–1428, 1431–1422.
Shaibani A, Sabbagh M (1998) Pseudoneurologic syndromes: recognition and diagnosis. Am Fam Physician 57:2485–2494.

8

Overutilizers

Overutilizers are usually highly dependent and manipulative.

RED FLAGS

1. Dissatisfaction with multiple caregivers.
2. Patient visits require excessive time.
3. Patients and families overadjust to problems and illness.
4. Functional status is more diminished than their symptoms explain.
5. Patient makes special requests that are uncomfortable to the physician, such as a letter regarding disability or medicines of questionable benefit.
6. Patient uses power tactics to gain control over medical care, such as an implied threat of a lawsuit.
7. Patient may have recruited one or more rescuers to be significant others.

ASSESSMENT

1. Description of symptoms in the context of their daily activity including things that attenuate or exacerbate the problem.
2. How significant others respond to the problem.
3. Narrow the focus to one or two problems per visit, as the patient may have many.
4. Explore how the patient and significant others have tried to alleviate the problem.
5. Obtain records of past medical care.
6. Explore what the patient and family has as their goal for treatment. Improvements in functional status should be the primary emphasis.
7. Goal of the physician should be to have dependence and other needs met in the community rather than in the medical setting as much as possible.

TREATMENT

1. Medical staff must recognize that the goal of the patient is to be taken care of and not to reduce symptoms and get well.
2. A highly structured plan must be developed that guides the patient toward having more dependency needs met by healthy behavior than by "sick" behavior. The structure should be defined as for the patient's own benefit. For example, "Patients, when sick, sometimes become overly dependent on medical staff; our program is aimed at preventing that." Appointments should not be contingent on symptoms; they should be time-contingent. Initially, frequent visits (e.g., weekly) for short periods of time (20 minutes) are a goal, including extra time for improved functional status with less time for symptom complaints. Specifically set the number of phone calls allowed. When enforcing these rules, it is important that the staff not show frustration or anger but be matter-of-fact. Threats should be ignored.
3. Elicit the family or significant others' help to provide distracting activities. Make sure significant others give more attention for functional status improvement than for sick behavior.
4. Prescribe new activities for having dependency needs met (e.g., support groups, volunteer work).
5. If patients complain about their medical treatment, prescribe the following: They should keep track of the complaints in written form and provide a list so the physician can examine them at a later time. At a follow up visit the physician should give a respectful, non-defensive but very brief response to the complaint list.

Patients who are overly dependent and manipulative (sometimes called the "problem" patient), although representing a small number in any physician's practice, often are the most time-consuming and frustrating. Physicians may be tempted to refer them to others, although the best opportunity for optimal care lies with the family physician, who can be open and caring yet set firm limits.

Assessment

These patients commonly present to the physician with a problem that has been chronic but in their view not adequately addressed. The patient initially is quite optimistic that the new physician can find the elusive cure. The complaint is often complex and vague, such as chronic pain or fatigue. Unlike patients with somatoform disorders, these people often have psychological problems as well, to which they readily admit (e.g., depression, anxiety).

A number of red flags may appear early indicating that this patient may be a one who overutilizes medical care. First, there is the history of being dissatisfied with multiple caregivers. Second, physicians find that they have spent much more time with the patient than they thought useful. Third, they recognize that the patient has overadjusted to the problems. That is, their functional status is much more diminished than their symptoms explain. Finally, the patient may make special requests with which the physician is uncomfortable, such as letters regarding disability or work excuses. There may be requests for medications of questionable benefit, such as tranquilizers or narcotic analgesics. If the physician denies the request the patient may take the denial as rejection despite exhaustive explanations. Sometimes these patients use power tactics to gain control over their medical care, such as a direct or implied threat of a lawsuit or being hypercritical of their care. The patient may have recruited one or more rescuers or perhaps has recently driven a significant other away with their neediness, exacerbating the need for professional attention.

A history of the problem should include their daily activities and how their problem is attenuated or exacerbated by these activities. How significant others are either helping or making symptoms worse is also important. It is useful to obtain this information from the patient and from the significant others if possible. If there are many complaints, it may be necessary to narrow the focus to the problem areas the patient and doctor see as most significant.

Attempted solutions should be explored. Specifics from both the patient and significant others, if present, on what helped and what did not should be obtained. It is helpful initially to obtain records of past medical care in as complete a form as possible and to spend time reviewing them before a long-term plan is developed. It is also important, while exploring the attempted solutions, to see what the sequence of improvement entailed, because often what occurs is an initial improvement, regardless of the new treatment, only to be followed by relapse. This most commonly occurs because initially the patient makes some changes to please the doctor. When these changes occur, however, the doctor provides less attention to the patient and less follow-up, and the patient regresses because the loss of attention is more important than any gains that might have been made for the presenting problem.

Explore the patient's and family's goals for treatment. These patients and family members frequently describe goals in utopian terms. That is, they expect all the problems to resolve completely. Another common response of these patients and their families is a vague description of what improvement would look like. It is important to establish some concrete goals that not only include some reasonable reduction in symptomatology but also some real increase in functional status. In fact, the emphasis should be on changes in functional status. For example, "What could you do that you are not doing now?"

The doctors should take note in their vision of improvement that most of these people are not going to change from highly dependent people to highly independent people. A realistic goal is to have their dependency needs met in the community rather than in the medical setting. The doctor and the patient can still see this as valuable improvement because it reduces the need of patients to exhibit symptoms to have their needs met.

Treatment

When developing a plan for these patients, it is useful to assume that they experience their neediness as the only way to gain attention. They feel most comfortable in a complementary relationship with a rescuer. They often come to rely on medical staff to take care of them when they have burned out significant others. Medical staff in response to this behavior may feel manipulated and angry, but these patients are usually not consciously aware of this pattern, as it is an automatic response that is self-perpetuating. The problem begins to diminish when the medical staff recognizes that the goal of the patient is to be taken care of—*not* to reduce symptoms and get well. Attempting to help the patient gain insight into this pattern is rarely helpful. Developing a highly structured plan that guides the patient toward having their dependency needs met by healthy behavior rather than "sick" behavior is most successful in the long run. Having dependency needs met outside the medical system is possible and leads to lessening of symptoms. It is helpful, when possible, to mobilize the involvement of significant others in this pursuit.

The first step is to develop a highly structured clinic program, which should include a set schedule of appointments for several months at a time. The appointments should be set initially at frequent intervals and then gradually spaced out (e.g., weekly for 20 minutes) for 2 months, followed by every other week for 2 months. The frequency and length of the appointments should be time-contingent only, *not* symptom-contingent. Frequency of telephone calls and other resource uses (e.g., emergency room) may also have to be specified to the patient. For example, "If you go to the emergency room, there is no need for me to see you that week."

Resistance to structure should be expected. One useful way to introduce the plan to minimize resistance is to state something close to the following: "When patients are having as many problems as you, it is quite common for them to come to depend heavily on medical staff. At times this can drift into your becoming overdependent on the medical staff. This may or may not be occurring in your case, but one thing we would like to do for you is to prevent any overdependence while still providing good care for you. Therefore for the next months I would like to see you on a schedule that allows us to follow your health closely while avoiding overdependence. I also believe that it would be useful for you to increase your activity. This increased activity will help you feel like you have some control over your life and not be totally controlled by your physical problems, and it will help distract you from your suffering."

Because most of these patients vehemently deny that dependence is a motivation, they act as though the plan is no problem for them, although they will then test its limits, claiming they are an exception to the overall rule. When this occurs, the rules should be enforced with the message, "We're doing this to help you be less dependent." When enforcing these rules, it is important for the staff to not show frustration or anger but be matter of fact. Showing emotion is a form of attention that encourages the behavior.

A slightly different structure can be used for these patients when they are hospitalized. The patients may continually make requests for nursing attention, leading to the nurses complaining to the physicians. A program can be set up whereby the patient is given a certain amount of nursing time per hour (e.g., 10 minutes per hour). Every time the patient turns on the call light there is a minimum time deducted of 4 minutes. This schedule is kept on the door of the patient's room so if they call the nurses more than three times in an hour they cannot call them again until the next hour. It is important to meet with the primary nurses involved to discuss this plan before implementing it so everyone is on the same wavelength. The best way to present this plan to patients is to tell them "that when in the hospital, it is not uncommon for people to become overly dependent on the nursing staff. "The program is being used to limit this overdependence." This explanation frames the structured program as being for the good of the patient, not for the staff's needs.

In either setting, when the patient begins to improve it is frequently useful to take a slightly pessimistic position, such as, "I'm not sure you're ready to reduce your contacts with the medical community. I'm worried that if you improve too quickly people will expect more of you, especially if your physical problems improve too quickly. Therefore don't do anything to improve too quickly lest the adjustment be overwhelming for you." This constructive pessimism often results in continued improvement.

The next step to prevent relapse is to guide them toward having their needs met outside the medical community. It is helpful, when possible, to elicit the support of significant others (remember, these are usually people who like to take care of others). The request is that patients need a great deal of help to overcome their problems. "But focusing on the problem such as depression or gastrointestinal distress only makes it worse. Getting involved in distracting activity is most therapeutic; it's the best medicine." Specific activities can then be prescribed as "medicine." It is important to encourage activities that are likely to give the patient care-taking social contact. Working in a nursing home or volunteering at a daycare center are examples. Support groups are sometimes good activities but should not be relied on solely, as they again focus too much on problems.

If the patient uses threats, a useful approach is to request that the patient be as vigilant of the care as they can be and to inform the doctor vigorously of any mistakes they see, even if the concern is minor. "In this way I can always be kept aware of how fearful you are of being treated poorly and not having enough control over your care." Whenever the patient subsequently makes threats the physician can say, "I hear you are worried you are not getting the best care; thank you for the information." The threat is then best ignored, as the more attention paid to it the more it is used. This reframes the communication into a more workable meaning.

Another variation of this approach is to prescribe behavior. For example, "Please keep a written list of all the mistakes I or any other medical staff make so I can use it to improve your treatment." Making the complaint a required task reduces its potential for attention and makes it an unpleasant chore. These patients will likely always need extra attention; but over time their symptoms can significantly diminish, and they ultimately require less attention.

Case Report

H.L. was a 78-year-old black female newly admitted to a skilled nursing facility. After a week in the facility the family physician who accepted her care was called by an almost tearful Director of Nursing. It seemed that the nursing home resident was constantly critical of virtually every aspect of her care and nursing home life. The food was bad or cold, the aides would not answer the call light on time, someone had spoken meanly to her. H.L. was constantly on the call light or at the nursing desk with demands about these complaints or with demands for some special treatment. The resident suffered diabetes mellitus type 2 and staff reported she was extremely noncompliant. As a result her blood sugar levels (by fingerstick) were in the 200–400 mg/dl range. Results were obtained only when H.L. allowed a fingerstick, which was less than half of the time.

Evaluating the problem, the family physician obtained a corroborating history from H.L.'s family, who reported that she had always been obstinate, demanding and difficult, although it was worse as she had become elderly and more feeble. The physician visited the resident and told her that he was receiving reports that she was unhappy and making complaints. He told H. L. that he believed she might be correct that "many things around this place are not right and need to be changed." "Unfortunately, you are complaining to the wrong people and at the wrong time. When you complain a lot people tend to tune you out. You need to tell the person in authority. Also, it is important not to make a complaint when the staff is trying to work. They probably won't stop and listen seriously to what you say even if it's a good idea because they are involved in their other duties. My plan is to arrange for you to meet with the Director of Nursing daily when she first comes to the building. At that meeting you can tell her all the things you need to express." This plan was shared with the Director of Nursing who, needless to say, was not particularly excited about it. However, the physician explained that by prescribing the complaining behavior the patient would not be able to obtain the secondary gain of attention and create frustration in the staff, which was her goal. The physician told the Director of Nursing to instruct her staff to simply hold up their hand in a stop sign gesture if the resident attempted to complain to them on an ad lib basis. Staff were then to say, "Don't tell me this now—save it for your meeting with the Director of Nursing." They were not to show frustration, make eye contact, or argue or linger further.

Within a short time the complaining behavior disappeared. The physician ordered a Geriatric Depression Scale, but it was negative. He undertook techniques to improve compliance with diabetic management.

References

Adams J, Murray R (1998) The general approach to the difficult patient, Emerg Med Clin North Am 16:689–700.

Gillette R (2000) "Problem patients": a fresh look at an old vexation. Fam Pract Manag July/August 7:57–62.

Groves JE (1978) Taking care of the hateful patient. N Engl J Med 298:883–887.

Schwenk T, Romano S (1992) Managing the difficult physician–patient relationship. Am Fam Physician 46:1503–1509.

9

Chronic Pain (Nonmalignant)

PREVENTIVE INTERVENTION
1. To prevent chronic pain, following an acute injury or illness develop a back-to-work plan with the goal of returning to work within 3–5 days.
2. Schedule a follow-up visit in a few days for patients if they are not working regularly. Partial return to work then is preferable to no work.

ASSESSMENT

Information about psychosocial factors regarding chronic pain must be gathered indirectly to minimize patients' defensiveness about their pain not being taken seriously.
1. History of patients' symptoms should include what makes the pain better or worse and how significant others have helped or exacerbated the pain.
2. Have them describe a typical day with a description of how the pain responds to the activities.
3. All medical or alternative treatments should be explored including all past medical records.
4. Work history, recreational history, and related litigation are items of useful information.
5. Some need must be met by the pain to diagnosis chronic pain disorder. The goal is to have needs met alternatively.

PLAN
1. Do all diagnostic work and obtain consultations as soon as possible to minimize the need for more workup later, which is usually counterproductive.
2. Give the patient the clear message that a positive medical workup is helpful, but a negative workup is just as useful for guiding therapy.

3. Once a full workup has been completed, the problem should be reframed for the patient and family. The pain should be defined as a likely lifelong problem and that functional improvement is the ultimate goal of treatment.
4. Develop specific goals for treatment with the patient and if possible the family. Work or other productive activity should be part of this goal.
5. Refer the patient to physical therapy, a work hardening program (occupational therapy), or both. Minimize passive treatment in the physical therapy program and emphasize active treatment aimed at increasing function.
6. Teach the patient pacing or have an occupational therapist do so.
7. Develop a plan for return to work and other normal activities.
8. Include the family in the plan and give them specific tasks to help the patient return to normal activities. This includes discussing how to distract the patient from their pain.
9. Alter medications from short-term medications to long-term chronic medications, such as a reduction of narcotics and benzodiazepines, changing to low-dose amitriptyline and nonsteroidal antiinflammatory drugs (NSAIDs) or occasionally time-release narcotics.
10. Schedule frequent visits that are time-contingent and focus on functional status improvement.

Chronic pain is often a frustrating problem for all involved, including the patients, their family, and the doctors. The behavior of these patients, which sometimes includes manipulative behavior and nearly always dependent behavior, sometimes alienates doctors. Although it is usually not a good use of time to delve into these patients' formative histories, many come from a background where getting attention from parental figures was difficult. Working hard at being successful rarely got noticed by the family, but when one got sick people paid attention. Under these circumstances the habits they developed for having their needs met are understandable. Insight into this dynamic is of little value to the patient, but when the doctor operates under the assumption that these dynamics are operating it aids treatment. Successful treatment is based on changing these dynamics. A strategic approach to treatment necessitates that the patient's dependency needs be met through healthy behaviors rather than through sick behaviors.

The multifactorial etiology of the pain makes it difficult to treat. The precipitant is nearly always an injury or illness, so the pain is almost never purely psychological. On the other hand, many studies have demonstrated that only approximately 5% of patients who have back injuries or headaches develop chronic pain syndrome. Physiologic variables generally do not differentiate between those who develop chronic pain syndrome and those who do not. In fact, studies show psychosocial factors to be the major variables associated with patients seen in chronic pain clinics. There are known social factors that contribute to the likelihood of chronic pain syndrome developing, such as a boring or noxious work situation the patient would prefer to avoid. Litigation related to an injury leading to pain leaves patients believing that they should be compensated for their suffering. Individual and family characteristics listed below have also been associated with the development of chronic pain syndrome.

Individual Characteristics

1. Dependent personality (often denied by the patient)
2. Poor stress resolution skills
3. Blames all problems on physical health
4. Uses symptoms to avoid conflict and anxiety
5. Life would be perfect if it were not for the pain
6. Alexithymia (no awareness of emotions, patients express emotions by complaining of somatic symptoms.)
7. Substance abuse
8. Long periods of boring activity or inactivity
9. Underachiever

Family Characteristics

1. Psychosomatic family profile
   a. Rigidity
   b. Overprotection
   c. Lack of conflict resolution with conflict detouring and triangulation
   d. Enmeshment (including a lack of generational boundaries)
2. Substance abuse in family members
3. Illness in the family (chronic pain and disability are common)
4. Family provides and/or receives secondary gain
5. Alexithymia

As noted above, most patients with pain from acute injury or illness improve, with only a small number suffering the sequelae of chronic pain. Therefore the initial challenge for the physician is differentiating who should get care directed toward prevention of chronic pain and who can be treated simply as having an acute problem. If the patient is well known to the physician, the characteristics listed above can be taken into consideration when treating the patient. The red flags listed below can help the physician more quickly recognize a patient prone to chronic pain.

Red Flags

1. Nonspecific aches and pains or multiple unrelated physical complaints
2. Repeated treatment failures or suboptimal therapeutic responses
3. Symptoms not associated with an explainable diagnosis
4. Chronic fatigue, insomnia, weakness
5. Anxiety or depressive symptoms
6. Recent loss
7. Misses work or school for minor somatic problems
8. Overadapted to chronic pain by family or other secondary gain
9. Litigation pending
10. "Gut feeling" that the patient wants more than the physician can give

The sooner the physician recognizes that the problem is becoming chronic and begins to treat the patient for chronic pain the better, as many treatments that are good for acute pain are counterproductive in the case of chronic pain. For the patient with acute pain, avoidance of strenuous activity but continued nonpainful activity, NSAIDs, and analgesics are often the mainstay. A few days after the pain onset, as-needed analgesics should be avoided. When used, they reward the pain experience. Furthermore, as-needed analgesics often lead to high dosing because once pain is established it requires more medicine to control it.

Pain at this stage of an injury or illness is an indication that time for healing is required. As time goes on, the likelihood of full resolution of the pain diminishes. The goal should then shift from resolution of pain to improved functional status. After this acute phase, inactivity and particularly narcotic medication is counterproductive. For nonmalignant pain in unusual cases, patients might benefit from long-term use of low-dose long-acting narcotics. Small dosages for these patients seem to allow them to get back to an acceptable level of functioning, and they do not escalate their demand for them. However, often when narcotics are used long term for nonmalignant pain, patients come to believe medicine can cure them and become angry with the doctor when they escalate their demand and the doctor does not comply.

Assessment

Chronic pain syndrome is not a diagnosis of exclusion. It can be dangerous to assume one has found the cause of a patient's pain simply by excluding the likely physiologic etiologies. Certain findings must be present to conclude that the patient has chronic pain syndrome: The patient must have had pain for more than 3 months, have had longer than expected healing of the injured tissue, exhibited great disparity between objective findings and the experienced pain, and must be found to have important needs met through the pain though not be consciously aware of it. Usually these needs are dependency needs, although avoidance of noxious activities may be primary. Additionally, there is often excessive use of the health care system and abuse of opiates, anxiolytics, alcohol, or similar substances. General deterioration of functional status as a result of the pain is usual. Most pharmacologic and surgical treatments lead to initial lessening of the symptoms followed by a gradual relapse to the pretreatment state.

Although it is important to understand the psychosocial variables related to the pain experience and behavior, many patients who have chronic pain syndrome are resistant to any direct inquiry, as it means to them that their physician is not taking their pain seriously and thinking it is "all in their head." The physician must therefore take precautions to make sure the patient believes the doctor is taking the pain seriously and so does not become defensive. An effective way to gather this information is to ask patients to describe a typical day and how their pain affects it; moreover, what would a typical day be like if they had no pain. Another useful question is about how others help them because they have pain. Obtaining a detailed description of how pain affects their day and their relationships with others provides most of the information necessary in the psychosocial history without alarming the patient. It is important to ask the patient for a description of all the attempted treatments and solutions already tried and to obtain this information through their previous medical records. This information prevents the doctor from trying things that have already failed. Litigation can also have a powerful effect on attempts to improve functional status and therefore must be explored.

Treatment

The decision about when to change the focus from acute to chronic treatment, where functional status is the focus, is often difficult. For those at risk, some special effort should be made to prevent chronic pain syndrome even while treating the acute problems. For work-related back injuries it has been repeatedly demonstrated that rapid return to work leads to less risk of chronic pain than long periods of rest and inactivity. Patients should be told at their initial visit to return to work in 3–5 days and to call and report how they are healing. This lessens the likelihood that the patient prone to chronic pain will go to bed for 2 weeks, then return to the doctor feeling worse and wanting a "note" for work. If the patient cannot yet tolerate full activity, light duty can be recommended for a specified period. Many employers now accept the value of gradual return to work for some patients.

When a patient is not improving as expected, it is easy to fall into the pattern of trying one diagnostic test after another. This only teaches the patient there is always one more test or consultant. If the patient does not respond to acute treatment, a more helpful approach is for the physician to decide what diagnostic workup and consultation is likely to be needed and to have it done at an early stage. It is helpful to tell patients when they are being sent for consultation or testing procedures that whether the test has positive or negative findings it will be useful for guiding treatment.

It is often also useful at an early point to tell the patient that stress can contribute to pain problems. Most patients accept stress as a contributing factor and do not believe the doctor is dismissing the problems as "in their head." Additionally, the patient can be informed that one true answer is unlikely, and several contributing factors may be discovered.

Once the physician has determined that the pain is chronic, the doctor should discuss with the patient, and usually the family, a shift in treatment goals and focus. It is helpful to empathize with the patient's desire for a definitive diagnosis and treatment while clearly stating that this outcome is unlikely. However, the doctor can offer help with improving the patient's functional status. It is not useful to proceed with treatment until the patient agrees to this change in focus.

Resistance to this switch is common. One approach is to acknowledge to the patient the difficulty of accepting chronic pain. "For some unexplained reason certain people develop chronic pain after an injury that is with them forever. I don't blame you for being reluctant to accept your diagnosis of chronic pain. It will likely lead to grief for your lost health so don't accept it until you're ready. Going to more consultants and doing more tests does keep up hope that the next test will find something new, but as we have seen that isn't happening in your case. It will take great courage to accept and face chronic pain, and I will be here for you when you're ready."

It is rarely useful to start a rehabilitation program when litigation is pending.

When the patient accepts the chronic pain diagnosis, rehabilitation can begin. Chronic pain, with a number of contributing factors, has been found to be best treated using multiple methods. Treatment should be guided by the following principles.

1. Medication is best used to prevent the pain from rising beyond a certain threshold and should therefore be scheduled. When patients have used narcotics or benzodiazepines, it is sometimes efficacious to maintain them on the current dose for the first 2-3 weeks of rehabilitation, then gradually taper them off.

2. Secondary gain for pain should be addressed in an indirect way to not anger the patient. To improve, patients must have their needs met more often through nonpain behavior rather than through pain behavior. This must include the care-taking behavior of others as well as alternative forms of attention.

3. Physical therapy is a central component of chronic pain treatment. Aerobic physical exercise is known to improve pain tolerance; and

stretching and strengthening exercises increase tolerance to overall activity, stabilize the injured area preventing further injury, and prevent deconditioning, which puts the patient at risk for further injury.

4. Pacing of activities should be learned by the patient to avoid over-exertion. Too little activity and boredom increase the pain focus.

5. Relaxation exercises help the patient avoid chronically tight muscles ("guarding against pain"), which contribute to pain.

None of the above treatments alone is likely to be effective, but combining them usually leads to improvement. Each of the above treatments is discussed in more detail below.

Medication is best given on a schedule rather than as needed. Avoid euphorics (e.g., narcotics and tranquilizers). Tricyclics have been studied the most for use against chronic pain. They are often helpful at about half the dose used for depression (e.g., 75 mg amitriptyline), which markedly reduces side effects. Unlike their use for depression where a single daily dose is administered, tricyclics for chronic pain often are more effective when given three or four times a day (tricyclics are contraindicated in patients with heart disease). SSRIs have also been studied in chronic pain patients but have not been found to be as helpful. Scheduled NSAIDs benefit some patients. Patients with headaches may benefit from specific medications designed for the type of headache they commonly have. However, this treatment usually has been maximized by the time the patient is identified as a chronic pain patient.

Physical therapy is a mainstay in the treatment of chronic pain. The patient should be warned that the benefits of physical therapy take up to 6 weeks to be experienced, and that at first they are likely to feel worse. The physical therapy program should involve close communication between physical therapist and physician. Its goals should be clearly defined as improved functional status, especially return to work. Active therapy, including aerobic exercise, strengthening, and stretching, should be primary with little use of passive therapies such as massage or ultrasonography. If passive treatments are used, they should be employed only at the end of an active program, which may further inspire the patient to work hard so as to receive this treatment. Work hardening programs (occupational therapy) are structured around these concepts and can be helpful.

With rare exception, it is more harmful than helpful to recommend disability status for patients with chronic pain. Being inactive at home often involves more stress and focus on pain than being active at a job. In some situations it is appropriate to recommend vocational rehabilitation, which allows the patient to become involved in some work for which they are more mentally and physically capable and more likely at which to succeed. It is also helpful to prescribe new activities that are "distracting from the pain" rather than more rest, which only allows the patient to focus more attention on their pain.

Simple relaxation exercises, biofeedback, meditation, and hypnosis are equally effective for pain patients. For some reason patients tend to respond better to one of the modes than another. Guiding the patient to experiment with these measures can be helpful.

It is important to involve the family in the treatment process. Helping the family redefine the problem from pain elimination to improvement in functional status is the first step. The family may deny providing secondary gain but usually accepts distraction as a way to help lessen the pain. It is helpful to guide them with specific suggestions for new activities they could do together that turn the focus away from the pain. In the physician's mind, these new activities must meet the patients' needs that are currently being met by pain behaviors. The new activities should not require that the patient maintain the "sick role." The family can be told that, rather than focusing on the pain, they can have a new activity that distracts the patient from the pain. Family members then feel like "helpers" without having to "take care" of the patient.

Follow-up visits to the physician should be scheduled frequently and are thus time-contingent, not symptom-driven. This again removes the sick behavior from having secondary gain in terms of physician attention. At visits, the physician should focus attention on the functional status (e.g., the new activities of the patient) rather than pain symptoms. When improvement has been firmly established, appointments can *gradually* be spaced out.

Case Report

E.B. was a 58-year-old Hispanic woman with a long history of healthcare-seeking for a variety of vague conditions. Her second husband, a 57-year-old caucasian man, was a practicing alcoholic, on disability with low back pain, and retired from the city maintenance crew. In January 1995 E.B. was involved in a pedestrian/motor vehicle accident and suffered a broken hip. Her intertrochanteric fracture was repaired surgically by a local orthopedist; and after an expected hospital stay and a period of home health with physical therapy the patient was discharged from the care of the orthopedic surgeon to the continuing care of a general practitioner with whom she had a long relationship.

Despite an apparently good result from the surgery, the patient reported continuing and severe pain along the lateral aspect of her left leg that was "burning and deep" in quality. The patient was treated with Vicodin 7.5/500 on an as-needed basis, receiving as many as eight doses per day. Her unrelenting pain returned her to the physician's office repeatedly, and she was sequentially placed on tramadol without success and then on butorphanol nasal spray.

With litigation pending, the patient underwent consultation by a neurologist, another orthopedist, and an alternative medicine practitioner before returning to her general practitioner. Episodes of intractable pain led her to the emergency room on many occasions where she received injections of meperidine, which provided temporary relief, or in some cases nonnarcotic prescriptions such as ketorolac, which she said "did nothing." E.B. never returned to her work as a nursing home aide following the accident. Finally, in 1999 she received a significant settlement from the accident in a judgment against the driver of the automobile.

Shortly thereafter. E.B.'s general practitioner died of a heart attack. At her next episodic visit to the emergency room she was assigned to a family practitioner from the primary care call schedule to receive follow-up care.

At E.B.'s first visit the family physician requested records from her prior caregivers. He reviewed her current pain regimen and sympathized with her lack of success in the past. He indicated that she was still receiving treatment as if she had acute pain, and he believed she was now suffering chronic pain, which is a different problem. He further indicated that although he did not believe he could take away her pain he was hopeful that he could reduce it over time to a point where she would be more able to live the life that she wished. The physician asked that E.B. describe a typical day and tell how the pain affected her daily activities. He then asked her to imagine what her days might be like if she did not have pain. He asked who E.B. had to assist her in activities the pain prevented her from undertaking. From these questions he learned that E.B. led a sedentary existence. Her husband was present in the home almost all the time and did almost everything for her unless he was inebriated. When she tried to do things for herself she would likely have an exacerbation of pain and either need to see her physician or, if it was not office hours, go to the emergency room. He learned that E.B. did not imagine a more active life were she to be free of pain.

By the next visit the physician had reviewed her prior records including various analgesic strategies that had been tried and failed, the tests performed, and the specialists seen. He found that the patient carried a prior diagnosis of chronic fatigue syndrome from one physician and fibromyalgia from another. The patient had been treated with alprazolam and diazepam, carisoprodol/aspirin, and various antidepressants in the past. Notes indicated that many interventions had briefly been useful only to have the patient relapse to a state of uncontrolled pain.

One thorough orthopedic consultant performed a good workup that failed to show low back problems or disc disease, and a trial of low back exercises had not been helpful. The neurology consultant also provided notes doubting the presence of neuropathy or radiculopathy.

The family physician told E.B. that by allowing her pain to increase before taking the butorphanol nasal spray as an "as needed prescription" she was allowing the pain to "get away from her." He recommended a scheduled dose of narcotic, which would prevent the pain from climbing to this level. He discontinued the butorphanol nasal spray and gave the patient a prescription for long-acting hydrocodone 10 mg bid with a short-acting hydrocodone/acetaminophen rescue pill to be taken as needed but not more than every 4 hours. She was asked to record the number of doses she required along with pain scores on a scale of 1 to 10 in a daily diary. He told E.B. that because she was having pain anyway it was a mistake to be sedentary. He recommended starting with some physical therapy to help her gain strength and mobility so she could begin to perform some activities that would help distract her from the pain. She was warned that initially she would feel worse. He recommended she attended Al-Anon both as an activity and to strengthen herself to help her husband with his alcohol problem once she "got it together."

At one point E.B. attempted to see the physician prior to her next scheduled visit. Although the physician did make a brief intervention, he was not warm in his mannerisms and did not linger. He provided little eye contact and in a matter-of-fact style reminded the patient of their prior plans.

At the scheduled visit the physician learned that E.B. had used six as-needed pain pills on average per day. He told E.B. that his goal was to give her enough long-acting pain medicine so she would never have to use the short-acting pill more than twice daily. He informed her that pain is not always the same; sometimes it is made worse by activities, the weather, stress, or other factors. Moreover, were he to give her enough long-acting pain medicine that she never needed a rescue pill, she would likely be sedated or constipated by too much medicine. He increased the long-acting hydrocodone to 20 mg bid and encouraged the patient to see if that would be enough so the rescue pill was needed less often than twice daily. He predicted that it would. He promised E.B. that she would be seen again on her regularly scheduled visit in 1 month. In the meantime she was to work on physical therapy, Al-Anon participation, and begin to seek out some other activity outside her home.

Subsequent visits with E.B. were undertaken at monthly intervals for a while and then stretched to 3-month intervals. There was gradual success in increasing E.B.'s functional status and socialization and in decreasing her inappropriate use of medical services. A careful record of her narcotic use was kept along with documentation of the improved functional status on this prescription to avoid any appearance of impropriety that might jeopardize the physician's narcotic's license.

Her participation in Al-Anon led to an alcohol intervention with her husband. Unfortunately, rather then undertake a third attempt at a treatment program her husband chose to leave, and they were later divorced. After a brief relapse with returning symptoms, E.B. showed additional improvement thereafter. If treatment for chronic pain had been started before she gave up her job, an even better outcome might have been achieved.

References

Caudill M (1995) Managing Pain Before It Manages You. New York: Guilford.
Daniels JM (1997) Treatment of occupationally acquired low back pain. Am Fam Physician 55:587–596.
Gatchel RJ, Turk DC (1996) Psychological Approaches to Pain Management: A Practitioner's Handbook. New York: Guilford.
Sullivan MD, Turner JA, Romano J (1991) Chronic pain in primary care: identification and management of psychosocial factors. J Fam Pract 32:193–199.
Wall PD, Melzack R (1999) Textbook of Pain. Philadelphia: Saunders.

10

Nonadherence

ASSESSMENT

It is important for the doctor to maintain a nonjudgmental stance with the nonadherent patient. If possible, the family is interviewed as well. When gathering the history, special attention should be paid to control issues.

1. What have the patients been doing for their illness?
2. Patients' view of the success and failure of their attempts. Have them describe attempts to comply with treatment in the context of a typical day.
3. Do the patients understand the cause of their illness?
4. What do the patients and families believe will help alleviate their illness most?
5. What bothers them most about their illness?
6. What is the most difficult and the easiest aspects of the treatment plan?
7. What do others do to help or hinder the plan?
8. What are the patients' goals for treatment?
9. How would they change the plan to make it more compatible?
10. Is there a financial problem?
11. How are they getting along with their doctor?

At the conclusion of the history, the physician should be able to assess why more of the patient's needs are being met through nonadherence than through adherence.

TREATMENT

1. If the patient does not understand the illness or treatment plan, reeducation should be attempted.
2. If forgetting to take medicine is the problem, developing associations with the task should help, such as putting birth control pills next to a toothbrush.
3. Any financial or cognitive deficits must be specifically addressed.

4. If the goals of the doctor and the patient are disparate, renegotiating acceptable goals is required.
5. If patients have only a low resistance to change, it is probably best to start with a three-step process: (1) behavioral self-management; (2) self-monitoring, (3) self-motivation. This process entails keeping a diary and a checklist each time they perform the task and then bringing the diary to their next doctor appointment.
6. When there is a major discrepancy between the health care views of the physician and the patient, family, or cultural experts, a meeting with the significant others should be scheduled to develop compromises.
7. When strong dependency needs are being met by nonadherence, the patient must receive more attention for adherence than for noncompliance. A family meeting is indicated.
8. When a power struggle between the doctor and patient develops, an attempt to develop a more collaborative relationship should be attempted initially. When the power struggle is extreme, using a restraining technique may be most effective: It may be suggested that patients should not or cannot comply because to do so they would have to accept the doctor's authority; therefore the doctor is willing to accept a less than desirable outcome.
9. The basic approach is to identify the needs being met by nonadherence and substitute a plan to help the patient have their needs met while exhibiting better adherence.

Doctors take care to communicate with their patients, carefully examining them, assessing the problem, and conscientiously developing an appropriate treatment plan. A week later the patient is no better. Upon further investigation the doctor finds that the patient had not adhered to the plan. The doctor naturally feels thwarted and cynical about attempting to help the patient further. The patient's behavior appears to be irrational and self-destructive.

This situation is far from rare. Studies show that whereas adherence to treatment protocols is relatively good for acute illnesses, such as antibiotic usage for a couple of weeks, for treatment of chronic illness adherence is usually only about 50%.

Often the physician's initial response to patients who do not adhere to treatment is to provide them with more education, assuming that rational understanding of the treatment benefits leads to improved adherence. Often patients are referred to an educator. In some cases, when patients do not understand the rationale for the treatment or are unclear about how to take care of themselves, further education does provide some benefit. However, as many studies show, once an adequate initial educational process has been undertaken, additional educational efforts are often disappointing. In fact, reeducation rarely is helpful with a patient who has valued beliefs different from those of the physician. Some studies have shown that when there is an implied threat— for example, "If you don't take your medicine you will die or get more seriously ill"— there is a boomerang effect, and resistant patients are less likely to follow the protocol. They become more interested in proving the health care provider wrong. According to studies, patients are least like to comply when treatment entails significant life style change.

In many cases, when a patient does not fully adhere to treatment it is not their specific intent to be noncompliant. In fact, several studies show that omitting medicine because the patient is busy and forgets is the number one reason for noncompliance. Often in this situation using good learning tools to create associations that help the patient remember to take their medicine (e.g., as putting their birth control pills next to their toothbrush) is all that is needed.

When the initial solutions, such as better education and making it easy for the patient to comply, do not work and there are no obvious factors that interfere (e.g., financial or cognitive deficits), it is best to view the problem as one of relative value to the patient. It is most useful to assume that the patient is having more needs met by nonadherence than they would by complying with treatment. A common circumstance, for example, is when the immediate consequences of adherence are uncomfortable (e.g., side effects) and the long-term benefits are difficult to foresee. This is easy in the teenage smoker who is especially prone to immediate gratification. Sometimes the gratification of noncompliance is subtle, such as having a sense of victory by not "giving in to the doctor." In this case, feeling in control may be much more important than the long-term health benefits. Patients who like to be taken care of may discover that by not following their diabetic regimen others provide much more caretaking behavior, which to them is much more valuable than the health benefits of a strictly followed diabetic protocol. Perhaps a patient is denying cancer is present and thereby avoids the pain of grieving for lost health.

Family and cultural belief systems play an important role in acceptance of treatment. For example, the view of a football coach who strongly promotes "playing hurt" may be much more important than a doctor who spends a few moments explaining the scientific likelihood that the players could have long-term sequelae from neglecting the treatment protocol for their injury. The rural donut shop where farmers gather in the early morning and brag to each other how they cut off their casts sooner than their neighbor after a fracture to get back into the field provides a powerful incentive to defy the treatment protocol. A family who sees medicine as the way people are cured take an antibiotic for an upper respiratory infection, seeing it as the only way to get better. In these situations it is all too tempting for the physician to respond by becoming argumentative and scientifically proving their point. Patients often accept the authority of their "cultural experts." Irrational fears are almost never overcome by education alone.

If the physician is to succeed in changing the patient's adherence to treatment protocol, they must find a way for the patient's needs to be better met by compliance than by nonadherence to a treatment protocol, and they must do it within the patient's frame of reference. Certain approaches to such assessment and treatment are helpful in this pursuit.

Assessment

When nonadherence is a problem, it is valuable to expand the history to include the following:

1. What does the patient believe is the cause of the illness?
2. What do the patient and their family believe will help?
3. What bothers them most about their illness?
4. What is the most difficult aspect and the easiest aspect of the treatment plan?
5. How do others help or hinder?
6. What are their goals for treatment?
7. How would they change the plan to make it more compatible?

It is important to have them describe any attempts to comply with treatment in the context of a typical day. This technique points a clear picture of behavior regarding adherence.

To appear nonjudgmental, it is usually best to start with what patients have been doing for their illness and their view of the success and failure of their attempts. When gathering the history, special attention should be paid to control issues. Is the patient feeling as if others are controlling? Examples include nagging by family members or statements such as "I know the doctor doesn't like it when I do this, but. . . ." This would indicate a great deal of sensitivity to issues of control and therefore the need for patients to prove they are in control and others are not. This history should also bring out the belief that alternative treatments are believed to be better for cure than the ones prescribed by the physician.

At the conclusion of the history, the physician should be able to assess why more of the patient's needs are being met by noncompliance than by compliance. If the situation is still unclear, the family should be interviewed as well.

Some common issues of nonadherence are as follows:

1. Not understanding the value of the treatment, or the treatment plan is too complex.
2. Immediate gratification is more important than long-term health including cost considerations.
3. Denial.
4. Patient gets more attention when sick.
5. Goals of the doctor and patient are disparate.

6. Expected life style changes lead to important needs being unmet.
7. Side effects are feared, even if irrationally.
8. Patient has a need for feeling in control by putting others down or proving them wrong.
9. Patient feels overly controlled by the doctor and so has to prove the doctor wrong.

After considering these possible explanations for nonadherence, the physician should be in a position to recognize the unmet needs engendered by the treatment plan and alter it to make it more satisfactory.

Treatment Plan

Patient adherence implies requesting that patients make some change in their life style even if it is simply to take medication with mild side effects. Change is difficult for people, and the more change required in someone's life style the more difficult it is.

The first step in working toward improvement of a noncompliant patient is making sure the treatment goals of the patient and doctor are compatible. Acceptable solutions must be negotiated. It is important to do this in a way that clearly communicates to the patient that the physician is not being judgmental. Remind the patient that you work for them; and if the original plan did not work for them, you can work together to find a better fit. In fact, it is often useful to begin by suggesting that the patient has good reason for their nonadherence. This helps them feel understood, not on the defensive; and they are much more likely to communicate more openly. For example, the provider might say, "I know there were a number of uncomfortable obstacles that got in the way of you adhering to the treatment program." It is also useful to establish a foundation on which agreement can lead to action. The provider might ask, "What, for you, are the most important reasons to take your medicine?" This question communicates that adherence is not an all or nothing situation but a compromise of differing, sometimes conflicting needs.

Take the case of the patient (Freeman, 1999) who was brought by ambulance to the emergency room following a motorcycle accident. A radiograph showed a cervical fracture that, although at that time led to no neurologic deficits, could easily lead to severe irreversible injury of the spinal cord. The patient refused hospital admission and was mentally competent to do so. He thought that he could not tolerate the degree of control a hospital would have over him. In the end, he did agree to not ride his motorcycle, which was totally destroyed anyway, and to wear a cervical collar and see the physician every few days. Without this compromise he was ready to walk out with no treatment at all. With the compromise, he wore the collar and followed-up regularly with the physician. His vertebrae ultimately fused.

If the patient has only low resistance to change, it is probably best to start with the most common interventions for compliance, that is, behavioral self-management, self-monitoring, and self-motivation. For example, it is well known that having patients keep a diary of their behavior or a checklist each time they perform a planned task and bring it to the doctor appointment leads to improvement. Frequent appointments by the provider, such as once a week, also encourage adherence particularly early in treatment. Having to report to the doctor and gain approval makes a difference to many patients.

When there is a major discrepancy between the health care views of the family or cultural medical expert, it is most helpful for an understanding and compromise to be worked out with the significant others. It is important to respect people's views and find an acceptable compromise (even if not ideal). This may require not only a family meeting but in some cases a meeting with other cultural experts as well.

For patients who respond to immediate gratification, a financial incentive such as free samples might help them begin treatment. For others, unless they pay for something it has no value. In this case not giving them free samples may be more conducive to adherence or having them pay in advance for something is encouraging. Once they have paid even a nominal fee, many people want to get their money's worth (e.g., diabetic classes). Sometimes it is useful to make something scarce and special for the person, "Lamaze classes are usually filled by this time, but I think if I make a call and talk with the person they will make a special place for you." For some patients this may be just enough incentive to get them over the initial hurdle of making a change.

Denial usually serves a useful function in reducing an overwhelming grief response, but when it interferes with treatment it must be overcome. In this case it is useful to start with an explanation for their denial in a respectful way: "I don't blame you for not following your cancer treatment protocol. To do so you would have to accept the severity of your disease, which would be painful. Even though the treatment could be helpful to you, perhaps we will just have to wait until you are strong enough to accept it." This reframing as "accepting disease" as a form of strength and not accepting it as a form of weakness often subtly encourages the patient to accept the disease and hence to accept the treatment. It must always include, though, a respectful reason for denial. It is also important to keep in mind that to use this technique to interfere with denial often leads to a strong affective reaction of sadness along with the improved treatment adherence.

When other short-term gratifications are more important to the patient than long-term health factors, a successful strategy is to find new reinforcers that can be experienced more immediately. For example, when an exercise program is the goal, it is well known that an enjoyable or group activity is much more likely to be undertaken consistently than a boring workout no matter how good it is for the patient.

In the more difficult cases, it usually takes family involvement for the short-term reinforcers to be significant enough to make a difference. For example, a teenager might be required to maintain excellent diabetic control to use the family car. This is a particularly good reinforcer as driving ability is a natural consequence of good diabetic control.

When the patient is having strong dependency needs met through non-adherence, family involvement is even more crucial. If improvement is to occur, patients must discover that they get more attention for adherence to treatment than for non-compliance. Often this requires a coordinated effort between the health care team and the family for optimal care. For example, a woman in assisted living frequently stops taking her seizure medicine, often leading to a seizure or pseudoseizure, which in turn leads to the staff at the assisted living center and the family performing caretaking activities for many days afterward. At a care conference, the family and staff agree to provide minimal necessary care following a seizure but determine a way to provide more attention when the patient is seizure-free. The patient discovers, perhaps unconsciously, that it is much more rewarding to take her medicine than to have seizures.

Probably the most difficult problems with adherence management are in the area of power struggles and control issues between patients and their families or patients and physicians. The very nature of health care interaction with patients puts the doctor and other health care personnel in a one-up position and patients in a subservient role. Many patients thrive on this, wishing to please the doctor and nurse, and this attitude can be used to improve adherence. For patients who cannot tolerate any sense of control by others, who would rather be sick or even die than feel controlled, this situation creates a difficult problem. Here it is important for the physician to create a collaborative relationship; and for certain patients even taking a one-down position may help. A collaborative approach might highlight the doctor's role as a resource. The physician then might offer patients several treatment options, with the patients choosing the plan that suits them. An example of a one-down approach is, "Your situation totally stumps me." The patient, knowing they've stumped the doctor may then feel free to take the treatment initiative. If this occurs, the doctor should not appear pleased but remain "stumped," continuing what has worked.

If the patient requests inappropriate treatment with which the doctor cannot in good clinical judgment comply, it is helpful if they blame it on some higher authority, "No, I cannot prescribe that medication because it is not considered appropriate treatment and could therefore get me into trouble." This moves the power struggle outside the individual patient–doctor relationship.

When the power struggle is extreme, it is useful to use a therapeutic paradox, suggesting to the patient that they cannot comply or that they are not ready to comply because to do so they would have to accept the doctor's authority. For example, "It is so important to you to feel in control of your life and feel as though nobody else is controlling you that you are incapable of going along with the treatment program. I can see that I, as your doctor, must accept this. You simply cannot follow your program." This may release the patient from the need to rebel by nonadherence. They can also rebel by proving the doctor wrong and be able to adhere.

In some situations it is the family where the power struggle occurs. Take, for example, the case of a university professor considered a standout in his area of science. In his early sixties he suffered a serious myocardial infarction (MI). His risk factors include obesity, high cholesterol, and hypertension, no doubt exacerbated by his weight. For a brief time following the MI, he followed his diet and exercise program, but over the course of several months he gradually reverted to his old ways. His doctors and his wife were constantly pressuring him, which he called nagging. Although he always agreed that he should adhere to the program, his effort did not follow.

With some encouragement from the doctor, the wife did the following. One evening she made all of his favorite foods, including several that had a high fat content. At suppertime she placed them all before him and told him, "I have been very selfishly wanting you to refrain from these foods. Obviously they are more important to you than anything else. I just wanted you to be around for me for a long time in the future, but I have to accept what is important to you. So, I've made this for you. It will make me feel too bad to watch you eat it, though, so I'm going for a walk. I'll be back in an hour." She returned an hour later to find that he had not touched any of the food, and his behavior began to change markedly.

The wife's intervention began the change of a number of behavioral interactions and reframed (created a new meaning) his behavior. Prior to this encounter his behavior was defined by him as autonomous. This intervention interactively and subtly shifted the meaning slightly to selfishness, or at least his not being charitable when it come to doing something for his family. The behavioral sequence of his doctor and wife trying to convince him to change was also altered to give him the opportunity to choose to change on his own.

This intervention is unlikely to work for many people. It was designed to fit this patient's and family's needs and style of living. The basic approach to identifying an unmet need that leads to compliance problems and then substituting a new plan that better satisfies these needs is a universal approach that helps many patients with compliance problems.

References

Fogarty J (1997) Reactance theory and patient noncompliance. Soc Sci Med 45:1277–1288.
Freeman J (1999) Personal communication.

McDaniel SH, Campbell TL, Seaburn DB (1990) Family-Oriented Primary Care: A Manual for Medical Providers. New York: Springer-Verlag.

Ruffalo R, Garabedian-Frufallo S, Pawlson L (1985) Patient compliance. Am Fam Physician 31:93–100.

Smith D (1995) Geriatric Psychopathology: Psychotropic Medication Compliance by Elders. Providence, RI: Behavioral Health Resource Press.

Smith D, Amundson L (1995) Psychotropic Medication Compliance by Elders Monograph. Providence, RI: Manissess Communications Group.

Stuart, RB (1982) Adherence: Compliance and Generalization in Behavioral Medicine. New York: Brunner/Mazel.

Weinstein R, Tosolin F, Ghilardi L, Zanardelli E (1996).Psychological intervention in patients with poor compliance. J Clin Periodont 23:283–288.

11

Insomnia

ASSESSMENT

1. For the patient with insomnia, obtain a detailed description of bed-time routine and sleep experience.
2. Identify recent changes in bedtime routine.
3. What has already been tried to make things better?
4. Screen for depression, anxiety, and substance abuse.
5. Screen for sleep apnea and restless legs. Explore symptoms of excessive drowsiness, morning headache, erectile impotence, frequent microarousal associated with lapses in breathing, snoring, leg jerks, or an arousal snort.
6. If possible interview bedtime partner as well.
7. Physical examination should rule out common physiologic causes of insomnia, such as asthma, reflux, or ulcer.

PLAN

1. If anxiety, depression, or substance abuse is present, treatment for this problem may alleviate the insomnia.
2. If physiologic illness is present or possible, treatment may alleviate insomnia.
3. For geriatric patients it is often enough to reassure them that night-time awakening, shallow sleep, and early awakening are normal for their age group.
4. Sleep hygiene program is often most effective. It entails changing the sleep environment and the pattern associated with sleep initiation. The circadian rhythm functions poorly in the face of frequent changes. The sleep environment should be structured to control for a comfortable temperature and avoid abrupt loud noises if possible. The bed should be used only for sleep and sex. The patient should wake up at the same time each day and if possible go to sleep at a similar time each night. Naps should be avoided even if the person

is not sleeping. Aerobic exercises should be encouraged but not be done an hour or two before sleep. If hungry, a light meal can be taken before bedtime, but avoid large meals. Caffeine, alcohol, and any other substance that alters sleep architecture should be avoided. Those who do shift work or travel to other time zones should be cautioned that changing the bedtime or waking up time more than 1 hour a day could lead to problems. Patients are told that when they go to bed they should allow no more than 30 minutes to fall asleep. If they have not fallen asleep after 30 minutes, they should get out of bed, go to a different room, and read a self-help book or do relaxation exercises for at least one-half hour. They can then return to bed; if they have not fallen asleep in 30 minutes they should again get out of bed and follow the previous pattern. This pattern is repeated as many times as necessary until they fall asleep. The program sometimes takes a number of days before it helps them achieve sleep consistently.

5. Drug therapy for the most part should be considered second-line treatment for sleep. Benzodiazepines can be used for situational disruptions that are likely to occur for 2 weeks or less. The patient is started on a dosage sufficient to achieve sleep and be maintained on that dosage for 2 weeks, followed by a week-long tapering process to avoid rebound insomnia. Zolpidem and zaleplon (benzodiazepine-like drugs) produce fewer side effects in most people and may be effective longer than benzodiazepines. In the rare instance where pharmacotherapy is needed long term, it is most effective to use a sedating antidepressant such as trazodone at low doses (e.g., 25–75 mg.).

Insomnia is a common problem. About one-third of all adults complain of insomnia each year, and approximately one in five report that it is a serious problem. The most common complaints are transient insomnia lasting a few days to a few weeks, often associated with a stressor, a major change in one's life, or a major change in one's daily routine.

For those experiencing chronic insomnia, more than half have an associated psychological problem, such as anxiety, depression, or a substance abuse problem. Primary physiologic problems also can lead to insomnia, including ulcers, reflux, and pain disorders. Sleep apnea accounts for 1–2% of sleep disorders. Restless legs account for about 10%. As people age they require less sleep and sleep less deeply. Snoring can become an increasing issue with age: By the time people reach age 65 nearly half snore regularly.

It is important when assessing sleep disorders to keep in mind that studies show that when objective observation of sleep is compared to a person's self-perception, most people sleep better than they think they do.

Assessment

A thorough sleep history is the most important diagnostic tool available. The doctor should explore the regular bedtime routine, the patient's experience falling asleep, and what they do to try to make things better. Any recent changes in the routine should be noted (e.g., moving to a new room, getting home from work later at night). Signs of depression, anxiety, and substance abuse should be explored. It is useful, if possible, to interview the bed partner. Attention should be paid to snoring, leg jerks, or lapses in breathing rate. The bed partner might have noticed a regular "arousal snort" typical of sleep apnea. The history also should include excessive drowsiness, unusual morning headaches, erectile impotence, and frequent microarousals associated with lapses in breathing. The physical examination should rule out common physiologic causes of insomnia, such as asthma, reflux, or an ulcer. Obviously, if there is a component of anxiety, depression, or substance abuse, focusing treatment on these problems often ameliorates the sleep disorder. However, a good sleep hygiene program can serve as both a primary treatment for insomnia and an adjunct treatment when the insomnia is secondary to another diagnosis.

A frequent cause of difficulty falling asleep is what is referred to as a "be spontaneous paradox." The pattern begins when a patient does not fall asleep as soon as usual. The patient then begins *trying* to fall asleep, becoming more and more frustrated when sleep does not come. The frustration ensures sleeplessness. The next night the patient is even more determined to sleep and more frustrated when sleep does not come. Sleep is a spontaneous reaction; and the very act of making an effort predisposes one to failing in the attempt.

Aging causes changes in sleep. Sometimes it is reassuring to the older person to understand that waking early, having nighttime awakening, and experiencing shallow sleep is normal for their age.

Sleep Hygiene Program

The body's circadian rhythm functions poorly in the face of frequent changes. It functions best in an atmosphere of consistency.

A sleep hygiene program should begin with a plan to structure the sleep environment and help the circadian rhythm. Regarding the sleep environment, the room should be maintained at a comfortable temperature, and abrupt, loud noises should be avoided if possible. The bed should be used only for sleep and sex, so the person is conditioned to those activities when in bed. Reading and watching television should be done elsewhere. Structuring the circadian rhythm begins with waking up at the same time each day and, if possible, going to sleep at the same time each night. Naps should be avoided even if the person is drowsy from lack of sleep. A regular aerobic exercise program has been associated with a quicker onset of sleep and deeper sleep, although such exercise should be avoided 1–2 hours before bedtime. Being hungry sometimes makes sleep difficult. On the other hand, being overly satiated also can lead to problems with sleep onset. Therefore if the person is hungry a light meal can be taken before bedtime. Stimulants such as caffeine should be avoided. Alcohol should also be avoided because although it can encourage the onset of sleep it distorts the sleep cycle, and frequent nighttime awakenings commonly occur.

Those who do shift work or travel to other time zones should be cautioned that changing bedtime or wake-up time more than 1 hour a day can lead to problems.

When the patient is in a pattern of having difficulty falling asleep (the "be spontaneous paradox," as described above) the following program is often helpful. If patients are not sleeping within 30 minutes of going to bed, they are to get out of bed, go to a different room, and read a self-help book for 30 minutes. They are not to read a highly stimulating book, nor are they to watch television or engage in any physical activity. A book on relaxation exercises or stress reduction is an excellent choice. Those with an interest may read scriptures. After reading for a half-hour they then can go back to bed but should not stay there again for any more than 30 awake minutes. If they are not sleeping within one-half hour, they should repeat the process as many times as necessary until they do fall asleep. The next morning they should wake up at their usual time, no matter how much sleep they have had. It sometimes takes a number of days for this program to lead to a more regular sleep pattern. The use of pharmacologic intervention during this process is usually not helpful and should be avoided.

Drug Therapy

Pharmacotherapy is rarely useful for chronic insomnia. It should be reserved for situational disruptions such as during a hospitalization. If this form of treatment is chosen, over-the-counter medication (usually comprised of antihistamines) can be recommended (except for geriatric patients), although efficacy rarely lasts longer than 2 weeks.

Because of their safety and efficacy, hypnotics such as benzodiazepines are the primary treatment of choice for short-term insomnia. They are useful only for short-term treatment primarily when patients have become so frustrated and fatigued by their lack of sleep that a brief period of treatment seems essential. They are not intended for chronic insomnia or for the depressed patient. They are contraindicated for the patient with a history of substance abuse. Their use should be kept to a maximum of 2 weeks followed by a week-long tapering, as insomnia rebound is common. There are significant drawbacks with hypnotics, including next-day hangover, although this occurs less often with short-acting medicines. Short-acting benzodiazepines have been associated with amnesia. An overall loss in mental functioning on IQ tests has been demonstrated when people are on even low doses of benzodiazepines. Along with rebound insomnia there are alterations in the sleep cycle that may lead to less efficient sleep; and there is a significant risk of addiction. Zolpidem and zaleplon, benzodiazepine-like drugs, have fewer side effects for most patients and may be effective longer.

In the rare instance where pharmacologic treatment is needed longer term, it is safest to use a sedating antidepressant such as trazodone at low doses (e.g., 25–75 mg). This is especially true if depressive symptoms are also present.

References

Eddy M, Walbroehl GS (1999) Insomnia. Am Fam Physician 59:1911–1916.

Morin CM, Colecchi C, Stone J, Sood R, Brink D (1999) Behavioral and pharmacological therapies for late-life insomnia. JAMA 281:991–999.

National Heart Lung and Blood Institute Working Group on Insomnia (1999) Insomnia: assessment and management in primary care. Am Fam Physician 59:3029–3037.

Neubauer DN (1999) Sleep problems in the elderly. Am Fam Physician 59:2551–2557.

Slama K, Smith D (1995) Sleep Disorders in Old Age Monograph. Providence, RI: Manissess Communications Group.

12

Substance Abuse

SCREENING

To screen for substance abuse, ask them:
1. When was your last drink or beer?
2. How many drinks or beers did you have at that time?
3. How many drinks or beers did you have last Friday night?
If the patient has had three or fewer drinks on both occasions, quit questioning; otherwise continue with the revised Cage questions.
4. Have you thought you should cut down?
5. Has anyone complained about your drinking?
6. Have you felt guilty or upset about your drinking?
7. Was there a single day when you had five or more (revised)?
If one or more answers are positive, further evaluation should be attempted. If two or more are positive, treatment is recommended. Further evaluation includes a 30-day period of abstinence to explore the patient's ability to control usage. Both family and patient should provide feedback.

ASSESSMENT

1. If the patient has not had a physical examination, one should be done to rule out associated sequelae of substance abuse.
2. Obtain a specific step-by-step description of when in the person's day the alcohol is commonly used, including how others respond to the alcohol usage. When is the patient least likely to drink?
3. What are the patient's motivation and goals for treatment? For example, most patients stop because of fear of losing a job, a spouse, their health, or their freedom through incarceration. If possible, interview the family as well. Explore their view of the problem and what they have done to help.

PLAN

The primary goal for a family physician should be working through expected denial and increasing the patient's motivation for change.

1. Use the change readiness protocol. The five-step approach includes the following.
   a. Precontemplative stage
   b. Contemplative stage
   c. Preparation stage
   d. Action stage
   e. Maintenance stage
2. If family members or significant others are more motivated for treatment than the patient, the motivated family members can be directed to a plan whereby they provide more attention when the patient is sober and become withdrawn and absent whenever the patient begins to use substances.
3. Once patients have agreed to the need for treatment, they can be directed to the appropriate level of care.
   a. If they are functional at work and do not drink daily, refer them to Alcoholics Anonymous (AA) for regular attendance. Referral to a substance counselor is an alternative option.
   b. If they are drinking regularly but still have a job that is not threatened by their alcohol use, a partial day or evening program may be suitable.
   c. If their drinking is interfering with work or they drink heavily daily, refer them to an inpatient program.
4. The physician should encourage the substance abuser and their family to explore what needs are being met by substance usage and become involved in new activities that can satisfy these needs in new ways.

Successful treatment of substance abuse nearly always requires a team approach. The family physician is in a key position to identify abusers and guide them into treatment. Rarely do patients seek out a physician because of substance abuse problems. It is usually identified when evaluating patients for other problems (e.g., ulcer, insomnia, accidents, abuse). Identifying substance abuse is challenging. Family physicians may also make valuable contributions to treatment as the patient and family progress.

Assessment

The health care maintenance examination provides an excellent opportunity to screen for substance usage. The best initial screen for substance abuse is to ask specific questions related to when the person had drunk or used substances last and how much. For example, the physician might ask, "When was your last drink or beer?" If the patient answers, "More than a week ago," alcohol screening can cease. If it has been less than a week, the patient should be asked, "How many drinks or beers did you have at that time?" The patient should then be asked, "How many drinks or beers did you have last Friday night?" If the patient has had three or fewer drinks on both occasions, the screening can conclude. If the patient has had more than three drinks on either occasion, the four Cage questions should be asked. The revised Cage questions are as follows:

1. Have you thought you should cut down?
2. Has anyone complained about your drinking?
3. Have you felt guilty or upset about your drinking?
4. Was there a single day when you had five or more?

One or more positive responses indicate a need for further evaluation. Two or more positive responses indicate a need for some level of treatment. One way to evaluate further is to request that the patient refrain from drinking for a 30-day period. Not only does the physician gain insight from their response to this request, but it is often the first step in helping the patient face denial.

Often patients deny the need to pursue anything related to their substance abuse despite it being clear to the physician that they have a problem. This denial and resistance to change are not necessarily cause for pessimism about ultimately successful treatment, as most people who engage in substance abuse initially offer significant resistance. Success is not related to denial or resistance but to how much stake patients have in getting over their substance abuse problem; that is, how much they can lose by not pursuing treatment.

Intelligence, as is well known, has nothing to do with denial or resistance to change. Like all well established behavioral patterns, if patients continue the pattern they are meeting important needs. There may be some physiologic needs being met by the alcohol, but most often other needs are being fulfilled as well. For example, anxiety may be self-treated through the use of alcohol, and alcohol can serve as a social lubricant. Alcohol may also be an excuse for one's failures, which then leads to rescuing. This care-taking pattern is common in substance-related co-dependent relationships. If alcohol has been a long-standing problem, one can be assured that some needs have come to be met through its use, and the psychological distress of not having these needs met leads to resistance.

The most common motivators for accepting the need to change is fear of losing something important (e.g., a job, one's marriage, money, one's freedom such as by incarceration) or fear of the consequences to one's health. For treatment to be successful it is essential to begin the treatment process before these losses have occurred. Most successful approaches to initiating treatment are organized around the principle that the only way for the patient to avoid the loss of one of these important factors is to obtain substance treatment. In family medicine where there is a long-term relationship with patients, the process of working toward the initiation of treatment for substance abuse can be dealt with over a period of time.

Sometimes patients argue that they cannot face their alcohol problem until other problems are resolved (e.g., marital problems). The physician should take the position that other problems cannot be addressed until after drinking has stopped.

It is a refreshing but rare occurrence for patients to come to the physician stating that they have an alcohol problem for which they need help. When this does occur the physician can simply explore the treatment options with the patient and make a referral. These options are addressed in a later section. Once the patient has agreed that a substance abuse problem exists, if they have not had a physical examination it should be done at this time to rule out associated sequelae of alcohol abuse. It is useful when exploring the problem to obtain a specific step-by-step description of when in a person's day the alcohol is commonly used, including information about how other people have responded to the alcohol use. For example: is the spouse continually nagging at the subject to not drink, so the alcohol serves the function of proving autonomy from the significant other. Understanding the sequence of events can help the physician develop recommendations that can alter social factors maintaining the alcohol usage.

Finding out when the patient is least likely to drink may also help treatment planning, as encouraging these experiences is often helpful. Finally, it is important to have a clear view of the patient's goal for treatment (e.g., save a job). This information provides the physician with motivating factors for change. It is useful to explore what patients and families have already tried for solving the problem. Perhaps they have tried not to drink when other people are around. Perhaps they have tried periods of abstinence when the pressure to quit has been great. Perhaps they have tried to convince other people they really have no problem, or perhaps they have attempted to put the blame on others, stating that they would not drink if the others did not bother them so much. The family members may have tried nagging, put-downs, idle threats, and brief periods of ignoring. Whatever the attempted solutions have been, it is important that a new plan be different in some significant ways. It is extremely helpful to include the family or at least one significant other in the assessment process to provide more accurate information and to prepare the family to help with treatment.

Plan

When developing a plan certain principles are important to further the chances of success. First, avoid blame. All recommendations for treatment and change should be placed in the context of doing things that are helpful but not necessarily related to who is at fault. Second, it is important for the patient to see and feel a sense of control over the solution, even though it is helpful to get the whole family involved in the solution. For example, for one patient who clearly was using alcohol in part as a tranquilizer for a stressful job, the wife agreed that when he came home from work he would be given an hour of free time to go jogging to unwind before making any demands on his time. Finally, it is essential that whatever plan is developed, it must address the needs of the people motivated to change. For example, if the patient's primarily complaint is stopping the spouse's nagging behavior, any effort made in the direction of controlling substances should be put in the context of stopping a spouse's nagging so patients can feel their needs being addressed.

One approach to helping a patient move toward change is based on Prochaska's model of change readiness (see Chapter 13). In this context the decision to take action occurs as part of a five-step process. It first starts with the precontemplative stage, when there is absolutely no urge to change. It then moves to the contemplative stage, where the person is considering change but in the distant future. The preparation stage is next, where persons by rehearsing it in their mind or by actual behavior are developing a plan to change in the near future. During the action stage the person is working at making changes. Finally, the maintenance stage is where the patient has made positive changes but must fight to not slip back into old patterns. With this approach to change the goal is to help the patient move from one stage to the next.

If persons are in the precontemplative stage, the physician can discuss with them what needs the alcohol is meeting. This helps the patients believe that the doctor understands them, and it encourages receptivity. The physician can then discuss with them how their needs can be addressed in other ways. They may also discuss road blocks to their making changes. To help them move to the contemplative stage, the doctor can ask them to think about what might occur that would make them interested in really making a change. The physician should avoid sounding like he or she is nagging the patient to make a change.

If patients are in the contemplative stage, the physician can discuss the advantages of the change, how they might go about making changes, what the roadblocks might be, and how they might negotiate ways around the roadblocks. The doctor can suggest that they think about what the first step to change might be. This process encourages them to action.

If patients are in the action stage, helping them choose the best treatment option is the central focus. This area is discussed later.

In the maintenance stage, the primary focus is on problem-solving. Determining the point at which temptation to relapse is likely to occur and alternative actions that might be taken to have the patient's needs met in new ways helps avoid relapse.

Another approach to change is family-based. Not infrequently it is a family member who is motivated to make a change despite the substance abuser's resistance. However, family members may believe there is nothing they can do that could affect the alcoholic's behavior. If one considers that the reason alcoholics begin treatment is to avoid a painful situation, a family member often can do much to promote change. It is important to keep in mind, however, that despite family members' eagerness to change, they may also have considerable resistance to change themselves. Some of their needs may be met through the substance usage. For example, it may make them feel important to be a rescuer when the person gets into trouble; perhaps they have a fear of closeness, and the substance abuse contributes to distance; maybe there are control issues, and they can pretty much run the family when the spouse is drinking.

If family members present with a desire to help the substance abuser, there is much they can do. First, to help them deal with their own possible resistance to change, suggest that they attend Al-Anon meetings or read a book on the topic of co-dependency. This background helps them prepare for changes they may have to make themselves, such as not rescuing the substance abuser. Also, it is difficult for the alcoholic to remain in denial if the wife/husband and children are regularly going to Al-Anon and Al-A-Teen.

Once they have attended Al-Anon or read a book on co-dependency, they are ready to begin the next step. They should be informed that this plan may take 3 months to start showing results, and that it may be extremely stressful during certain periods. It is based on making substance usage painful while making abstinence a better way for the alcoholic to have his or her needs met. The family member starts by telling the substance user, one time only, that they care for them but cannot stand to be around them when they drink. Therefore they will no longer be around when they are drinking. At this point family members must avoid any arguments but simply state that at any point the substance abuser would like to seek counseling they can go together to their family doctor. Once this is said, all argument regarding the subject should be avoided despite the fact that often the substance user attempts to initiate arguments. From that point on, whenever the user has even one drink or the first instance that the significant others become aware the patient is using, they should leave the scene if possible. For example, if they are at home in the evening they should go to some safe place, perhaps a family member's home, perhaps the library. If there are school-age children, taking them to the library to study evenings when this occurs can be helpful. When it is time to go to bed they can come home and go to bed without saying a word to the user. When the others cannot leave the house, at the very least they should ignore the user when drinking. Often the user attempts to engage the significant others in argument. This is a way to overcome being ignored. Family members should avoid arguments or any interaction when substances have been used. In fact, the attempt to engage in arguments should be explained to the significant others as a sign that this intervention is working. Often the initial response of the alcoholic is to become angry. When anger does not work to return the situation to the usual atmosphere, the user is likely to attempt ignoring the family as a way to deter the process. When ignoring does not work, often the substance user becomes dysphoric and tries to elicit rescuing behavior. However, until the drinking stops or the person asks to go to the doctor, this program should be continued. At the same time, the positive reinforcement side of the program encourages the family to heap attention on alcoholics whenever they are *not drinking*. This makes it clear to the user that it is not they who are being rejected, only their usage. The attempt here is to break the usual pattern surrounding the alcohol usage, which it can be assumed is contributing to maintaining the pattern. Many family members are so angry with the user it is difficult for them to provide the positive reinforcement. The doctor can help by giving encouragement with regular appointments.

It usually takes weeks to a few months for this program to have an impact. It often, however, leads users to agree that they need treatment or at least to reduce their usage markedly. An alternative to this protocol is to refer the significant other for an "alcohol intervention" procedure, which is similar to the above but much quicker.

Once users have agreed to the need for treatment the physician can guide them into the therapeutic protocol that is most likely to be effective. The following is a basic breakdown of options available in most areas. For the patient who is a daily user and it has affected both the home relationships and job performance, an inpatient program is probably necessary. For those who have some days of abstinence and it has not markedly affected their job performance, a partial day or evening program may be as effective, or even more effective, because they can continue at their job. Usually these programs require persons to keep working, but they can attend the program during most of the time they are not at work. Less intense programs for those who are binge drinkers or maintain fairly long periods of sobriety when required can be referred to attend AA meetings on a regular basis. For those who do not find AA helpful or perhaps the spiritual requirements are not in keeping with their belief system or life style, a substance abuse counselor or family therapist is an alternative. For those who are using alcohol to treat anxiety, interpersonal problems, or some psychological symptoms, referral to a therapist may be most effective. The family physician may still provide important therapy during or after treatment because they are likely to know the family well and can be useful in helping guide the family in new directions to have needs met in a new way, without alcohol. Often people who are addicted to substances fully recover only when they become addicted to some other healthier activity, such as exercise or a hobby.

Medications

Medications have little use in the treatment of substance abuse. Tranquilizers and other drugs, which might lead to dependence or addiction, are especially to be avoided, as co-addiction is common. Our previous comments on nonpharmacologic treatment of anxiety and depression are especially germane in the context of the psychiatric problems accompanying substance abuse. Patients with substance abuse should not learn that relief comes from a pill. Occasionally, in the face of serious mental illness (especially major depression with psychotic features, bipolar illness, or schizophrenia) accompanying substance abuse (known as a dual diagnosis) appropriate psychotropic medication is indicated.

In the elderly the family physician often encounters "secondary alcoholism," or alcoholism as self-treatment of anxiety or more often depression. This is the exception to the clinical rule that "no problem can be solved until the alcohol problem is solved." Appropriate treatment, whether it be with nonpharmacologic methods or antidepressants, must be undertaken in this case before working on the alcoholism. In fact, when treatment of the underlying psychopathology is effective, the alcoholism usually vanishes without specific treatment.

Antabuse is effective in certain circumstances to allow alcoholics to make a morning decision whether they will remain sober and then enforce that decision for the rest of the day by taking the pill. This is best accomplished under the supervision of a family member, in an alcoholism program, or in a work release from jail program. Antabuse, when used alone, is not effective treatment.

Several other substances have been researched in regard to decreasing the "cravings" associated with various addictions. Some have shown a positive effect, but they are considered experimental and at this point have no place in the treatment of substance abuse in the community by family physicians. The exception is the use of bupropion (Zyban, Wellbutrin, Wellbutrin SR) for treating nicotine/smoking addiction. As part of a well constructed plan for smoking cessation, this drug has shown a slight increase in efficacy over the same plan without the drug. Nicotine replacement also may be helpful for smoking cessation.

Case Report

B.B. was a 52-year-old caucasian woman who presented to her family physician with headaches. In the process of performing brief mental health screening the family physician learned that the patient was distressed by her husband's abuse of alcohol. When under the influence her husband was verbally abusive, although he had never been physically abusive. He never abused their infant granddaughter, for whom they regularly cared to help their divorced daughter.

The physician asked B.B. to fill out a headache questionnaire and performed a brief examination. She quickly determined that the headaches were of the tension type and prescribed gum chewing, relaxation techniques, and some range of motion exercises for the neck. She discouraged frequent use of analgesics, even aspirin and acetaminophen.

The physician pointed out to B.B. that the stress of living with a family member who suffered substance abuse was probably at the root of her headaches. She briefly discussed the history of the husband's substance abuse and found that it had been going on for a number of years though not as bad as lately. There had been no interventions at any time in the past. She learned that B.B. had often begged her husband to stop drinking and had threatened to leave him many times, though she had never carried through with these threats. Her adult children had often tried to convince her to leave.

The physician referred her to the local Al-Anon program with the intent of learning about alcoholism and how she might help him stop. She briefly educated B.B. about enabling and co-morbidity. The physician indicated that once B.B. had gained strength and educated herself on these matters the physician would be ready to assist with an alcohol intervention. In the meantime she asked if B.B. could convince her husband to come for an office visit. B.B. doubted it.

After a number of weeks the physician met again with B.B., this time along with her daughter and two sons. They discussed undertaking an alcohol intervention and set a time for a home visit, as B.B. had been unable to convince her husband to come to see the physician. The physician outlined an agenda for this confrontation and instructed the family on what they might say to their father/husband.

Three days later the physician drove to the family's home at 5:30 p.m. The family was gathered, and B.B.'s husband was surprised to find this meeting ongoing when he arrived home from work. The physician explained why she was there with the family, and each family member in turn made a prepared comment to the father/husband. They explained how his alcohol usage had affected them. At first Mr. B denied that he had a problem; then when confronted with a number of family recollections and a reminder of his two episodes of driving while intoxicated, he acquiesced and agreed that sometimes he "let things get out of hand," but he specifically denied "being a drunk." The family stood fast and unified in their insistence that Mr. B obtain some help. As agreed at the preliminary meeting, they insisted that Mr. B either begin to see the physician on a regular basis and to go to Alcoholics Anonymous (AA) or they would be forced to undertake an alcohol commitment to an inpatient program. The physician added that even if Mr. B came to her office and attended AA but was unable to remain abstinent he might still need to enter an inpatient program. Mr. B bargained and at one point became verbally abusive, but he eventually agreed to this plan "just to get people off my back."

At the end of the week the physician met with Mr. B. He was hostile and uncooperative, providing little history and showing little motivation for change. He had not made contact with AA. The physician asked the Cage

questions, and the answers probably indicated denial and lack of cooperation, given the history Mrs. B had provided that undoubtedly was reliable.
The physician told Mr. B, however, that because it was his word against his
family's whether he was an alcoholic that she wished him to prove that he
was in control of his drinking and undertake a 1-week period of "controlled
drinking." She explained that what she meant was that Mr. B would have
one drink and no more each night. Both he and Mrs. B would monitor this
intake. Mrs. B would call the physician with the results from her point of
view, and Mr. B could tell the physician how he had done at their next weekly
visit. Furthermore, the physician said that she wanted Mr. B to agree to sign
himself into an alcohol treatment unit if he were unable to limit himself in
this way during the 1-week period of "controlled drinking." He agreed.

At the next visit the physician was prepared with a report from Mrs. B
that the patient had been unable to restrain himself to a single drink nightly.
He had done well for 4 days and then become severely inebriated nightly
thereafter. When confronted with this record the patient had first tried to
rationalize it; but when the physician reminded him that Mr. B's family was
ready, willing, and able to undertake an alcohol commitment he recanted
and agreed to go on his own. The physician and he went over a list of nearby
facilities, and a choice was made.

The physician received a telephone call from the alcohol treatment center
5 weeks later explaining that Mr. B would be returning home soon and
needed to schedule an aftercare visit. The treatment center indicated that Mr.
B would be attending AA, and Mrs. B would continue with Al-Anon.

References

Baird MA (1984) A protocol for family compliance counseling. Fam Syst Med
2:333–336.
Burge SK, Schneider FD (1999) Alcohol-related problems: recognition and interven-
tion. Am Fam Physician 59:361–367.
Cooley FB, Lasser D (1992) Managing alcohol abuse in a family context. Am Fam
Physician 45:1735–1739.
Del Toro IM, Thom DJ, Beam HP, Horst T (1996) Chemically dependent patients
in recovery: roles for the family physician. Am Fam Physician 53:1667–1673.
Kaufman P, Kaufman E (1979) Family Therapy of Drug and Alcohol Abuse. New
York: Gardner.
Mallin R, Tumblin M Am. Fam. Phy. (2000) Addiction Treatment in Family Medicine
Monograph (249th ed). Leawood, KS: American Academy of Family Physicians.
Miller NS, Gold MS (1998) Management of withdrawal syndromes and relapse pre-
vention in drug and alcohol dependence. Am Fam Physician 58:139–146.
O'Farrell TJ (1993) Treating Alcohol Problems: Marital and Family Interventions.
New York: Guilford.
Stanton MD, Todd TC, et al (1982) The Family Therapy of Drug Abuse and Addic-
tion. New York: Guilford.

13

Habit Problems

CONDITIONED RESPONSES

Assessment

1. For those with habit problems, obtain a description of the sequence of events preceding, during, and following the problem behavior.
2. Explore the reinforcements (i.e., what needs are being met). What is pleasurable to the patient?
3. Explore past attempted solutions to avoid repeating them.
4. Identify noxious or extinguishing responses.

Plan

1. Each time patients alter their behavior in a way that demonstrates a small improvement, a reward should be supplied.
2. Rewards should at first be frequent and expected improvement gradual. Patients should keep a diary of target behavior and reinforcement history to measure progress.
3. As improvement occurs, expectations can gradually become higher and rewards less frequent (although larger).
4. Once desired change has occurred, offer intermittent reinforcement (e.g., every third time).
5. Negative reinforcement helps (e.g., immediate withdrawal of attention in response to some behaviors).
6. If absolutely necessary, an aversive response can be used initially. Aversive response, however, should not be harmful or disrespectful.
7. Ultimately, the new behavior should be able to meet needs sufficiently that the patient does not revert to the problem behavior.

LIFE STYLE HABIT PROBLEMS (e.g., smoking)

Assessment

1. Assess the sequence of events preceding, during, and following the problematic behavior.

2. Assess what needs are met by the problematic behavior.
3. Assess the patient's level of readiness to make a change.
4. Assess past attempted solutions.

Plan (using the following five-stage approach)

1. *Precontemplative stage.* Patients are in denial. The doctor should acknowledge that their needs are being met by the problematic behavior; ask them to define these needs; ask them what might be altered to make them more interested in change. Use a scaling technique to have them place themselves on a readiness-to-change scale.
2. *Contemplative stage.* Patients at this point recognize the problems but see change at some unspecified time in the future. Therapeutic strategy begins with helping patients define the advantages and the roadblocks to making changes. Ask them to think about how they would decide when it was time to change and request that they think about or get more information about what it would be like if they decided to change.
3. *Preparation stage.* Patients are committed to change but procrastinate, still feeling overwhelmed by potential obstacles. Ask patients to begin to develop a specific plan on how they would go about the change when ready. The more specific the better, particularly in regard to dealing with obstacles. Determine if they are ready to set a date to start change.
4. *Action stage.* Patients are beginning to follow a plan of change. The goal should be to reinforce the change and recognize when the change is most difficult and develop specific responses to obstacles.
5. *Maintenance stage.* Patients have achieved their goal for a significant length of time. Explore when they are most apt to regress; develop specific plans for dealing with these difficult periods. Also develop alternative plans for having needs met that were once met by the problematic behavior. For example, if alcohol usage was used to provide socialization, they should find other ways to get their socialization needs met.

   NOTE: If the patient relapses (i.e., with a full return to the problematic behavior) rather than an occasional slip, the doctor should define it as a temporary setback, explore what the patient can learn from this setback, and develop a new plan for confronting it.

All animals whose behavior is not totally instinctive develop habits. Habits, no doubt, have evolved because they are useful to the individual. They allow the animals to develop repetitive behaviors that satisfy needs without having to expend energy. Habits become a problem when circumstances change their value or they become so exaggerated they are more harmful than helpful. For example, self-grooming behavior, which in all primates tends to lower anxiety, can lead to nail biting, which causes the person problems. Smoking brings immediate pleasure from nicotine and perhaps social acceptance but in the long run has obvious health consequences. Because habits at one point satisfy some need, they become difficult to alter. The longer they have gone on and the more needs that have been satisfied by the behavior, the more difficult it is to change. Habits that are intermittently reinforced are particularly difficult to extinguish (e.g., playing slot machines).

It is useful for the purpose of treatment to divide habits into two broad categories: conditioned responses (those that are largely unconscious reactions that have become habituated, e.g., thumb sucking) and more cognitively learned, complex behaviors, such as smoking or a sedentary life style.

Pavlov's experiments are the most famous of the conditioned responses. Pavlov rang a bell while at the same time presenting the dog with some meat; the dog salivated and ate the meat. Soon Pavlov could simply ring the bell and the dog salivated with no meat present. The dog associated the bell with the pleasure of eating the meat but no longer needed the meat for the salivation response. In fact, "thinking" interferes. A child, for example, gets a good feeling when mom cuts his fingernails. The body's natural association with grooming behavior relaxes the body. The child experiences this as pleasurable. The next time the child is anxious, the child bites his fingernails and experiences the relaxation response, which becomes an ingrained habit. When the child's parents try to interfere with the nail biting, the child experiences it as their taking away a good feeling. Furthermore, even if the child wants to stop, it is difficult. Similar problems, such as a demented patient who makes repetitive noises when anxious, can be seen as conditioned responses.

Assessment and Treatment of Conditioned Responses

A description of the sequence of events preceding, during, and following the problematic behavior should be detailed. It helps to identify the reinforcements or how the needs of the individual are being met in a way that is maintaining the behavior. The therapeutic strategy then is to alter the sequence of events so the reinforcement is no longer associated with the problematic behavior. In some cases even a noxious or extinguishing response might be used to deal with problematic behavior. It is most effective to replace the problem behavior with something that meets the person's needs effectively. In some cases, in addition to original needs being met by the behavior, there are secondary rewards as well. For example, a 5-year-old who continues to suck his thumb may have initially done so simply because he enjoyed the sucking behavior and associated it with the pleasure of drinking milk from a bottle. However, as this child gets older there may also be the reward of winning the power struggle with the parents. For this behavior to be extinguished, both of the need-fulfilling experiences must be addressed. In the case of a dementia patient, similarly repetitive behaviors such as yelling might provide some anxiety reduction or relief from boredom; if this behavior also brings added attention from a nursing home staff, it is an additional reward that maintains the behavior.

For a 5-year-old the process of reducing the thumb-sucking behavior might include the following program. First, to win the child's support rewards should be frequent and the expected improvement gradual. For example, each time children go longer than usual (e.g., 15 minutes) without sucking their thumbs, they would be rewarded with something from the parents. Perhaps doing something special with the parent, such as reading a book for 5 minutes, would be rewarding. If the child is eager to earn this reward but keeps forgetting, an aversive association can be applied to the thumb, such as some bad-tasting substance, as a reminder. As the child improves, the rewards can become slightly larger and the time needed to attain the reward can be extended.

The same approach can be used with the dementia patient. For example, a dementia patient who strikes the staff when they walk by their room clearly does it for attention (when other needs such as attempts to communicate pain have been ruled out). Whenever this dementia patient happens to not strike out when a staff goes by them, the staff can make a special effort to interact with them in some pleasant way (e.g., to stroke their hair if that is pleasurable or give them candy). Because improvement usually comes slowly, good records must be kept so it is clear that the target behavior is improving. As the patient goes for longer and longer periods of time, the rewards can be increased (e.g., the staff spending an even longer time with them but not as often). The less memory the patient has, the more frequent the rewards must be given.

Once improvement is established, it is also helpful to use intermittent rewards. For example, use the reward every second or third time the improved behavior is evident. Negative reinforcement may also be used. This method differs from punishment or aversive therapy, though the term is often misused to mean the latter. With negative reinforcement a desired stimulus is withdrawn if a behavior occurs. This also illustrates the point that an appropriate reward or need (attention or love) is often achieved by the patient through undesired behavior. We may use this very need as the reward for a new, appropriate behavior through negative reinforcement.

For example, a nursing home resident calls for staff assistance to toilet or adjust her lap blanket to the point of being a demanding nuisance. When the staff reacts by ignoring the patient, she screams her requests and complaints. When the staff shows irritation, she gets the attention albeit negative and the behavior escalates. If a token system provides five poker chips per shift and one is spent each time the resident seeks attention inappropriately, she has no chips to spend for a half hour of tea and conversation with her favorite staff member. If she has one, she enjoys the attention that every human needs and deserves in an appropriate way and at reasonable times. As the behavior improves, the "price" of tea and talk may go up until tokens are not needed.

If absolutely necessary, an aversive response can be used initially. This response, however, should not be harmful or disrespectful; for example, a loud shout at a child or elder sometimes discourages behavior. (If it is experienced as attention it could have the opposite effect.)

Life Style Habit Problems

For life style problems (e.g., smoking) classic conditioning often does not work effectively. It is essential to work with patients to develop their own motivation toward change.

A common error sometimes made by physicians when attempting to encourage patients to change life style habits is that they get ahead of the patient. They talk with patients about specific ways they could improve their health while the patients are still struggling with whether they will work on a change. The doctor in these circumstances usually is dismissed by the patient as not understanding them and not being helpful.

Prochaska and his associates studied the way people go through the process of deciding to make a change and then making a change successfully. They used their findings to design therapeutic tools that enable clinicians to help move people along more quickly toward useful behavioral changes. Wildenhaus and his associates have specifically adapted this model to family practice, using it to battle such things as smoking and substance abuse and to initiate exercise programs. Their work has been well integrated with a brief therapy model in general and forms the basis of what we present here.

Readiness to change can be divided into five stages: precontemplative, contemplative, preparation, action, and maintenance; and for some there is a sixth stage, relapse. We discuss each of these in turn, including the patient characteristics and therapeutic strategies. A realistic goal for the clinician is to help the patient move to the next stage rather than to achieve immediate change.

During the precontemplative stage patients are essentially in denial. They see no problem or admit to no problem. The patient can be highly argumentative and resistant to any discussion about the problem. The therapeutic goal then is to move the person to the contemplative stage, where at least they are cognizant that a change may be beneficial.

Therapeutic strategy begins with empathy and getting patients to recognize that the doctor can appreciate their viewpoint. It is helpful to point out what gains they are getting from their habit and the difficulties they face if they change. For example, in the case of smoking, the physician might say,

"I know that smoking relaxes many people during a time of stress. It is also an extremely difficult habit to eliminate and so in many respects avoiding it makes things easier." The doctor may then ask the patient about warning signs that might occur that would make them feel it is worth it to make a change in tobacco use despite the difficulties. If the patient then identifies one or more warning signs, the doctor can then ask about what advantages there might be to "cutting down." Finally, it may be useful for the doctor to conclude with a scaling question regarding change, such as, "On a scale of 1 to 10, with 1 being no desire to change and 10 being a plan to do it tomorrow, where would you put yourself?" Scaling reframes the decision to change as lying on a continuum, rather than an all-or-nothing decision. If at any point the patient becomes argumentative, the physician should conclude by simply requesting that they think about it.

Patients in the contemplation phase see their behavior as a problem that at some point in the future they would like to change. They do not see it as an immediate imperative, or they see many deterrents in the immediate future. At this stage they usually have become more open to discussing the problem. The goal of the physician at this stage is to move them toward making a commitment to action.

Begin by asking the patient what has led them to decide to change. What are the advantages of making the change? What are the roadblocks? How would you decide it is time to change? With this information, the physician can encourage the patient to speculate on a specific plan. How might they meet the challenge of the roadblocks when they do decide to change? What support system can they use? What might occur that would make the difference in their deciding that the time to change is soon? If the doctor senses the patient is close to action, he or she might encourage the patient to begin to experiment with change (e.g., go one-half day without smoking or cut down from drinking 4 days a week to 3 days, or perhaps call up a number of exercise programs and find out what they would cost if they did decide to join an aerobics class). This should be done in the spirit of simply gathering more information to help them decide whether they are ready to make a change. Studies show that the more actions people take to explore change, the more they become committed to making the change.

The next step is the preparation stage. At this point the patient is committed to making change but may procrastinate about when it might occur. The potential obstacles still might be overwhelming them. At this point the physician wants to move them to the action stage. The best way to pursue this step initially is to discuss setting a date when change will begin. It is then useful to talk about the specific ways they will go about making the changes and the roadblocks and specific plans for dealing with these roadblocks. If the patient is a smoker, use of nicotine replacement might be discussed; if the smoker is worried about weight gain, discussing diet might be useful. If it is someone altering their alcohol habit, beginning an alcohol treatment program or getting involved in some new activities during the time they would usually go to the bar may be helpful. It is useful to program a follow-up appointment for a few days after the "date" the patient plans to begin the change. This helps motivate the patient to follow through with the change no matter how uncomfortable it might be because most patients want to report positive results to their doctor. It is helpful to tell patients that even if they do not have full success with their plan and relapse, it is still useful to make follow-up appointments.

The action phase commences when the patient begins to follow a plan of change. During this phase the goal of the clinician is to reinforce and maintain the changed behavior. It begins with liberal praise. Even when there have been minor slips, it is important to focus on the positive changes that have occurred. A slip should be defined as a learning opportunity to improve the treatment plan. The primary focus of therapy then becomes specific problem-solving, discussing what difficulties are arising while maintaining the changed behavior and developing specific alternatives to overcome these problems. It is also helpful to focus on what needs the problem behavior once satisfied that are now going unsatisfied and then develop a specific plan for having these needs met in new ways. For example, if a smoker found the habit relaxing, developing new relaxation techniques might be helpful. If drinking was a way to engage others, finding other ways to socialize might be explored. If smoking was one way teenagers asserted their independence, finding alternative actions to meet this need might maintain the behavioral change.

The maintenance stage begins once the goal has been achieved for a significant period (e.g., exercising or not smoking for 3 months). The basic therapeutic process during the maintenance stage is similar to that for the action stage. The doctor gives positive reinforcement for changes and offers problem-solving devices for the times patients have difficulty. For major changes such as cessation of substance abuse, new habits must be worked on if relapse is to be avoided. For example, if individuals have given up their drinking buddies, they must learn to socialize around other activities. If they had received attention from their spouse by rescuing behavior, they must find other activities that lead to care-taking behavior (e.g., a message to relieve stress).

Dealing With Relapse

If the patient relapses (i.e., with a full return to the problematic behavior) rather than having just an occasional slip, they may try to avoid the doctor. It is useful for the physician to make contact by phone or letter if necessary to prevent the relapse from becoming long term. When contact is made, it is important that the physician focus on the positive gains and what was learned by the attempts to make a change, rather than on the failure. Defining the relapse as a temporary setback frames it as something that can be gotten past, rather than as a failure, which supports "giving up." Admonishing patients leads only to their being more defensive. If the doctor takes the approach that we can learn something from the relapse, the patient might be more easily returned to either the preparation phase, or a new date may be scheduled for change with a return to the action phase.

Throughout these stages, when the physician meets with major resistance from the patient it is best to not be confrontational but to acknowledge the difficulties. The physician can then discuss with the patients the next *small* step or at least encourage them to think about it.

References

Prochaska J (1994) Changing for Good. New York: Guilford.

Prochaska J, DiClemente C, Norcross J (1992) In search of how people change: applications to addictive behaviors. Am Psychol 47:1102.

Sierles F, Blom BE (1982) Conditioning. In Sierles F (ed) Clinical Behavioral Science. New York: SP Medical & Scientific Books.

Wildenhaus K, Jordan M, Bellg A (1995) Patient Empowered Readiness Model (PERM). Detroit: Henry Ford Health Sciences.

14

Relaxation Exercise Training

Patients should begin relaxation exercises by making themselves comfortable. Patients are told to focus on being in touch with the muscles in their feet in as many ways as possible, such as sensations of touch, temperature, visualization, and kinesthetic sensation (body position), among others. The doctor instructs them: "I will count first from 1 to 5. Gradually tighten the muscles of your feet so by the count of 5 they are as tight as you can get them. I will then count back from 5 to 0 while you relax the muscles so that with each count the muscles in your feet are more relaxed than the count before; when I get to 0 the muscles in your feet should be totally relaxed, like a rag doll. During this process maintain your focus on nothing but the muscles in your feet."

1. "I am beginning the count now (counting very slowly): 1, 2, 3, 4, 5, 5, 4, 3, 2, 1, 0. Your feet are totally relaxed; totally let go, like a rag doll."
2. "Go to the next set of your muscles, such as from the ankles to the knees, and repeat the process. Continue this process with each set of muscles until you have covered your entire body."
3. "While experiencing your body as being totally relaxed and comfortable, next visualize yourself in a warm, comfortable place (there are many associations with warmth, relaxation, and comfort). For example, "Visualize yourself on a warm beach with the sun beating down, or in a hot tub with warm water flowing over you, or perhaps floating on a cloud with a warm breeze coming across you as you allow yourself to sink deeper and deeper into a relaxed state. Now comfortably and slowly breathe in through your nose and out through your mouth several times."
4. "Focus on how your body is feeling: all the relaxed muscles, the easy slow breathing. Become aware of how you have learned to control your relaxation and your body so fully, and be aware that you can return to this relaxed state any time you want. Let's practice

how to do this: "Begin by curling both fists, tightening the biceps and forearms, and wrinkle up your forehead. Then take a deep breath, hold it, and in a relaxed way exhale very, very slowly while relaxing your arms, forearms, biceps, fists, and forehead. Just let them go, returning to a totally relaxed state. Practice this several times at the end of each relaxation session so it becomes easier and easier to return to the relaxed state that you have come to experience."

5. "Practice the above exercise at least twice a day for 2 weeks, then daily."

Progressive relaxation exercises have a beneficial effect for a wide variety of problems. Although relaxation exercises are rarely the sole treatment used, as an adjunct treatment they can be helpful for any disorder in which a hypersympathetic response is part of the problem, such as stress disorders, anxiety disorders, pain disorders, and musculoskeletal problems. Related treatment approaches, such as biofeedback, meditation, and hypnosis, have also been found to be effective for these disorders. In fact, these methods have been found to be equally effective, but relaxation exercises are much simpler to learn, much easier for the physician to help the patient master, and require no equipment such as biofeedback instruments. Some patients do not respond well to relaxation exercises but do respond well to meditation, biofeedback, or hypnosis. Because it is, for the most part, unpredictable as to who responds best to which of these measures, using relaxation exercises as part of first-line treatment makes sense as they are simple and cost-effective.

As is well known, arousal of any specific sympathetic area (e.g., muscle tightness or rapid breathing) of the autonomic system excites the entire sympathetic system. The converse is also true and is the foundation of the relaxation response. For example, if one causes a reduction in electromyographic activity by relaxing one's muscles or learns to breath more slowly and rhythmically, a corresponding decrease in sympathetic activity occurs in the entire autonomic system.

The physician can teach the patient progressive relaxation exercises themselves often in 5–10 minutes or can recommend a book or tape. Many such books and tapes are available at the bookstore and library. Often it is best to try several until one is found that works well for the individual and then purchase it. Suggesting that the patient visit the library and try several works well.

What follows here is a relaxation exercise that works for many people and is simple to learn and teach. There is a learning curve related to relaxation exercises so one does improve with practice. Usually it is recommended that the patient practice for 15 minutes twice a day for at least 2 weeks prior to using the relaxation exercises in a therapeutic manner, such as in reaction to increasing anxiety. This point is important, as patients may lose confidence in the process if they try it before they can use it effectively.

Instruction in Relaxation Exercise

A guiding principle when coaching someone through a relaxation exercise is that distractions, particularly negative thoughts, can make achieving a relaxed state more difficult. It is therefore useful to guide the patient to concentrate on several sensations at a time. This effort to focus keeps stressful distractions away from the area of concentration, making the relaxation exercises more effective.

Patients should begin the exercise by making themselves comfortable. Ask them to visualize the muscles in their feet and establish a mental image of seeing and feeling the muscles. Tell the patient to focus on being as in touch with the muscles in their feet in as many ways as possible (e.g., by sensations of touch, temperature, visualization, kinesthetic sensation).

The doctor should instruct them: "I will count first from 1 to 5. I want you to gradually tighten the muscles of your feet so by the count of 5 they are as tight as you can get them. I will then count back from 5 to 0. I want you to relax the muscles so that with each count the muscles in your feet are more relaxed than the count before, until I get to 0, when the muscles in your feet should be totally relaxed, like a rag doll."

Instruct them now to try it. "Visualize the muscles in your feet and I will begin the count now [counting very slowly]: 1, 2, 3, 4, 5, 5, 4, 3, 2, 1, 0. Your feet are totally relaxed, totally let go, like a rag doll. Now focus on the muscles from your ankles to your knees. Again visualizing in your mind and feeling with your whole awareness where the muscles in your leg are tight and where they are relaxed. Again, I will count up to 5 and then down to 0. Again, tighten as I go up, then relax more and more with each count from 5 down to 0 until your leg is like rag doll. Visualize and we can begin. 1, 2, 3, 4, 5, 5, 4, 3, 2, 1, 0." Repeat this process from the legs up to the top of the head for broad muscle groups (e.g., knee to hip, abdomen, chest, lower back, upper back, shoulders to fingers, neck to front of head, back of head). Take each in turn using the visualization process, initially tensing the muscles and then relaxing them as one counts slowly.

Once patients have gone through their entire body in this way, I suggest that they can experience their entire body as being totally relaxed and comfortable. They can then see themselves in a warm, comfortable place (as there are many associations with warmth, relaxation, and comfort). For example, "Visualize yourself on a warm beach with the sun beating down, in a hot tub with warm water flowing over you, or perhaps floating on a cloud with a warm breeze coming across you as you allow yourself to sink deeper and deeper into a relaxed state. While maintaining this comfortable, relaxed experience let's next focus on breathing."

Instruct the patient: "Place one hand on your abdomen and one hand on your chest. Inhale very slowly and deeply through your nose into your abdomen to push up your hand as much as feels comfortable. Your chest should move only a little and only with your abdomen. When you feel at ease with this process, smile slightly, inhale through your nose, and exhale through your mouth, making a quiet, relaxing whooshing sound like the wind as you blow gently out. Your mouth and tongue and jaw are relaxed. Take long slow, deep breaths that raise and lower your abdomen in a rhythmic manner. Focus on the sound and feel of your breath as you become more and more relaxed. Continue this process for a few minutes."

Then tell the patient to "focus on how your body is feeling: the relaxed muscles, the easy slow breathing, becoming aware of how you have learned to control your relaxation and your body so fully. Be aware that you can learn to control this state and allow yourself to return to such a relaxed state any time you want. Let's practice how to do it. Begin by curling both fists, tightening the biceps and forearms, and wrinkle up your forehead. Take a deep breath and hold it. Then in a relaxed way exhale very, very slowly while relaxing your arms, forearms, biceps, fists, and forehead. Totally let go, returning to the totally relaxed state. Practice this several times at the end of each relaxation session so it becomes easier and easier for you to return to the relaxed state you can experience it more and more completely. The more it is practiced, the better you can do it."

Some physicians find it useful to make a cassette tape of the above and distribute it to their patients. By practicing the exercises 15 minutes twice a day for 2 weeks most patients become effective enough to use the technique in the face of stress.

For people who are athletes or have performance anxiety, the end of the relaxation session can be concluded with some guided imagery exercises. The guided imagery exercises consist of visualizing oneself performing a skill in slow motion, seeing and feeling it, experiencing it in as many ways as possible in one's mind while maintaining the relaxed state. Combining the visualization of a difficult experience with the sense of relaxation allows persons to be more in control and feel more comfortable the next time they face the challenge. Practicing this exercise at least twice a day makes it increasingly effective. It takes most athletes 1–2 weeks of practice before benefit is realized. Once they have mastered the guided imagery at home, they should practice it in the athletic arena. Regular practice is necessary to maintain benefit.

References

Cox RH (1994) Sport Psychology: Concepts and Applications. Madison, WI: Brown & Benchmark.

Davis M, Robbins Eshelman E, McKay M (1998) Relaxation and Stress Reduction Workbook. Oakland, CA. New Harbinger.

Fischer-Williams M (1986) A Textbook of Biological Feedback. New York: Human Sciences Press.

Wallace KG (1997) Analysis of recent literature concerning relaxation and imagery interventions for cancer pain. Cancer Nurs 20(2):79–87.

15

Crisis Intervention for the Suicidal Adult

ASSESSMENT

1. For suicidal patients, maintain a safe environment throughout the interview, if necessary having security personnel involved.
2. If significant others are offering support, include them in the interview. If there appears to be antagonism between the patient and their significant others, separate them initially; they can be included later.
3. Crisis interview often must be more structured than the usual clinic encounter. Begin with easily answerable closed-ended questions. When good control is established, address the presenting complaint.
4. Describe the sequence of events that led up to the crisis, a description of the crisis, and how the crisis is different from the usual life situation.
5. Explore the attempted solutions, including the role of significant others. If patients describe a significant degree of hopelessness or helplessness, they should be specifically asked whether suicide ideation is present.
6. Recent losses, physical illness, substance usage, relationships with significant others, depressive symptomatology, and past suicide attempts should be discussed. Consider other risk factors if appropriate (see Table 15.1).
7. If suicidal ideation is present, ask about the plan, the expected outcome, and how significant others would be affected. See Figure 15.1.

PLAN

1. If the patient is at high risk of suicide, hospitalize in a facility capable of maintaining suicide precautions.
2. For most patients, consider an outpatient program. The primary goal of the program is to develop a sense of hope and control for the patient.
   a. Review the coping mechanisms that were helpful for past stressors.

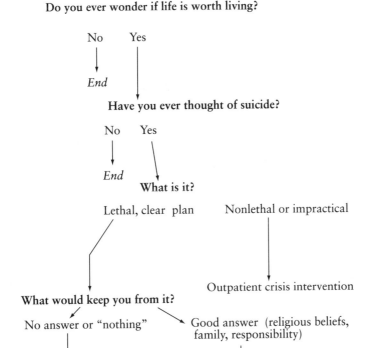

FIGURE 15.1.

b. Develop a specific plan that allows patients to feel as though they are moving toward their goals, at least making a small first step.
c. Evaluate if the patient and significant other believe that this plan has a possibility of achieving success.
d. Plans should avoid long periods of inactivity and social isolation, which exacerbate suicidal ideation.
e. Have written "no harm" contracts between patients and physicians stating that the patients will not harm themselves at least until the next appointment.
f. Medication is usually not helpful, although occasionally benzodiazepines or one of the newer agents can be used short term if a severe sleep disorder is present. If severe anxiety is preventing the patient from maintaining a healthy level of activity, benzodiazepines can be used short term as a negotiating tool to gain agreement to return to activity. Antidepressants, although inef-

fective for crisis intervention in the short term, can be offered in
selective situations where the patient would develop a greater
sense of hope if the drugs are prescribed by dated prescription.
Give only enough medicine to last a few days, with refills as
needed. Dangerous drugs such as tricyclics should be avoided.

3. Once a plan is developed, suicidal ideation should be reevaluated.
If the patient and significant others now have a degree of hope and
feel more in control, hospitalization can be avoided. Establish a
lifeline (i.e., someone to call if things go badly).

4. Schedule a definite return appointment, or at least a phone call, the
following day. *If the patient is hospitalized and remains suicidal or
hopeless for more than one day in the hospital, consultation by a
mental health specialist may be indicated.*

A suicidal adult can be a vexing problem for the physician. The core of the
problem usually entails a sense of helplessness and hopelessness. These feelings commonly develop after a loss or disappointment in one's life and all
attempts to cope with the tragedy seem to fail. The loss may be a loved one
or a job, or someone may be threatening to leave. For example, a farmer
thought that by the time he was 50 years old he would be out of debt; but
now he is 50 and believes it will never occur, leaving him with a subjective
loss of his future. Social isolation, anger, guilt, subjective feelings of loss of
control, or manipulation as a way to recapture control is often a part of the
picture. Sometimes depressed patients develop the hopeless belief that they
can never feel better. The most useful interventions usually entail guiding the
patient to some action they can take so they believe there can be a difference
in their life, restoring a sense of control and hope.

Studies have shown that a visit to a doctor often precedes a suicide attempt. When family physicians, after taking the history of the presenting
complaint, conclude that the reason for the visit is still vague, they should
consider suicidal ideation.

Assessment

A crisis interview often must be more structured than the usual clinical encounter. It is frequently best to not address the most emotionally laden topics
until a sense of control has been established. Therefore the doctor should
start with easily answerable closed-ended questions rather than with the
presenting complaint. For example, it is often useful to start with the name,
the type of work they do, where they work, their birth date, and so on. This
type of questioning establishes a sense of organized control during the interview. Once this question/answer set has been established, the doctor can
address the presenting complaint. Although the affect related to the problem

area at some point must be addressed, it should be postponed until the physician believes the patient is in good control. Therefore if the patient becomes emotional, the doctor might say, "I want to understand your problem, but when you scream and cry it makes it difficult for me to hear you. Therefore, I would like you to explain while controlling your emotions." This gives the message that the doctor expects that they can and will control their emotional expression during the interview.

A decision should be made as to whether significant others should stay or leave the examination room. It is important at some point to interview the significant others involved, but if there is obvious antagonism between family members they should be separated initially. If the significant other is providing emotional support, it is best to interview them conjointly. Also, do not promise full confidentiality because if the patient presents a danger to himself/herself or others it may be necessary to inform someone.

When the interview environment seems secure to the physician, the presenting complaint can be addressed. The patient is asked to describe in concrete terms the sequences that led up to the crisis. This should include how the crisis is different from the usual life situation. For example, if patients state they are feeling like they are losing control, the doctor should ask, "What is going on that gives you the view that you are losing control?" The sequence of events leading up to the crisis and the attempted solutions that have been tried since the crisis began should be explored, including the role of significant others. How have they been helpful in their attempts, or how have they made matters worse? Significant others should not be allowed to speak during this part of the interview until the patient has completed his or her explanation. The same questions should then be asked of them.

The next topic should be whether suicidal ideation is present. Physicians sometimes erroneously believe that asking about suicide gives the patient ideas. Research has repeatedly shown this not to be true. Patients are usually open and relieved when asked. If suicidal ideation is present, the patient is asked to describe the plan, the expected outcome, and how significant others would be affected. Recent losses, physical illnesses, substance usage, relationships with significant others, depressive symptomatology, and past psychological history should be evaluated (Table 15.1).

The first four characteristics in Table 15.1 should be used as the prime factors when evaluating the need for hospitalization. The subsequent factors in Table 15.1 are important if the physician is still questioning the need for hospitalization. The physician should take note of the characteristics of the presuicidal syndrome: (1) the patient feels "boxed in," believing that no action appears useful; (2) values seem useless; (3) they see all relationships as empty and meaningless; (4) they experience a sense of overwhelming depression, which they see as endless; (5) they experience time as standing still; (6) all decisions appear to be black and white with no compromise possible; and (7) patients state they feel restless although outwardly they may appear calm.

TABLE 15.1. Signs Comparing People Who Complete or Attempt Suicide with the General Population

Sign	Suicide	Suicide attempt	General population
Suicide plan[a]	Specific, with available, highly lethal method; does not include rescue	Less lethal method, including plan for rescue; risk increases if lethality of method is increased	None or vague ideas only
History of suicide attempts[a]	About 65% have history of highly lethal attempts; if rescued, it was probably accidental	Previous attempts are usually low-lethal; rescue plan included; risk increases if there is a change from many low-lethal attempts to a highly lethal one	None or low-lethal with definite rescue plan
Resources[a] (psychological, social)	Limited or nonexistent; or person perceives self with no resources	Moderate or in psychological and/or social turmoil	Intact or able to be restored through nonsuicidal means
Communication[a]	Feels cut off from resources and unable to communicate effectively	Ambiguously attached to resources; may use self-injury as a method of communicating with significant others when other methods fail	Able to communicate directly and nondestructively for need fulfillment
Recent loss	Increases risk	May increase risk	Is widespread but is resolved nonsuicidally (e.g., through grief, work)

Sign			
Physical illness (especially chronic or terminal)	Increases risk	May increase risk	Is common but responded to through effective crisis management (natural and/or formal)
Drinking and other drug abuse	Increases risk	May increase risk	Is widespread but does not in itself lead to suicide
Isolation	Increases risk	May increase risk	Many well adjusted people live alone; they handle satisfactory social contacts
Unexplained change in behavior (including religiosity)	Possible clue to suicidal intent, especially in teenagers	Cry for help and possible clue to suicidal ideas	Does not apply in absence of other predictive signs
Depression	About 65% have a history of depression	Large percentage are depressed	Large percentage are depressed
Social factors, problems	May be present	Often are present	Widespread but do not themselves lead to suicide
Mental illness	May be present	May be present	May be present
Age, gender, race, marital status, sexual identity	Statistical predictors that are most useful for identifying whether an individual belongs to a highly lethal risk group, not for clinical assessment of individuals	May be present	May be present

Source: Hoff LA: *People in Crisis*. Jossey-Bass, a subsidiary of John Wiley & Sons, New York, 1995, by permission.
[a]If all four of these signs exist in a particular person, the risk for suicide is high regardless of all other factors. If other signs also apply, the risk is increased further.

Many alcohol-intoxicated patients who are suicidal no longer have suicidal ideation upon achieving sobriety. If they can be maintained in a safe environment until sober, hospitalization can be avoided.

The first consideration during crisis intervention for suicidal patients is safety. The desperation of a patient in crisis on rare occasions leads to dangerous behavior in the clinic or hospital setting. Although rare, it is important to be prepared with a structured environment, so the safety of the patient and others can be maintained. If the individual at first appears to have tenuous self-control, proper backup, such as hospital security or even the police, should be called immediately. The authorities should be kept in visual contact but, unless necessary, should remain out of the examination room. When entering the examination room the doctor should leave the door open until there is a sense of control. When the situation is threatening, the patient should be told by the doctor, "I am concerned about us both feeling comfortable and safe; therefore I am leaving the door open and have people available to help us if the need arises." The doctor should have access to the door and not turn his or her back to the patient. Paranoid patients are more likely to attack when they feel boxed in. If possible, the doctor avoids blocking the door. It is also helpful to patients in crisis to reduce stimuli, particularly if the patient is psychotic; so a quiet, out of the way place is best.

Plan

For patients who have expressed suicidal ideation, the doctor's first step when developing a plan must be to decide on the level of supervision required. It may include a locked inpatient psychiatric unit, an acute care unit in a community hospital, an open inpatient unit, at home with significant others, or in the case of intoxicated patients a temporary holding unit. Many patients with suicidal ideation can be successfully treated as outpatients. Some studies show that fewer than one-third of patients with suicidal ideation require hospitalization. In fact, in some cases hospitalization has negative effects; for example, a highly dependent patient can easily become hospital-dependent, and for some the stigma of hospitalization lowers self-esteem. The use of hospitalization should be based on the degree of suicide risk based on the criteria in Table 15.1. Patients who feel hopeless and helpless, who have a specific suicidal plan that is lethal with little chance of rescue, and who feel cut off from everyone are likely to require hospitalization. This is especially true if they have a history of dangerous attempts.

For the person who needs it, hospitalization offers several benefits. The decision to undertake suicide usually takes great energy. Just a few days' respite can lead to lessening of this goal for a time. The patient may feel more connected to people and have an opportunity to see problems from a different perspective. This situation usually allows the patient to develop some greater sense of hopefulness, and their suicidal intent markedly decreases. Patients hospitalized for suicidal ideation should be required to be active and social in the hospital, or they cannot benefit from it. *If the patient does not respond to treatment in the hospital in a day or so, consultation from a mental health specialist should be considered. This is particularly true if the patient remains hopeless and suicidal.*

Most patients can gain enough from an outpatient crisis intervention to not require hospitalization. Hope and control are the primary goals. The past attempted solutions must be altered in some way to give the patient renewed hope and a sense of control. It is important to prescribe specific activities for the subsequent several days that are new or have had a positive benefit in the past and will likely lead to at least a small step in the resolution of the problem. For example, if a marriage is about to break up and the suicidal spouse has continually tried to pursue the estranged spouse, the doctor might prescribe alternative activities that connect the patient with others who can serve as a support system (e.g., joining a church group, starting an exercise class, or attending Alcoholics Anonymous). Such efforts may help avoid escalating the situation and using self-destructive behavior in an attempt to bring back the estranged spouse. If support persons are present, they should have input into the plan's specifics, especially helping to decide whether the plan has a chance to work successfully. If they are pessimistic, the plan must be altered enough that the patient and the support person present believe there is some likelihood of success. The plan must avoid long periods of inactivity and isolation, which usually exacerbate suicidal ideation. It is often helpful to include a written "no harm contract" between the patient and the physician. Patients often refuse to agree to "no harm" forever but usually agree to a contract that lasts until the next appointment.

Medication

The use of medication in a crisis intervention for nonpsychotic patients is limited. Patients in crisis might dramatically alter their mood state in a matter of days. Because antidepressants take 2–4 weeks to reach significant levels of effectiveness, they are not a good crisis treatment and are certainly not a solution to the crisis. If the patient is suffering from severe sleep deprivation, the use of benzodiazepines, zaleplon, or zolpidem may be helpful short term. The use of benzodiazepines in the crisis situation is at times helpful for agitation, although these drugs are sometimes overused, with the disadvantage of reducing impulse control, reducing cognitive functioning, increasing depressive symptoms, and reducing the confidence gained from self-efficacy. The risk of becoming dependent on them is heightened during crisis as well.

If there are certain activities the patient cannot be brought to do unless they are given a medicine, the medicine might be used briefly as a therapeutic tool to increase positive activity. Sometimes when patients exhibit depressive vegetative signs, offering them an antidepressant might help them feel hopeful that a positive change can occur. However, if the suicidal risk does not subside over several weeks, an antidepressant might energize them enough to carry out a suicide plan. The potential benefit of antidepressant medication is usually better considered at the next follow-up visit when the initial crisis has subsided. Certainly dangerous tricyclics should be avoided in the suicidal patient. Only enough medicine should be given a suicidal patient to last a few days, with dated refills as needed to prevent impulsive acting out.

Reevaluation

Once a plan is developed the suicidal ideation must be reevaluated. Does the patient now have some degree of hope and sense of being in control? Is the significant other more hopeful? Will the patient agree to a "no harm" pact at least until the next follow-up visit? Can a lifeline (someone to call if things go badly) be agreed upon?

The follow-up plan must include a definite return appointment or at least a phone call at a specific time the next day to set up a follow-up appointment. Often daily phone calls until the next appointment can be reassuring to both doctor and patient.

References

Beebe JE (1975) Treatment of the suicidal patient. In Rosenbaum CP, Beebe JE (eds) Psychiatric Treatment: Crisis/Clinic/Consultation. New York: McGraw-Hill.

Hoff LA (1995) People in Crisis, 4th ed. San Francisco: Jossey-Bass.

Olfson M, Weissman M, Leon A, Sheehan D, Farber L (1996) Suicidal ideation in primary care. J Gen Intern Med 11:447–453.

St. John D (1996) The suicidal patient: identifying, evaluating, and intervening. Home Care Provider 1:246–253.

Zealberg JJ, Santos A, Packett J (1996) Comprehensive Emergency Mental Health Care. New York: Norton.

16

Crisis Intervention for the Suicidal Adolescent

ASSESSMENT

In most situations the suicidal teenager has suffered a serious perceived loss within the past month or two, such as rejection from a family member, the end of a romantic relationship or other close friendship, a humiliating experience, or a family crisis. The youngster has been unable to relieve the pain of this situation, which has led to hopelessness and helplessness. A plan should be aimed at helping such individuals gain a sense of having more control over their lives and some sense of hope.

1. If parents are supportive of the teenager, the family can initially be interviewed together. If they are antagonistic, they should be separated. Under all circumstances at some point in the interview the teenager should be interviewed alone, and the parent and teenager should be seen together particularly during the planning stage.

2. Before exploring the presenting problem, establish rapport with youngster while developing an understanding of the overall context of the teenager's life by asking about five areas.
   a. School performance
   b. Extracurricular activities
   c. Peer relations
   d. Relationship with family including parental rules and consequences (child abuse should also be queried)
   e. Substance usage

3. The crisis situation should then be addressed in terms of the sequence of events leading up to it, what made it a crisis, what has been done to try to cope with it, and how significant others have attempted to help or have made things worse.

4. Evaluate signs of hopelessness, helplessness, and depression. If suicide ideation is present, the teenager should be asked if there is a plan and if so what it is; the expected outcome of a suicide attempt; how hopeful the teenager is that his or her problems can be ad-

dressed. If teenagers have a specific plan, if dying is the expected outcome, if they have made steps to carry it out, and if they expect that others would not care or would be relieved, the suicide risk is high.

5. If the patient is psychotic or highly impulsive, it raises the risk.

PLAN

1. If the adolescent has significant risk factors, hospitalization is likely necessary. Otherwise outpatient treatment may be superior. If hospitalization is the plan, a drug screen is almost always indicated. Hospitalization should take place where suicide precautions can be put in place.

2. If outpatient treatment is contemplated, the discussion should begin with alternative ways to deal with the loss, conflict, or other situation that has led to hopeless feelings. A plan that gives the teenager a sense of hopefulness and empowerment to confront the problem is the goal.

3. The above plan includes being in a structured situation at all times, such as being at school, engaging in an activity, or being at home under the supervision of a parent or some other parental figure until the teenager is feeling better.

4. The plan should avoid secondary gain, such as the teenager getting some added power from the suicidal behavior.

5. A "no harm" written contract between the doctor and the teenager, considered binding until the follow-up visit, should be agreed to. The removal of weapons and drugs from the household should be agreed upon.

6. Medications in the immediate crisis situation are usually not indicated except in the case of psychosis.

7. A return appointment should be scheduled (or at least telephone follow-up, at which time an appointment is scheduled) should be made within 1 day. Daily phone calls are sometimes helpful until the follow-up appointment.

Suicide is among the top three causes of death among adolescents. There appears to be a greater than 100:1 ratio of attempts to completed suicides. Reports show that more than 50% of teenagers at some point have thoughts of suicide, and about 10% develop a suicide plan. Boys succeed in killing themselves more often than girls because they more frequently use violent means such as guns, which account for 61% of all teenage suicides, and hanging, which accounts for 16%. Poisoning is responsible for 9%, and 83% of all such attempts are overdoses. Gas (primarily carbon monoxide) accounts for 6%.

Although suicidal ideation is common, making an actual attempt or even developing a serious plan is not. Certain risk factors predispose the teenager to move from thinking about suicide to planning it.

Adolescents who are at risk often have family problems, such as lack of parental control, serious rejection beyond angry confrontations, high levels of ongoing interparental conflict often despite being divorced, substance abuse by one or both parents, or parents not giving the teenager any attention. Domestic violence and sexual abuse is more frequent in the backgrounds of suicidal adolescents. The teenager frequently has no close friend in whom to confide. The teenager may have substance abuse problems, depression, or a personality disorder. The adolescent may have identity conflicts, particularly concerns about homosexuality, or might be failing at activities important to him or her, such as athletics or school.

Commonly preceding a serious suicide attempt there is a perceived loss of something important to the adolescent, usually within the past 2 months. This loss might be serious rejection by a family member, a romantic relationship, or a close friend. It could be a humiliating experience, such as a dramatic failure at school or athletic event or an arrest. Other common precipitants include a family crisis such as parental separation. Social withdrawal and withdrawal from usual activity usually precedes a suicide attempt. Recent escalation of antisocial behavior, such as running away or extremely defiant behavior toward parents, is common among suicidal teenagers. A sense of hopelessness is probably a better predictor than depression preceding a serious suicide attempt and in fact is almost always evident.

Teenagers who make serious suicide attempts often follow a similar pattern prior to acting out. Long before any suicidal behavior these youngsters have usually had suicidal ideation; when there is a major life stress the suicidal ideation intensifies. A plan begins to emerge. Sometimes it is at this point that the physician becomes aware of the teenager's troubles, as frequently this exacerbation of suicidal ideation frightens the teenagers enough that they directly or indirectly allow their troubles to be known. If no intervention occurs and the situation does not improve, a sense of hopelessness develops. This leads to a more specific plan, especially by those who make the most dangerous attempts. Finally, if the process is not interrupted a crisis occurs, such as an argument with a parent, friend, or romantic partner. The teenager might become intoxicated, and the attempt is made. Often following an attempt teenager is frightened and communicates the act to parents or friends.

Easy access to firearms, especially for impulsive or intoxicated teens, can be disastrous in this circumstance. It does not allow for a second chance by telling a friend or relative about it.

A suicide attempt can meet a number of needs of the teenager, which is important to keep in mind because it helps us understand the motivation. The teenager is in a painful situation and wants out. He or she frequently tries to communicate these feelings to a significant other, which is often a cry for help. Perhaps these teenagers are trying to manipulate to gain control of a situation, such as getting a lover to not leave them. There is usually some expression of anger: They know somebody will be hurt by their suicide or attempt, and they indeed want to hurt them. Also to be considered is the iatrogenic contribution; that is, if there have been past attempts that have led to considerable secondary gain (e.g., attention seeking) these attempts are liable to lead to future attempts when the teenager again craves attention. Now, however, he or she often feels the need to escalate the dangerousness of the attempt to obtain the desired response. Many completed suicides by adolescents appear to be gestures that did not go as planned.

Because the peer group has a strong influence on adolescents, schoolmates and suicide pacts among teens can influence the behavior of an adolescent already experiencing suicidal ideation. It is unlikely the peer group could influence this behavior in a youth who has no suicidal tendency.

Assessment

When evaluating a teenager who is possibly suicidal, it is important to remain nonjudgmental. Teenagers are unlikely to speak openly about their concern to someone standing in judgment. It is extremely important during an evaluation session for the physician to be in control. For example, if parents are antagonistic toward a teenager or vice versa, it is useful to separate them initially. At some point during the course of the evaluation the physician must see the teenager alone to explore any concerns about which the teenager may be uncomfortable when discussing them with the parents, such as an unplanned pregnancy or a failure at school. Often when separating teenagers from parents it is important to lay down ground rules of confidentiality. The physician should say, "There may be some things we discuss that will remain confidential to the doctor-patient relationship. Issues that are dangerous are not confidential and will be talked about if I believe there is a need to." It is usually useful to talk to parents alone as well because sometimes they are reluctant to talk about issues such as suspected drug abuse. It is also important to have some of the interview take place with the parents and the teenager together to examine their interactions and to discuss the plan.

Exploring four areas—school performance, extracurricular activities, peer relations, relations with family including parental rules and consequences—usually provides an overall picture of the teenager's functioning. It provides a context for the crisis behavior being evaluated. When examining these areas the physician should pay close attention to signs that teenagers have withdrawn from their usual close associates and activities. Substance usage must be investigated and, if questionable, a urine drug screen applied. A drug screen should nearly always be done when a teenager is to be hospitalized. Abuse in the home should be investigated.

Talking about overall functioning before discussing the crisis situation allows adolescents to step back for a moment and view their life situation, which can be helpful when discussing the presenting problem. This crisis situation should then be addressed in terms of the sequence of events. It should not be addressed just as symptoms. For example, if the teenager says, "I just got more and more depressed," the interviewer should ask "When you are depressed how is your day different from usual?" The answer should include how close associates respond. Attempted solutions can then be addressed. The physician should be watchful of indirect suicide communication, such as giving away valued possessions.

When discussing these issues with a teenager and the parent(s), if there is any suspicion the youngster is suicidal he or she should be asked directly if there have been any thoughts of suicide. At the same time the doctor should be vigilant for any subtle message of suicide intent, such as "I don't need to worry about next week anyway." If teenagers are having suicidal ideation and the physician has developed at least some rapport, the youngsters are almost always open about it. The physician then needs to ask specifically if they have developed a plan for suicide and, if yes, what the plan entails, including the expected outcome and the impact on others. Most worrisome is if they specifically state that they expect to die and that others would be relieved or unconcerned or they are not sure if the others would be concerned. The teenagers should also be asked how hopeful they are that their problems can be solved at some point in the future.

If there is any question about psychosis or other cognitive changes, a formal mental status examination should be performed. Psychotic suicide is unpredictable, so warning signs are often not present.

The parents should be asked to give their perspective on all areas covered above, including school performance, extracurricular activities, peer relationships, how the youngster is getting along with family including compliance with rules, and any changes in the family. Withdrawal from activity, antisocial activities, failures, losses, rejections, and substance abuse should be explored. If there are significant risk factors for suicidal behavior, parents should be asked directly if they are aware of any suicide communication or if they have concerns about it.

In a crisis situation it is usually necessary for the physician to take a more direct stance. On the other hand, doctors must be careful not to make declarations on which they cannot follow through. The physician, for example, should never say to an adolescent, "I will control you if you do not take control of yourself" unless the physician is willing to take all the necessary steps to do so, including using physical restraint if necessary, which usually entails a hospital setting. Teenagers are likely to challenge limits at first. Deciding on the need to hospitalize according to the following criteria is the first task.

First, was there a suicide plan? If there was, does the teenager have the means available to carry it out? Was the intent to die? What was the expected effect of any self-destructive activity on others? Specifically, did they expect that it would not affect others [which is quite serious]? What was the likelihood of discovery? Was a note left? Have there been past suicide attempts with increased dangerousness? The latter would indicate a serious pattern and the need for hospital admission.

Second, what is the teenager's level of hopelessness? Is there flexibility in the sense of hopelessness and helplessness so he or she could see the potential for a change in their environment for the better?

Third, what has been their history of impulsive acting out? Do they have extreme swings in their moods and activities where they go from feeling quite good about things to immediately acting self-destructively or dangerously? Impulsive behavior or substance usage requires greater structure during times of suicidal ideation.

Fourth, what is their mental status? Are they seriously intoxicated, or is there a question of an overdose having already occurred, which could be dangerous? If they are intoxicated, are the parents in a position to maintain control over them until they have become detoxified? Is the teenager psychotic? Suspicious of suicidal intent in a psychotic patient should nearly always result in hospitalization.

Fifth, in general, what is the parental or parental figures' ability to oversee the situation and provide enough structure for the teenager through the crisis?

Plan

If the above criteria lead the physician to believe that a dangerous situation exists, hospitalization should occur. Once physicians have made the decision to hospitalize, they should proceed without equivocation. Whatever means necessary should be taken to hospitalize the teenager including police force if necessary. Along with the proper structure of suicide precautions in the hospital, a drug screen should be done immediately, preferably a urine drug screen; if there is immediate need and the teenager is not willing to cooperate, a blood sample should be obtained for the drug screen. More often than not hospitalization is not required, but close follow-up is.

If outpatient treatment is contemplated, the physician, with the teenager and parents, should explore changes that will have the teen's needs met in new ways. Often simply agreeing to a future counseling program to work on problems is enough of a change to reduce suicide intent sufficiently. For example, if a conflict between parents and the teenager or the teenager and a significant other is the central issue, a plan to work on resolution of the problem should be developed. In the case of a romantic breakup, a plan on how to grieve a lost love successfully should be developed. If substance abuse is involved, a plan or several alternative treatments should be explored. The new plan should provide a sense of empowerment to confront problems and inspire hope.

Such a plan should include proper structure and supervision for several days, including proper parental authority. This is not a time for the adolescent's threats of suicide to be used as a tool to reduce authority and structure. In fact, care should be taken to avoid secondary gain for suicidal behavior. If teenagers gain attention or power from threats of suicide, they may be more suicidal in the future, leading to escalation of the problems. In fact, teenagers must know that while feeling suicidal they need greater supervision. Although adolescents may protest, they should be required to be at school or at home with a parent for a couple of days until they "feel better." This directive often provides noticeable relief to everyone involved.

Often a "no harm" written contract between the doctor and the teenager is reassuring. The agreement must be considering binding until the follow-up appointment, when it can be renegotiated.

The physician should insist on removing all lethal weapons and drugs from the household, or at least they should be hidden or locked away where it is certain that the adolescent does not have access. Teenagers may complain that you are not trusting them, but the issue is one of safety, not trust.

With the exception of psychosis, drugs are not indicated for the immediate crisis situation. A return appointment should be scheduled. If a definite time cannot be scheduled (e.g., in the emergency room) a time for a telephone follow-up should be scheduled at which time a specific appointment can be set up. This should be within just a few days of the initial evaluation. If an appointment cannot be scheduled for as long as a week, regular telephone calls should be made. Daily phone calls are sometimes needed to allow everyone to feel secure enough to avoid hospitalization.

Finally, the question should be asked of the teenager and the family whether they have confidence in the plan that has been worked out. No matter how good the plan from the physician's perspective, if the patient and family have no confidence that it can be followed, it will not work and a more dangerous situation may develop. In that case the plan can be altered in such a way as to raise the confidence level or hospitalization can take place.

References

Bell CC, Clark DC (1998) Adolescent suicide. Pediatr Clin North Am 45:365–377.

Berman AL, Jobes DA (1991) Adolescent Suicide Assessment and Intervention. Washington, DC: American Psychological Association.

Buzan RD, Weissberg MP (1991) Suicide: risk factors and therapeutic considerations in the emergency department. J Emerg Med 10:335–343.

Pallikkathayil L, Flood M (1991) Adolescent suicide: prevention, intervention, and postvention. Nurs Clin North Am 26:623–634.

Pfefferbaum B, Geis H (1995) Adolescent suicide: implications for primary care. J Okla State Med Assoc 88:523–530.

Shaffer D, Garland A, Gould M, Fisher P, Trautman P (1988) Preventing teenage suicide: a critical review. J Am Acad Child Adolesc Psychiatry 27:675–687.

17

Behavioral and School Problems of the Child and Adolescent

Behavioral and school problems are most often caused by inconsistent discipline or lack of positive reinforcement for good behavior.

BEHAVIORAL PROBLEMS

Assessment

1. Parents give the history first, followed by the child/adolescent. Evaluate adolescents both with and without parents present.
2. A detailed description of a representative misbehavior is elicited, including the sequence of events leading up to the behavior and following it.
3. A description of the child's school progress, peer relations, extracurricular activities or interests, and relationship with the family is obtained, including how discipline occurs and what the family members enjoy together.
4. For teenagers, evaluate substance abuse and sexual activity.
5. Ask the child/adolescent to describe their goals for treatment, which can serve as motivators.

Plan for the child

1. Make it clear to the parents that they are not to blame for the child's problems.
2. Have the parent or parents develop a specific list of rules with specific consequences for misbehavior and specific rewards for good behavior. It should be put in written form. It is essential that in two-parent households both parents compromise so they can support the plan. In divorced families, it is most important that they not undermine each other's discipline.
3. Because parental attention is the most effective motivator, timeouts in the room should form the basis of consequences for misbehavior. Timeouts should average 3 minutes per year of age. Rewards comprise parental attention unencumbered by distractions.

4. Work on one or two target behaviors at a time.
5. The parents must accept temporary rejection and worse behavior before improvement occurs.
6. If there is a lack of self-esteem, encourage the child to become involved in some new activity with a small group or club in a potential area of interest.

Plan for the adolescent

1. Because independence for most teenagers is a more significant motivator than parental attention, consequences for misbehavior should be built around taking away freedom, such as having earlier curfews, removing their use of the car, and grounding. Rewards are centered on increased freedom. Parental attention should be offered as well.
2. In two-parent households, both parents should develop a written set of rules with rewards and consequences clearly spelled out. In divorced families, parents should be advised to not undermine the other parent's rules even if they disagree.
3. Avoid escalating arguments that can lead to serious problems, including threats. To do this the teenager can have 5 minutes to argue their case after which point the parents do not respond and ignore the teenager if he or she continues. The parents should not alter consequences as a result of this discussion.
4. If there is a lack of self-esteem, encourage the adolescent to become involved in some new activity with a small group or club in a potential area of interest.

POOR SCHOOL PERFORMANCE

Assessment

1. Only grades below C are defined as a problem. It is often helpful to obtain the school records in addition to the grades.
2. Beyond grades, in the areas of reading and mathematics, skill development should be specifically investigated at least by the parent's history. If there is a question regarding these skills, past standardized tests should be examined or the youngster referred for testing.
3. The home environment should be evaluated regarding support for academic subjects. For example, how much television do the children watch? Do the parents read to their child?

Plan for the child

1. Request that the school send reports home. From sixth grade on, they can be weekly reports. The reports can simply state whether children completed their assignments adequately for that day.

2. For each subject that children have not completed the assignments, they are required to do one-half hour of homework under the parents' supervision. The parents can help them with the assignment if they truly do not understand it. Once the assignment period begins, children should not be allowed to do anything else until they have completed their tasks. Sessions should be limited to 30–45 minutes depending on age.
3. After the child has completed all the assignments from the teacher, the parents should spend special recreational time with him or her, giving at least as much attention for completing the assignment as they would have for a deficiency.

Plan for the adolescent

1. On Fridays teenagers should bring home a progress report from each class in which they are deficient. If they forget to bring the report home, it should be considered a failure in that subject for the week. The teachers should be requested to report only on that particular week's work.
2. For each class in which adolescents do not complete work for that week, they should be required to do 1 hour of work on Saturday and 1 hour of work on Sunday before they are allowed to participate in any free or recreational time, including watching television.
3. For completing all schoolwork for that week they should be allowed some increased freedom, such as a curfew that is a half-hour later.
4. If they do not understand the assignments a tutor should be secured.

One well known child psychiatrist described children as "fishermen." He says they try various baits until they find one that snags their fish, and then they keep using it until it no longer gets the fish. Most often the biggest fish for the prepubescent child is parental attention, and for the postpubescent child it is freedom. Behavioral problems occur most frequently when the child has more (fish) needs met by misbehavior than by prosocial behavior.

The most common problems are related to inconsistent parental discipline. Here the rules for the child are unclear or the consequences for violating of the rules are not consistent. For example, the parent might tell a child that if he hits his younger brother he will not be able to watch television that evening. The child tests the limit, hitting the younger brother. The parent turns off the television for a few minutes. The child complains, cries, and makes promises so the parent gives in and the television is turned on. The child has learned he can hit his brother and by crying avoid taking responsibility—plus get lots of attention. One of the most common reasons parents do not consistently follow through on discipline is that the parent is fearful of being rejected by the child and therefore is not able to tolerate the child's anger.

Another common cause of behavioral problems is a marked discrepancy between the two parents' rules or between home and school rules. For example, one parent strictly enforces a set of rules, but the other parent is lax and provides no consequences. In divorced families this can occur even when the noncustodial parent rarely sees the child. Sometimes the extended family, such as grandparents, interferes with disciplinary consistency. If the child gets into trouble primarily at school, it is often because the child is aware that the parents do not support school rules.

Problems also occur with children who attempt to get attention from their parents by acting badly. Though the attention may be in the form of discipline, even harsh discipline, they find it more rewarding than being ignored. This often occurs when a new sibling is born or if there is some distraction at home such as marital discord, substance abuse, or workaholic parents.

Not uncommonly a single parent becomes "best friends" with the child, making discipline difficult. Suggesting ways for the parent to find alternative support for himself or herself may help a clearer child-parent relationship to develop. The family physician, using brief therapy intervention, is likely to be able to develop a successful treatment program for cooperative parents.

Prepubescent Behavioral Problems

Assessment

When parents talk about misbehavior they often do not provide the data necessary for treatment. When obtaining the history it is important to have a detailed description of a representative misbehavior, including the sequence of events leading up to the behavior and following it. It is preferable to have both parents present. Often even divorced parents agree to meet for the child's good. When both parents are present it is important to have each parent describe his or her perceptions without interruption by the other parent. This allows the clinician to understand the viewpoint of each parent and makes each an equal authority on the child. When parents interrupt to correct the other's view of the problem, it can be pointed out, "It is helpful for me to understand each parent's perception of the problem."

It is useful to obtain a picture of children's problem within the context of their life style. Information on the child's school progress, peer relations, extracurricular activities or interests, and how the child is getting along in the family is helpful. This includes what family members enjoy doing with the child and how discipline occurs.

It is helpful but not always essential to interview the child as well. Interviewing the child even when the parents have provided enough information helps establish the doctor as an authority on the child's problems. When the child is interviewed along with the parents it is important to have the child speak last, which may be the opposite of what the doctor does during normal health care maintenance visits. In this circumstance, however, it begins to correct the common problem of the parent not having enough power, as the person chosen to speak first is usually seen as the family *authority* on the problem. It is helpful to have the child describe what he or she wants to get better because these factors can be used as motivators for the child to change.

Plan

The most common mistake made when counseling parents is not taking enough care to communicate to the parents that they are not being blamed for the problem. If parents feel blamed they expend more energy disproving their guilt than making useful changes.

It is important for parents to understand that although they are not to blame for the problem they are responsible for the solution. For example, one approach is to say to them, "Your child is characterologically stubborn, which means it will take unusual effort and teamwork on both parents' parts to provide highly structured discipline that makes it more rewarding to the child to act appropriately than to misbehave." The first step is to request that the parent(s) prepare a specific list of rules with specific consequences for misbehavior and specific rewards for good behavior. Having the parents put this in writing tends to increase its importance. In two-parent households, parents are told that it is essential that they compromise with each other so that neither believes they are "giving in" but that the rules reflect both their views. In shared custody circumstances it is ideal but not necessary for the parents to have the same rules in each home. Consistency within each set of rules matters more. It is essential that divorced parents not undermine the authority of the other. The trusted family physician can sometimes serve as intermediary to broker agreeable compromises on the issues.

Some general education on setting up a structured discipline program is all some parents need. The guiding principle for the prepubescent child is that getting or losing parental attention is most motivating. Therefore the most effective consequence is being sent to their room (3 minutes per year of age, e.g., 15 minutes for a 5-year-old) without discussion. The timer should not start until the child is quiet in the room. Use of television, video games, or a computer is not allowed during timeouts. These instruments should be removed from the room if there is difficulty with enforcement. The most motivating rewards are having activities with the parents (e.g., playing a 10-minute game with the parent for improved behavior). In the young child consequences and rewards must follow the behavior swiftly. As the child becomes older delays can be extended.

It is more effective to work on just one or two target behaviors at a time. The rules and consequences should be discussed only *once* before implementation. No attempt should be made to win agreement with the child. Initially, there must be rigid adherence to the rules by the parents, with no exceptions.

When parents ask specifically about the use of corporal punishment, although we never recommend it we also do not tell them it should never be used. There is no research stating that when used infrequently and not with excessive force it has caused children any harm. Parents can be told that there are better disciplinary approaches.

Most importantly, one recommends that whatever rules they do chose to impose on their child, they must follow through on the consequences and the rewards as consistently as possible. It is usually best to develop as few rules as they think are necessary so that whatever rules they have they can follow as absolutely as possible. The physician should warn parents that they must accept temporary rejection by the child until things improve and that problems get worse in the short term (owing to the child initially escalating limit-testing) before they get better.

Sometimes parents blame misbehavior of their child on a lack of self-esteem. There may be something to this; but before that issue can be addressed, control of the child must be established. When the doctor addresses self-esteem, it is useful to keep in mind that before school age self-esteem comes from parental praise. Once in school, successful accomplishment compared with that of other children becomes increasingly important.

Given the opportunity, all children can find some activity they do well. With some investigation, the parent can help the child find something to try that has potential. Academic subjects and athletics are often all that has been tried; and if children are below average at these activities they see themselves as failures. Perhaps the child can try something artistic, build and race a go-cart (mechanical), engage in a 4H project in agriculture or cooking, join a chess club. There is nothing like a 4H ribbon or Cub Scout merit badge to raise self-esteem. These activities also help the child establish a good peer group.

Case Report

Jason is a 5-year-old who is seen because of tantrums. Jason's single mother reports he throws tantrums most often at the worst times. She might be just home from work trying to fix supper for him and his 3-year-old sister. He requests something, and if she has to put him off he hits his sister or throws things. She asks if medicine might help. She says she has tried many times to explain that if he would just wait she would fulfill his request. She comes for help now because his tantrums are more frequent and worse. She says she has tried "everything" to make things better: ignoring, yelling, spanking, and timeouts on a chair or in another room. When asked to describe these punishments in more detail the doctor learns she has tried them about three times each. She admits she yells at him all the time. Jason's kindergarten teacher has said he occasionally gets in trouble.

To avoid having the mother feel blamed for her son's problems, she is told her son does not appear to have attention deficit hyperactivity disorder

(ADHD) but is manipulative and stubborn. Therefore it will take unusual parental skill to help him. She is told that Jason is taking attention away from his sister and that she could use this motivation to control him; he will dislike her at first, which could be painful for her. She is told she was on the right track when she put the boy in his room, but this action usually leads to problems worsening before they get better. She had good maternal instincts but did not stick with it long enough. Also, good behavior needed a reward of her attention soon after it happened. It is suggested that if he throws a tantrum he should be put in his room for 15 minutes and that the time does not start until he is quiet; moreover, it starts over if he comes out prematurely. If he refuses to stay in the room, the door should be held shut, but nothing should be said to the child until after he has served his time. On the other hand, if he shows improved behavior (e.g., does not have to be sent to his room for a full hour after his mother gets home from work) she will find something for his sister to do (e.g., listen to a book on tape) while she spends 15 minutes of special time with him reading him a story in addition to his regular bedtime story. Although she was told to expect him to behave worse for several weeks, as expected things improved by the fifth day. Both Jason and his mother can be complimented for turning things around so quickly. Jason's mother can now begin to address tantrums at bedtime using a similar approach.

Adolescent Behavioral Problems

Although there are many similarities between adolescent and childhood behavioral problems, there are also significant differences. First, as is well known, adolescent rebelliousness serves a useful function as it helps the teenager move toward a greater sense of independence from parents. A lack of rebelliousness leads to overdependence in some. For the teenager it is a problem of extremes. Another difference is that because the teenager is more able to delay gratification than a child rewards and consequences for misbehavior can be less immediate and spread out over a longer period of time (e.g., a day or week—but not much longer) rather than minutes or hours. Also, although parental attention is important, independence is often an even more significant motivator of adolescent prosocial behavior. For the adolescent, altering freedom is the most effective motivator. Curfews, use of the car, phone privileges, and money for activities can be used to promote appropriate behavior.

The underlying difficulties associated with adolescent misbehavior are often similar to those in children: inconsistent discipline because parents are uncomfortable with their teenager's anger toward them, the teenager manipulating one parent against the other, or the teenagers getting into trouble to be noticed by their parents because they are getting so little attention otherwise.

Teenage manipulation sometimes escalates to frightening levels. To get their way, teenagers may threaten to hate their parents, to run away, or to quit activities good for them. In extreme situations they escalate to threatening suicide to get their way. These threats usually come in the midst of heated arguments. Once verbalized, however, teenage pride can get in the way of backing down. Hurt and fearful after these episodes, parents often give up control of their children before they are ready to handle the freedom. The family physician, by helping the parent at an early stage, can often prevent problem behavior from escalating to this point. Because the rejecting and threatening behavior usually starts out much more benign and gradually escalates over months or years, confronting the problems early often prevents more serious escalations, which may require referral. Success comes from not over- or underreacting to the misbehavior. Maintaining a consistent plan over months can ultimately achieve positive behavioral change.

Assessment

The evaluation process for adolescents is similar to that for young children. One parent should be present and ideally both. The parents speak first, each describing common representative behavior, including events preceding and following the problem behavior. Evaluating the teenager includes examining such factors as their relationships with peers; school performance, including relations with teachers; extracurricular activities; at what they excel; and family relationships, including accepting the rules of the parents. Substance usage should also be explored. The physician should determine if the youth is sexually active and, if so whether birth control is being used. Once sexually active, teenagers rarely return to abstinence. Some but not all of this information is better gathered without parents present.

Plan

When a teenager is in trouble, one must start with a behavioral program that is initially overly controlling. Appropriate behavior is gradually rewarded by allowing greater independence, but not too quickly.

A simple behavioral program for a 16-year-old with curfew violations and alcohol usage might be as follows: Curfew is at 5 p.m. on weeknights and 9 p.m. on Saturday. For each week of compliance, 30 minutes is added to the 9 p.m. time on Saturday until it reaches midnight. If late, 2 minutes are lost for each minute late up to 30 minutes, after 30 minutes the teenager is grounded for the weekend. If the parents even suspect drinking, no proof is needed. The teenager is grounded 1 week and loses use of the car for 2 weeks. If the car was used after drinking, driving privileges are lost for a month. These restrictions comprise only one example. It is important the parents primarily decide what the rules should be. It is critical that whatever plan is use it is devised by both parents. Rules should be in writing, as should be the rewards and consequences.

To avoid escalating arguments when the rules are enforced, parents are instructed to allow teenagers 5 minutes to state their views (timed). The parents should then proceed to telling them the consequences *without* trying to prove to the teenager that the consequences are justified because the youngster is unlikely to agree and the argument would escalate. Once finished, the teenager is ignored until the situation calms down.

The peer group is commonly blamed for the adolescent's problems. Usually teenagers seek out peers to support their rebelliousness. If parents provide enough structured discipline (e.g., curfew, consequences for drinking) the teen ultimately must decide to make new friends or be in trouble all the time. They usually opt for new friends, but not overnight. If teenagers become involved in a new activity (e.g., sports, church group, new job) they may be more open to developing new relationships. This change usually takes months.

Case Report

Dorene is a 15-year-old tenth grader. She was seen at her parent's request, and both parents came to the initial evaluation. The parents described the problems as her grades having dropped from A's and B's to C's. The parents feared that she had poor self-esteem. She had recently changed friends, and the parents blamed the friends for much of her difficulty. She had stopped playing soccer during the past year; and although she was still in the band, she was talking about dropping out of that as well.

The parents had tried to correct these difficulties by convincing her that this was wrong, that her new friends were not good for her. On occasion when she would come in late for curfew, they had grounded her and taken away use of the car. When given these sanctions she argued intensely, and ultimately the parents would at least partially rescind the sanctions. The final straw was her coming home several hours past curfew, obviously drunk two evenings in a row.

Dorene stated she did not believe there was much of a problem except that her parents were treating her unfairly compared to the parents of other children who had a lot more freedom. She blamed her low grades on having bad teachers. When interviewed alone she denied alcohol or substance abuse and sexual activity. She believed that things would overall be better if her parents simply left her alone more. When interviewed alone, the parents said they were fearful that their daughter was sexually active but they had no evidence to prove it.

Dorene's misbehavior can be viewed as an example of an overly rebellious teenager. The parents were uncomfortable maintaining firm enough limits.

The parents were asked to spend the next week working together to decide on rules and consequences for Dorene. It was emphasized that the two of them needed to come to a mutual agreement they both could support. The parents were told, in front of Dorene, that they could expect Dorene to hate them for a while, as it was a normal response. When the doctor expresses this expectation in front of the teenager it defuses the rebelliousness somewhat. Teenagers do not want to do what the doctor expects. The one specific recommendation in this case was that Dorene be grounded for the next week because of her recent misbehavior. Dorene responded to this angrily, but after expressing her anger the topic was changed.

The parents were also told that they should not have lengthy arguments. Specifically, it was recommended that Dorene be allowed to state her case in 5 minutes, and after that the parents would simply cut off the discussion and ignore any further statements.

It was recommended to the parents that they not try to control specifically who her friends were as it was impossible. Regarding her school performance, it was suggested to the parents that anything below a C should result in a behavioral program for school (see Poor School Performance below). However if her grades remained above a C the teenager could decide if she needed help. Finally, it was recommended that each parent offer to spend some quality time with their daughter during the next week. Dorene did not have to take them up on this offer, but it was important to make it.

At the follow-up appointment a week later we reviewed the rules and developed a specific plan on how the parents would make them work. If they had not developed adequate rules and consequences, we would have done so at this appointment. Dorene's behavior improved a great deal over the next 6 weeks, which is a bit faster than usual.

Poor School Performance

Parents frequently approach their child's doctor with questions regarding their child's poor school performance. Sometimes these queries come in the form of concerns regarding possible attention deficit disorder or learning disabilities. Although these factors are sometimes the source, most commonly the problems are behavioral or environmental. For example, the highest variable found to correlate with reading skill in young children is whether parents regularly read to their children early (by age 3). The most helpful interventions usually require good cooperation between parents and school.

Assessment

Assessment should include the grades the child is receiving. If the child is receiving at least C's and B's the problem should be defined as nonpathology, even if it represents underachievement. Children at this level are likely progressing adequately so it does not inhibit their potential for success academically or vocationally. In fact, parents can be reassured that the correlation between very high grades (e.g., A's) and a C+ average predicting future vocational success is minimal. The two important skills needed in elementary school are the ability to read and to do mathematics well.

Information regarding whether the child is known to be reading and doing mathematics at their age level should be specifically requested; grades are only part of this information. The home environment regarding academic subjects is useful information. Specifically, do the parents read to their children? Does the child read outside of school? Do parents assist with homework? Do they enforce homework rules (e.g., no television until homework is done)? Math skills can be broadly evaluated because by the time children are in second grade they should have a pretty good understanding of addition and subtraction, and by fourth grade they should have the basics of multiplication and division. The ability to understand fractions starting in sixth grade often distinguishes those who do well in mathematics from those who have trouble, as this is something of an abstract ability. If there is still a question of ability, standardized testing can be requested. Attempted solutions to the problem should be investigated: how the school has tried to improve things and how the parents have tried to help.

Related factors affecting the child should also be reviewed, including significant changes in the child's life such as a change of school, marital separation, how the child gets along with the teacher, and discipline and peer relations. If attention span is a concern, see Chapter 18. The number of hours per day of television watching by the youngster is also significant. More than 2 hours per day can affect children's academic performance. Not eating breakfast has also been found to compromise school performance. If the problem is primarily related to academic performance, a structured behavioral approach is usually most effective.

Plan

First, it is important to have the cooperation of both parents, especially if the child resides with both parents. Even if the child is in the custody of one or the other, it is still generally a good idea to obtain the cooperation of the noncustodial parent by talking with them on the phone or, most effectively, have both parents present when the plan is drawn up. The plan should include frequent evaluation of the child's progress. For the younger child (e.g., grades 1–3) evaluation reports should be obtained daily; for the older child (e.g., the sixth grader) weekly reports are adequate. Usually the school system, primarily through the school counselor, is willing to provide these evaluations. If not, the physician may have to call the school counselor directly.

The program works as follows: If the child has not completed the expected work, during the evening (not right after school) at a set time the child completes the work under the guidance of the parent. If the child is able to do the work but simply did not, he or she should do it alone. If the child does not understand the work, the parent should help. The child is not allowed to engage in recreational activity until time is spent at serious work. These sessions should be kept to no longer than one-half hour for the young child (first or second grade), one hour for the older child (fifth or sixth grade), or two one-hour sessions for the adolescent. If there is still work to be completed after this time, it should be completed on the weekend under the parent's supervision.

It is important that there be rewards for good performance. When children have completed work at school, they should be given parental attention for the same amount of time, but they can choose whatever activity they like. It is essential that the child get at least as much attention when completing work at school as when they do not complete their work.

Children should be expected to try to manipulate the system (e.g., "forget" the teacher reports). If this occurs, it should be assumed that the child flunked all of the work for that day and so is required to do assignments in all classes. Usually it is best to make children work at least a little harder if they "forget" their evaluation than if they remember. When the parents have proven to the child that they will rigidly stick to this program, the child usually no longer manipulates as much. Once this occurs it is not long before positive results from this program are achieved.

Academic Problems of the High School Student

A similar program works for teenagers with some adjustments. Teacher reports can be obtained weekly (e.g., Fridays) and used to determine the amount of schoolwork for the weekend. The reports can be targeted to the classes that have been given a grade of C or below. The high school student should be required to do 2 hours of work on the weekend for each class they received a grade below C for the week's work. The time can be divided into half on Saturday and half on Sunday. The teenager should not be allowed to do anything recreational (including watching television) until the schoolwork is done for that day. When the overall grade for the course is above C, weekly reports can stop.

Once children enter pubescence, it becomes difficult for parents to tutor their own offspring. An independent tutor can be helpful to the adolescent, particularly for mathematics. One-on-one tutors in mathematics can understand how the student is comprehending the subject and target their teaching to help the student understand the concepts. This is critical in mathematics skill development but is often ignored in favor of a quick fix (learning the process approach). If the student goes to college this approach is a disaster. Professional tutors are expensive, but college students can often be recruited by calling the college department and having them post a bulletin asking for a tutor. College students often tutor for work-study wages (just above minimum wage) and can do an excellent job.

References

Amatea E (1989) Brief Strategic Intervention for School Behavior Problems. San Francisco: Jossey-Bass.

Christophersen ER (1992) Discipline. Pediatr Clin North Am 39:395-411.

Haley J (1980) Leaving Home. New York: McGraw-Hill.

Leung AK, Fagan JE (1991) Temper tantrums. Am Fam Physician 44:559–563.

Leung AK, Robson WLM, Lim SH (1992) Counseling parents about childhood discipline. Am Fam Physician 45:1185–1189.

Novak LL (1996) Childhood behavior problems. Am Fam Physician 53:257–262.

18

Attention Deficit-Hyperactivity Disorder

Symptoms of attention deficit hyperactivity disorder (ADHD) should be distinguished from behavioral problems, anxiety, and academic problems including boredom.

ASSESSMENT

1. What are the child's usual activities?
2. What are the child's favorite and least favorite activities?
3. How long does the child typically spend on each of these activities? When pushed, how long will the child spend on them?
4. How well is the child learning to read?
5. How well is the child learning mathematics?
6. What are the behavioral problems? Where do they occur? What is the sequence of events that leads up to the problems, and what occurs after the problem behavior? (Does the child exhibit attention problems in more than one setting, e.g., school, home, scouts, sports, church?)
7. What types of discipline/rewards are employed by parents and teachers? What are the results? (Is discipline consistent and appropriate with clear rules and consequences?)
8. What do the parents and child enjoy doing together? (Does the child get adequate attention for appropriate behavior?)
9. What are the attempted solutions to problems by the parents, teachers, others? What are the results?
10. Are there major changes in the child's life or serious stresses, such as a recent move, death in the family, divorce, loss of a parent's job? Are there contributing major stresses, or is there a chaotic environment?
11. Is attention span or hyperactivity a problem? Does it interfere with academic endeavors, important activities, and social interaction? Is discipline, a stressor, or lack or parental attention contributing to the problem or the major source of the problem?

12. If ADHD is likely, obtain school records and have the teacher fill out a questionnaire three times a week at noon for 3 weeks. Parents are to collect and bring this information to the doctor weekly.

PLAN

1. If the problem is primarily a behavioral one, see Chapter 17. The child should be given attention for prosocial behavior and lose attention for problem behavior.
2. If recent stress is high, work on reducing the stressors and reevaluate the results later. If the child is highly anxious because of a chaotic or chronically stressful environment, a referral may be necessary.
3. If ADHD is the primary diagnosis and confirmed by the teacher questionnaires the first week, consider the treatment options.
    a. Benefits, limitations, and risks of medication should be discussed with the parents.
    b. Methylphenidate is most commonly prescribed. Start at 5 mg in the morning and increase in 5 mg increments as recommended later in the chapter. Have the teachers continue to submit evaluations three times a week at noon. Keep them blinded to when the medication is started and the titration. Based on teacher feedback, adjust the morning dose. When a proper morning dose has been achieved, add the same dose at noontime.
    c. Develop a highly structured discipline program with parents as described in Chapter 17.
    d. Develop reinforcers to improve the attention span, such as attention given during evening story time and a chart to reward progress.

The diagnosis of attention deficit-hyperactivity disorder (ADHD) defines a child who has an extraordinarily poor attention span, is hyperactive and impulsive, or has both problems. It is often difficult to distinguish between symptoms of ADHD and other childhood problems. The differential diagnosis includes anxiety, oppositional defiant disorder, conduct disorder, mood disorder, and learning disabilities including dyslexia. Often the diagnosis is a combination of these entities. An ADHD child has difficulty paying attention and completing tasks, being aware of details related to a task, and is easily distracted by external stimuli. The hyperactive impulsive child is constantly moving, is interested in everything, has trouble keeping quiet and is constantly on the go, has trouble waiting his or her turn, and often interrupts.

Considered a developmental disorder, the diagnosis of ADHD must be apparent early in a child's life. It can interfere with normal and usual activities, especially school. A number of factors are involved in the development of attention span, impulse control, and motor activities, including a biologic contribution. One must keep in mind that all children start out with little attention span, and that as they grow older their attention span increases (about 3–5 minutes per year) through at least pubescence and perhaps beyond. One's ability to control one's self (i.e., the development of self-control) is affected by such factors as age, parental authority and discipline, a highly structured versus chaotic environment, the expectations of the social structure (e.g., school), and the opportunity to engage in regular physical activity. Certain factors can negatively affect these characteristics. For example, when children are highly anxious and stressed, they have a great deal of difficulty paying attention and often become fidgety. Self-control then becomes difficult.

When evaluating a child for this disorder, it is important to conduct a comprehensive evaluation. This evaluation should include how the child behaves in school and social settings. It is best to gather this information from both parents wherever possible, although school records are also important. It is often helpful to have information from other settings if possible, such as from athletic coaches or Sunday School teachers. Because attention span and self-control increase with age and development, developmental delay can account particularly for early problems in this area. The child may grow out of these problems just as they grow out of enuresis and other problems associated with developmental delay. Therefore waiting to evaluate children until they are kindergarten age is most often the rule of thumb.

Assessment

A useful way to begin the evaluation is to ask the parent(s): What are the child's usual activities? What are the child's favorite and least favorite activities? How long does the child typically spend at each of these activities? When pushed, how long does the child spend on these activities? How well is the child learning to read? How well is the child learning to do mathematics? What are the behavioral problems? What is the sequence of events that leads up to the behavioral problems, and what occurs as a result of the behavioral problems? What types of discipline and rewards do the parents, teachers, child-care workers, and baby-sitters employ? What do the parents and child enjoy doing together? What solutions have been attempted by the parents, teachers, and others? What are the results of these attempted solutions? Finally, have there been any recent major changes in the child's life or serious stresses, such as recent moves, a death in the family, divorce, parental job loss?

When reviewing the above information the following areas should be considered. When the child is motivated, how long does he or she engage in a particular activity? Intense activities such as Nintendo are not a useful evaluative tool, but activities where children themselves are motivated to pay attention are useful. For example, does the child play board games? Does the child sit and draw? Does the child put together Legos for an age-appropriate period of time? Does the child sit and listen to the parents read an interesting and exciting story? If the child spends an age-appropriate time at an activity (increasing at about 3–5 minutes per year) the physician has an idea of what the child can do if motivated sufficiently. Motivation can be enhanced by a positive reward (e.g., parental attention) or negative consequences (e.g., removing something desirable, such as the parents' attention by placing the child in his or her room). An evaluation of how a consistently structured discipline program in various environments, such as home and school, can help the clinician understand how children are being motivated to reach their potential for self-control and involvement in an activity that might not itself be pleasurable, such as school work. Comparing various environments, such as home, school, church activities, and scouts, helps us to understand how different environments affect attention span and self-control.

Because self-control and delay of gratification is learned to a large degree, it is essential to understand the efforts already made to teach the child self-control. If the child has been exposed to a chaotic environment with few reinforcers for staying on task, the child cannot be expected to learn these behaviors within a short period of time when 6 years old and in first grade compared to children who have had adequate preparation in these areas. Frustration by this inappropriate preparation frequently leads to the child and the teacher giving up, which only solidifies the child's inability to improve self-control and pay attention to task. Sometimes these children do quite well in a highly structured environment with clear rewards and consequences, such as school; but at home, where there is less structure and perhaps a high level of stress, the child becomes out of control. If environmental factors are significant contributors to the child's problems with attention span or impulse control, it likely is more useful in the long run to introduce a behavioral/interpersonal intervention rather than pharmacotherapy. In this circumstance, although drugs may more immediately help control their behavior, it obviates children's chances to learn to control themselves.

Treatment

A significant number of children referred for ADHD evaluation are ultimately diagnosed as having a primary behavioral problem, school performance problem, or family problem (see the appropriate chapter for treatment). Many parents are more comfortable with the diagnosis of ADHD because it clearly removes the onus of responsibility for the problems from them and defines the problem as lying within the child's genetics. Therefore when framing the assessment (diagnosis) for the parents it is important to avoid blaming them for the problems if one is to achieve a cooperative relationship. A useful way to frame it is, "I am not surprised you are having difficulty with your child. He [or she] is headstrong and a real handful. I believe you'll benefit from some special approaches to parenting to which most parents don't have to resort." This definition of the problem often allows parents to be less defensive about a behavioral/interpersonal approach.

If after interviewing the parents and child and obtaining school records, it is apparent that there is substantial ADHD symptomatology, for which the environment clearly does not account, the next step is to gather as much objective information as possible from the school. An effective way to do this is to have a brief questionnaire for the teachers that can be filled out in a few minutes (Table 18.1). The teacher is asked to complete this questionnaire for a 3-week period on Mondays, Wednesdays, and Fridays at noon. Each Friday the parent picks up the questionnaire and brings it to the physician's office. It takes less than a minute to calculate the results of the questionnaire (see footnote to Table 18.1 for this information). When the parent brings the questionnaire in after the first week of school and the scores are evaluated, a decision can be made as to whether to place the child on medication.

If the child clearly falls into the ADHD classification, medicine can be tried. If the results are equivocal, alternative ways to help the child gain better self-control can be attempted, particularly if the parents are not eager to start medications and are willing to put forth some effort. (See Table 18.2 regarding the risks and benefits of methylphenidate usage.)

If the child is clearly diagnosed with ADHD and the parents wish to start a medication, the physician can prescribe 5 mg of methylphenidate each morning. The first week it is taken Monday and Tuesday just before going school and then increased to 10 mg each morning on Wednesday, Thursday, and Friday. The teachers continue to fill out the forms at noon Monday, Wednesday, and Friday. Neither the parents nor the child should tell the teacher that the medicine has been started.

Although this is not a perfect approach, it is an opportunity for a blinded evaluation of the medicine's effectiveness. The half-life of methylphenidate is relatively short, so most of the effects have disappeared by afternoon; therefore it is essential that the teacher fill out the form at noon so the evaluation is based on the morning session of school. The next Friday the evaluations are again picked up by the parents and taken to the physician's office. If the child's evaluation now lies close to average, the 10 mg dosage can be set as the standard. If it is headed in a positive direction but is still above the ADHD threshold, the dosage can be increased to 15 mg in the morning and the evaluation continued until the teacher questionnaire falls

TABLE 18.1. DSM IV-Based Teacher Questionnaire

Criterion	Rarely	Sometimes	Often	Very often
1. Fails to pay attention to details or makes careless errors				
2. Has trouble keeping attention on tasks or play				
3. Does not appear to listen when being told something				
4. Does not follow through on instructions				
5. Has trouble organizing activities and tasks				
6. Dislikes or avoids tasks that involve sustained mental effort				
7. Loses materials needed for activities				
8. Is easily distracted by external stimuli				
9. Is forgetful				
10. Squirms in seat or fidgets				
11. Inappropriately leaves seat				
12. Inappropriately runs or climbs				
13. Has trouble quietly playing				
14. Appears driven or "on the go"				
15. Talks excessively				
16. Answers questions before they have been completely asked				
17. Has trouble awaiting turn				
18. Interrupts or intrudes on others				

Source: Adapted from DSM IV criteria (American Psychiatric Association, 1994).
To diagnose inattention, six of the first nine items should be in the "often" or "very often" range. To diagnose hyperactivity/impulsivity, six of the next nine should be in the "often" or "very often" range. There are many other ADHD Teacher Questionnaires that are known to work well.
Note: The student's name, the date, and the teacher's name are noted at the top of the form. There is space left on the bottom of the form for comment by the teacher.

TABLE 18.2. Benefits and Risks of Methylphenidate

Benefits
   Global rapid symptom improvement
   Teachers and parents need to use less discipline
   Less negative feedback to child
   Academic performance improved short term
   Relatively safe

Risks
   Global performance long term related to nonmedicinal variables
   Less opportunity for learning self-control
   Child/parent ascribes improvement to medications
   No benefit proven for long-term performance
   Tics, hypertension, insomnia, short-term growth retardation may diminish
     athleticism

below the ADHD threshold or the medicine is demonstrated not to be useful. Once an appropriate dosage has been found, the methylphenidate can be given twice a day: once in the morning before school and once at noontime. A 20 mg sustained-release form is also available, but its benefit is controversial.

Some parents advocate an afternoon dose at 3:00 or 4:00 p.m. so the evening hours are easier on the parent and child. There are distinct disadvantages to this practice, as many children do not sleep well or eat dinner well. This medicine does have side effects, so it is best to have as much drug-free time as possible. For this reason, it is beneficial to have weekends free of medicine as well, allowing the child to practice impulse control and attention to task without drugs.

Even when medicine is used, a highly structured environment with clear discipline and rewards should be established. There is one other exercise that can help the child develop a better attention span. It takes time and effort on the parent's part, but motivated parents have helped these children improve. The parent reads to the child three times per night for a week and charts how long the child listens to them read with encouragement, be it 1, 5, or 10 minutes. The average of these times then becomes the starting point. The child is given a reward for listening to the parent read 20% more than they had averaged the week before. For example, if the child averaged 4-minute blocks, there would be a reward for listening 5 minutes. This reward, which should include parental attention, is given soon after the success. The book should not be a schoolbook but one the child has chosen. It is important to work on this protocol when the child is not being affected by the medicine, such as during the evening, 6–7 hours after the last dose of methylphenidate. In many children, if it is done consistently, there is significant improvement in the length of time spent on task over a several month period. When children are older (e.g., 10 years of age), they can read to the parent.

Case Report

G.C. was a 7-year-old boy brought to the family physician by his mother at the advice of the principal of the elementary school. G.C. had been taken to the principal's office for disruptive behavior several times each week during the first month of this school year. The physician learned that Mrs. C was a single parent, and her ex-husband was currently incarcerated in the state penitentiary for breaking and entering and possession of a controlled substance with intent to distribute. Mrs. C gave a history that her son had been a difficult child since he was a toddler, defying parental authority, unfocused, and "into everything." From his early years he took household items apart and, of course, did not put them back together. School problems were apparent from the beginning, and recently his behavior had become worse as the new school year began. G.C. created a great fuss at bedtime and then was difficult to arouse and motivate to go to school the following day. His teacher reported that he fidgeted, talked out of turn, and blurted out answers to questions that had been directed to other children. He was argumentative with the teacher and regularly had to be removed from the classroom because of his disruptive behavior.

Mrs. C was observed during this interview to reprimand her son frequently for disturbing the physician's tongue blades, tearing the paper on the examination table, and fingering the equipment. Her verbal reprimands were strongly worded including threats of corporal punishment but were either totally ignored by G.C. or were answered with a similar insolent and threatening statement.

The physician entertained the possibilities of oppositional defiant disorder, anxiety, and ADHD. He provided Mrs. C with several copies of the ADHD Teacher Questionnaire, requesting that they be filled out sequentially as outlined earlier in the chapter. The physician learned that G.C. had no problems with enuresis, encopresis, fire setting, or cruelty to animals. The physician set up an interview with Mrs. C alone on another day and excused her to interview G.C. alone. As the physician and child talked, G.C. was disrespectful and oppositional to the physician as well, but when the physician, in a firm but quiet tone, simply repeated his request that G.C. sit down and talk with him the child complied.

The physician asked the child about his friends at school, what he did after school, whether he had one close friend or many friends, what he wished to be when he grew up. In this way he hoped to build rapport and gain some general information from the child. He then asked who was the boss at home. G.C. replied emphatically that he was. The physician asked what G.C. would wish for if he were to be given three wishes by the genie in the lamp. The child replied "$1 million, a dog, and a racing car."

After further interviews with Mrs. C and G.C. and a review of the teacher questionnaires followed by a telephone call to the teacher, the physician suspected some degree of oppositional defiant disorder or anxiety. The teacher questionnaires were also suggestive but not diagnostic of ADHD. The physician discussed the possibility of medication with Mrs. C, but together they decided to try other methods. Mrs. C was told that G.C. either had a mild case of ADHD or simply was a difficult, headstrong, especially energetic child. Furthermore, because she had no parenting partner she might have to use parenting methods that were more structured and well thought out than would be used by other parents. She was encouraged to enroll in a local parent effectiveness training course.

A call was made to G.C.'s teacher while Mrs C. listened in. The physician requested that the teacher make a brief note about the acceptability of G.C.'s behavior daily and send it home with the child. Mrs. C was asked to promise the child a 30-minute activity together after supper if the teacher's report for the day was a good one. If there was a poor daily report G.C. would not be allowed to choose a game, book, or other activity to enjoy with his mother. Mrs. C. was encouraged to accept that her son might sulk or carry on but that she should exert appropriate parental authority in this matter. In addition, G.C. was to begin to receive an allowance of $2 each week contingent on good reports the entire week. The teacher was asked to continue filling out the teacher questionnaire at 1-week intervals prior to scheduled visits with the physician; these, along with quarterly report cards, were reviewed by the physician with G.C. at office visits. The physician praised G.C. for each incremental improvement in his grades and comments about his behavior, and he expressed disappointment with continued failures.

When impulsiveness and poor attention span continued to be a problem, the evening reading activity was instituted by his mother as described earlier in the chapter. Over time G.C. was able to improve his reading attention span from 10 minutes to 30 minutes, and these improvements seemed to carry over to his school activities.

At future visits Mrs. C explained that she had learned to be firm without being theatrical when exerting authority over her son. In addition, she expressed an awareness that in the past she had been inconsistent and had promised consequences for misbehavior but had not followed through, so G.C. had learned that she was a "paper tiger." She thought that her discipline was now much more consistent and reasonable, and it was usually effective.

The physician suggested that Mrs. C get her son into Cub Scouts and particularly that she ask around and see what Scout leaders seemed to have a knack for dealing with children with problems. He also suggested she either look into the Big Brothers program or check with her relatives to see if one of the adult men might befriend her son on a regular and ongoing basis. Visits to the physician became less frequent and more positive. Eventually, physician visits were required only for ordinary health maintenance appropriate to the child's age.

References

American Psychiatric Association (1994) Diagnostic and Statistical Manual of Mental Disorders, 4th ed. Washington, DC: American Psychiatric Association.

Barkley R (1990) Attention-Deficit Hyperactivity Disorder: A Handbook for Diagnosis and Treatment. New York: Guilford.

Carlson CL, Bunner MR (1993) Effects of methylphenidate on the academic performance of children with attention-deficit hyperactivity disorder and learning disabilities. School Psychol Rev 22:184–198.

Dunne JE (1999) Attention-deficit/hyperactivity disorder and associated childhood disorders. Prim Care 26:349–372.

Elia J, Ambrosini PJ, Rapoport JL (1999) Treatment of attention-deficit-hyperactivity disorder. N Engl J Med 340:780–788.

Higgins R (1997) ADHD: the role of the family physician. Am Fam Physician 56:42, 44.

Johnson T (1997) Evaluating the hyperactive child in your office: is it ADHD? Am Fam Physician 56:155–160, 168–170.

Kendall PC, Braswell L (1993) Cognitive-Behavioral Therapy for Impulsive Children. New York: Guilford.

Stein DB (1999) Ritalin Is Not the Answer: A Drug-free, Practical Program for Children Diagnosed with ADD or ADHD. San Francisco: Jossey-Bass.

Taylor MA (1997) Evaluation and management of attention-deficit hyperactivity disorder. Am Fam Physician 55:887–897.

Zametkin AJ (1999) Problems in the management of attention-deficit-hyperactivity disorder. N Eng J Med 340:40–46.

19

School Phobia/Separation Anxiety

ASSESSMENT

1. Children commonly present with either a somatic complaint or fear of going to school.
2. The usual pattern is that on school mornings the symptoms become increasingly worse, subsiding when the child is allowed to stay home. There are usually fewer symptoms on weekends.
3. The parents' attempts to improve the situation usually entail trying to convince the child that it is okay to go to school, trying to understand their physical complaints, or repeatedly taking their child to the doctor for medical treatment.
4. The parents erroneously believe that the child's symptomatology must diminish before returning to school.
5. Exploration of the child's overall functioning finds associated characteristics of perfectionism, shyness, self-consciousness, dislike of physical education, and unstructured social situations with peers, such as recess.

PLAN

1. Reframe for the parents that avoidance is the problem and that return to school is the ultimate solution. After children return to school their symptoms are more likely to resolve.
2. For the child in kindergarten or first grade, often the solution is simply reassuring the parents that if they leave the child at school (even when experiencing stress or physical symptoms) the symptoms soon diminish or disappear.
3. If this does not work, change the sequence of events surrounding preparation and going to school, for example, have the other parent take responsibility.
4. If this does not work, the next approach is to gradually desensitize the child, such as the parent taking the child to school despite the distress and then staying at the school to provide support for a

period of time; for example, start with 2 hours and gradually decrease the time over a week or two.

5. When the child acceptably attends school, on return home that day the parents should give special attention as a reward.
6. If the parents are unable to decide if the child's somatic complaints are significant enough to keep the child home, the child can be brought immediately to the medical clinic in the morning. If the physician declares the child healthy, the child should go directly to school.
7. The physician should communicate with the school the assessment and plan for the child, in some cases following up with a letter.
8. When the child and family are unusually recalcitrant, an outside authority must be brought in to transport the child from home to school.
9. Once school attendance is regular, to prevent relapse it is helpful to focus on peer relations. It is often helpful to have the child become involved in a small group activity with peers to improve socialization.

Children with separation anxiety/school phobia most commonly present during their kindergarten and first grade years. When this disorder presents later it usually reflects a more difficult problem. In the young child it most often manifests as refusal to go to school or to separate from a parent, whereas in an older child it may manifest as somatic symptoms. Common symptoms are headaches, stomachache, and sometimes more unusual symptoms such as weakness or "spells." The symptoms often have a pattern of improvement over the weekend and exacerbate during the early mornings before school, although this is not always true. The child may have an underlying fear of something happening to the parent when they are not home. This frequently develops after an infectious illness requires time away from school.

There are other commonly associated characteristics, such as the child being a perfectionist, shy, self-conscious, or disliking physical education and any other aggressive activity. Children may be overly mature, desiring to spend most of their time with adults rather than their peers. At school the child may be spending time seeking attention from the teacher, wanting to be in close proximity to the teacher. The child feels most comfortable in familiar surroundings with parents and most uncomfortable in public, unstructured places with peers, such as during recess at school.

Assessment

When parents are asked to describe the sequence of events leading to the problem, they most commonly state that the child is expected to go to school but he or she complains of being fearful or of having a somatic complaint. The parent responds by trying to be understanding and explaining why it is okay for them to go to school. This leads children to escalate their complaints of distress until the parents give up and accept the child's need to stay home or to be protected from their fear or somatic symptom. In some circumstances the child goes to school, but a teacher or nurse calls informing the parent of the child's distress or "illness." The parent then rescues the child from school, and takes him or her home or to see a physician to find a cure for the somatic disorder. In either case the parent is convinced that the suffering from the fear or somatic complaint must resolve before the child can return to school.

Most commonly the parent overempathizes with the child's physical or emotional distress and tries to cure the problem through understanding discussions and education or frequent trips to the doctor. When this method does not work, the parent protects the child from discomfort by avoiding the outside activity. The primary view of the family in this instance is that the symptoms must be alleviated before the child can be expected to return to usual activities. In most cases the parent identifies returning to school and other activities as signs of improvement. However, in some circumstances the parent identifies improvement as being better able to handle anxiety or curing their physiologic symptoms. This attitude must be addressed when the intervention is framed. The child often does not commit to any need for treatment.

Plan

Getting the child to attend school regularly is the centerpiece of nearly all treatment approaches. The parental resistance to this resolution is frequently the idea that the child's distress must diminish before going back to school. In fact, quite the opposite usually occurs: Once the child attends school regularly the distress diminishes. In many instances, particularly for the child in kindergarten or first grade, all that may be needed is to reassure the parents that firm direction to go to school, no matter what the symptoms, can help alleviate the child's symptoms. In other circumstances, particularly in the adolescent, a more compelling intervention is usually necessary before the child returns to school.

Sometimes the least intrusive approach is to change the sequence of the morning activities in preparation for school. One of the most successful ways to do this is to have the parent who formerly was not the morning authority take responsibility for getting the child to school. When proposing this solution, one must be careful not to give the message that the other parent has failed to do an adequate job because this would only lead to resistance. The parent might unconsciously have to make the other one fail equally to avoid being blamed for the problem. Sometimes a way to avoid this dilemma is to ask the parents if they have ever had to overcome a fear or distressing situation in their past. You can choose the target parent you would like to take the child to school as having had an experience that you find particularly beneficial as a model for their child. This parent then is responsible for getting the child ready for school, providing transportation, leaving the child at school, and not responding to the child's distress signals.

Another approach is to frame the child's problem as avoiding distress. The solution is teaching the child to approach problems gradually rather than running away from them. The doctor can institute a desensitization program as a solution. It may require gradual steps in expecting the child to separate more and more from home and parents. For example, have the child initially go to school for an hour or two during the time of day when the activities are most comfortable. Then, over the period of a week, gradually expect the child to stay in school for more time, ignoring the distress while giving some sort of positive reward for having success at school.

For the highly somatic child, it is usually not useful to tell the parents that the somatic complaint is not real or not important. It can often be successfully reframed by describing the somatic problem as an ongoing one the child must learn to overcome in a way that does not affect daily life. For example, if the child has headaches or gastrointestinal distress, the physician can state that it is likely to be an ongoing problem for them, that perhaps the child has a sensitive stomach or a tendency toward tension headaches and so needs to learn to live with the problem in a way that does not interfere with activities. It can be pointed out that distraction and becoming involved in other activities is one of the most useful ways to overcome somatic symptoms. When one sits around idly at home with time to focus on the pain, it worsens.

When parents overempathize with the child's somatic problem, it is sometimes useful to help the parents share some of their concern with the doctor initially. A protocol can be set up whereby if the child is sick and the parents believe the child is unable to go to school the physician or a colleague evaluates the child as early as possible in the morning. The child is brought to the clinic fully dressed and ready to go to school. If the physician determines that the child is not so sick he or she cannot attend school the next step is to go directly from the office to school. This process is usually required only once or twice because the parents do not go through such a hassle and expense many times before they realize the child will be going to school anyway.

Another approach that works in a small number of situations is to reframe the problem as a power struggle between the child and the parents. This works when the parents already are hinting at this view. A behavior program is set up for the child's return to school through a series of rewards and consequences. The consequences might be that if children stay at home, they must stay in their room doing their homework alone without parental aid, and because they are sick they must stay in bed and rest with as little stimulation as possible. This means no radio, no television, and no light on until they feel better. Because it is obviously a "very grave illness" it should be treated as such. On the other hand, if the child does go to school the parent from whom the child desires attention and close proximity engages the child in some pleasurable activity after school.

With all of the above approaches, it is important for the doctor to directly or through the parent communicate with the officials at school who are involved in the process of keeping the child at school. The best approach for school staff is to give children as little attention as possible for symptoms while making sure that they get some extra attention for positive interactions, particularly with peers. The school officials should be told not to send the child home because of somatic complaints unless there is objective evidence of illness (e.g., a high fever). Documenting this in the form of a letter from the physician may help school officials feel less threatened by fear of liability.

Once success has been attained for the child beyond first grade age, it is sometimes useful to focus on the power struggle between the parent and child. Many times once the child is back in school the parent is more open to this view of the problem. One way to introduce this concept in a playful way that diminishes potential resistance is to suggest a game where children choose 1 day during the week when they pretend to have their old symptoms. The parents' part of the game is to make sure they get to school despite the symptoms. The children are to do their best job of pretending to convince the parent to let them stay home. Whether the symptoms are real is to be kept a secret until their next appointment. This intervention can be explained to parents as the child needing to find out that the parents have the authority. Use of this plan can prevent relapse.

Follow-up should also address giving children some reward for their attendance at school. It may also be useful at this time for children who have difficulty becoming involved with their peers to address the problem in a broader prospective. This may be accomplished by placing them in a structured small group situation where they may have more opportunities for successful contact even though shy or uncomfortable with peers. Examples include a 4H group, model airplane group, or athletic team. A good adult leader can prevent "bullying" of a socially challenged child, draw a shy child into participation, and teach the group to work together toward a common goal. School-phobic children can gain confidence and positive rewards from the peer group interaction—the antithesis of their original problem.

For the highly recalcitrant child and family in unusual situations, it is sometimes helpful to bring in an outside authority to provide structure. For example, sometimes the police, child protective services, or a school official can be used to collect these children from home in the morning and transport them to school. This maintains the expectation for both parent and child that the child will go to school. In the most difficult situations hospitalizing the child or going to the juvenile detention center for a brief time is necessary. In either circumstance almost from the day they get there, even in the hospital program, they should begin school the next day at their regular school.

Someone other than a parent should transport the child to school for a few days and then back to the hospital after school, with consequences and rewards taking place within the hospital or other institutional setting. A visit with parents in the evening is a good reward. Once attendance has occurred the parents should be expected to transport the child to school from the hospital or detention center. When children are successfully attending school from the institution, they can be discharged, and one of the home programs outlined above can be instituted.

Case Report

V.S. was a 6-year-old girl just beginning her first grade year. She presented to her family physician with abdominal pain of approximately 2 weeks' duration. The physician performed a gastrointestinal and genitourinary review of systems and learned that the abdominal pain was intermittent, usually occurring in the mornings; it was unrelated to the type of food eaten, and there was no accompanying nausea and vomiting, constipation, or diarrhea. Pain was sharp and severe, causing the child to grasp her stomach with both hands and double over. Despite the severity of the pain, it was not well localized. Her mother could not explain any exacerbating or ameliorating factors except to say that if the child was allowed to rest the pain gradually subsided. There were no other gastrointestinal symptoms, no genitourinary symptoms, and no constitutional symptoms or fever.

On examination the physician found a well developed, malnourished girl appearing her listed age with normal developmental landmarks and normal behavior in the office, albeit somewhat shy. The head/ears/eyes/nose/throat (HEENT) examination was normal. Her lungs were clear, and the heart had regular rhythm and a normal rate with a grade 2/6 systolic murmur that was harsh, high-pitched, and best heard at the apex. The abdomen was mildly obese without mass, organomegaly, surgical scar, or hernia. There was diffuse, mild tenderness to palpation without rigidity or guarding; and normal bowel sounds were heard. There was no tenderness to palpation over the symphysis pubis. On auscultation, the physician appeared to listen intently and pushed the diaphragm of the stethoscope deeply into the abdomen in areas in which palpation formerly had caused some discomfort. There now appeared to be no such response.

The physician returned to history-taking, asking Mrs. S if symptoms were more likely on school days than on weekends. She responded in the affirmative. She asked about the child's adjustment to kindergarten the previous year and found that the child had attended half-day kindergarten with some separation anxiety at first but later without significant problems. There had been no significant life events in the family except that a much older brother had left home for the military service. The child and he had been close.

The physician suspected that the abdominal pain was a somatic symptom designed by the child to avoid attending school. When exploring this hypothesis with Mrs. S the physician noted some reticence on the part of the mother to accept it. She suggested they perform a blood count and urinalysis but predicted that they would be normal, corroborating "stress at school leading to abdominal pain in a child with a particularly sensitive stomach." She received permission to call V.S.'s teacher. A follow-up office visit was planned with a request that Mr. S be in attendance as well. Prior to that visit the physician spoke with the first grade teacher, a woman of many years' experience, who portrayed V.S. as clinging, shy, and easily intimidated by her peers, who sometimes teased her about her weight.

At follow-up the laboratory studies were reported as normal. While V.S. read a book in another room the physician discussed her problem with her parents. She asked each parent to recall a time, as a child, they had to overcome something fearful. Both were able to supply stories, but the physician purposefully chose Mr. S as sharing an experience that might make him particularly capable of shaping their child's behavior through his own experience. She asked if Mr. S might be made responsible for getting his daughter off to school each morning. If V.S. were to have abdominal pain her mother might check her temperature, but if it was normal Mr. S was to help his daughter get to school regardless of symptoms. At the same time, the physician wrote a note for the parents to give to the teacher and school nurse. It suggested that the teacher do what she could to involve the child in positive peer relationships and to use necessary discipline to decrease the teasing that had been going on. If V.S. had abdominal pain at school the nurse might perform an examination but in the absence of objective findings was not to send the child home.

The physician asked whether the mother might reward V.S. for school attendance with an after-school activity, especially something that might involved the child's peers. Mrs. S quickly agreed, adding that she had recently been asked to take leadership of a Brownie troop.

An appointment was scheduled for the following week. The following week, Mrs. S called and cancelled saying it was not needed as V.S. was attending school regularly.

When the child was seen months later for a U.R.I. the mother reported V.S. had, had a difficult time the first days back at school. She was seen by the school nurse several times but was not sent home. By the end of the week her symptoms were less frequent.

As the physician did not hear back about this problem, she presumed it had been solved. When she saw Mrs. S. at a community function she spoke to the woman briefly and found that this was so.

References

Jellinek M, Kearns M (1995) Separation Anxiety. Pediatrics in Review, 16(2), 57–61.
Schmitt B (1995) School Avoidance. In Parker S, Zuckerman B (eds) Behavioral and Developmental Pediatrics. Boston: Little, Brown and Company.

20

Eating Disorders

ANOREXIA NERVOSA

Assessment

1. Expect strong resistance from patients with anorexia nervosa. To improve accuracy gather the history from multiple sources.
2. History should include a detailed description of eating habits, including any bulimic behavior; patients' view of their body image; history of weight fluctuations; desired weight; history of menstrual pattern; laxative, diuretic, or diet pill usage; exercise habits; substance abuse; mood and anxiety problems; suicidal ideation.
3. History should also include the patient's school and work performance, peer relationships, relationships with the family, and extracurricular activities.
4. Have there been any attempted solutions by the patient and family?
5. The patient's weight should be measured while gowned.
6. A thorough physical examination and laboratory testing should be done. The laboratory tests should be directed at the secondary effects of starvation.
7. Diagnostic criteria include being 15% below ideal weight, having a distorted view of the body image, being preoccupied with weight, having three consecutive missed periods (girls and women).
8. Associated individual factors include perfectionism, eagerness to please others, anger inhibition, low self-esteem despite significant successes and a lack of movement toward independence from parents in a normal pattern, and avoidance of an adult sexual identity.
9. Family characteristics include overenmeshment, lack of generational boundaries, overprotection, rigidity, and poor anger resolution.

Plan

1. The initial goal of treatment should be directed at weight gain, with menstruation in women being a key target symptom.
2. The criterion for hospitalization is being 30% below ideal weight or if the weight loss is fulminant and the patient highly resistant to treatment. Family support for treatment should also be considered.
3. In or out of the hospital, a behavioral program should be used as primary treatment for weight gain. Restrictions on activity should be used as consequences, whereas more freedom and the ability to have increased activity should be used as rewards. Rewards and consequences should be based on gowned weights measured upon awakening. In the outpatient situation the weight should be measured with the patient gowned at least weekly. Medical personnel, not parents, should record all weights. The parents should be encouraged to ignore eating behavior, ensuring that they are informed of serious weight problems.
4. A nutritional counselor for the nutritionally naïve patient can be helpful.
5. Once weight gain is progressing, treatment goals should be directed at psychosocial issues.
    a. Involvement in social activities with peers.
    b. Increased independence from the family.
    c. Reducing perfectionism by joining a noncompetitive activity.
6. For athletes, a minimum weight should be set for participation.
7. Eating disorder support groups aimed at the isolated teenager may be helpful.

Medications

In general, psychotropic medications have not been found useful. Hormone therapy for prolonged amenorrhea to prevent osteoporosis may be needed. If nausea with fuller meals is an initial problem, medication is occasionally helpful.

BULIMIA

Assessment

1. History should include a detailed description of eating habits, including any binge/purge behavior; the patients' view of their body image; history of weight fluctuations; desired weight; history of menstrual pattern; laxative, diuretic, or diet pill usage; exercise habits; substance abuse; mood and anxiety problems; and suicidal ideation.
2. History should also include the patient's school performance, peer relationships, relationships with the family, and extracurricular activities.

3. What bothers patients most about their problem?
4. What makes the problem better or worse?
5. Have there been attempted solutions by the patient and family?
6. The patient's weight should be recorded while gowned.
7. Thorough physical examination and laboratory testing should be done. The laboratory tests should include electrolytes.
8. The central theme for bulimic patients is control issues: others controlling them and they controlling themselves. Control of weight is especially consuming.
9. Criteria for diagnosis include binge episodes, purging, or other inappropriate attempts at weight control such as laxative usage. Self-evaluation if often centered on weight; but unlike those with anorexia, they have a more realistic body image.

Plan

1. Hospitalization of patients with bulimia is rarely necessary unless there is profound hypokalemia or suicidal intent. If suicidal ideation is present in bulimic patients, they should be evaluated as any other potentially suicidal patient (see Chapters 15 and 16).
2. Frame the overall problem for the patient as being caused by feelings of being out of control and looking for appropriate ways to be in control of their food intake and their lives.
3. Begin with a self-observational task (SOT) directed toward food intake. They should maintain a diary, which includes their behavior before, during, and after food consumption including what they consume, how others interact with them, and the use of any substances such as laxatives. Initially they should not make an attempt to alter their eating behavior. Explain that this information is important for treatment.
4. Follow-up visits should be at least weekly at first. If in response to the SOT patients significantly reduced the bulimic behavior, they should simply be told to continue this program to obtain an even clearer picture.
5. If they have done the SOT but not improved, treatment should be directed to small alterations in the eating and purging sequence. Explain that attempts to gain more control should occur slowly. They should begin the attempt by each morning planning in great detail the bulimic episodes based on what they have previously written in their diary. Some small step should be requested of them as far as change. For example, "Wait 5 minutes more before purging, or eat 10% less during the binge."
6. Follow-up should continue with small changes in the binge/purge cycle. Continue with the SOT.

7. Because anxiety relief is part of the gain from the binge/purge cycle for many patients, alternative behavioral treatments for anxiety should be offered (e.g., relaxation exercises).
8. If substance abuse is an issue, it should be treated.
9. If patients live with their parents or have a significant other, a conjoint therapy session should take place to deal with changing the focus of conflict or control away from food and onto issues of normal control and independence.
10. Patients should find some new way to feel more in control of their lives (e.g., being more assertive with someone, making one change that would surprise everyone).

Medication

Medication should be limited to the treatment of depressive symptomatology in patients who do not respond to brief therapy with improved in mood. An antidepressant is chosen that does not cause significant weight gain or nausea.

The eating disorders anorexia nervosa and bulimia most often develop during adolescence or the early twenties. Commonly patients deny having a problem, particularly those with anorexia nervosa. Families are often in denial as well. The family physician is frequently the first person to see patients with these problems, as they are usually highly resistant to going to mental health specialists. Early intervention by the family physician can prevent the problems from solidifying, making the treatment much easier and effective. If anorexia nervosa goes untreated for more than a year, cure takes many years at best.

Anorexia Nervosa

The diagnostic criteria for anorexia nervosa include failure to maintain minimum weight for height. Fifteen percent below ideal weight is considered by many to be the cutoff criterion but a specific weight is not absolutely diagnostic. These patients have an intense fear of obesity and are preoccupied with weight and body image, seeing themselves as fat. Females are affected about 20 times more often than males. Three consecutive missed menstrual periods due to weight loss are also required for diagnosis.

If the problem has gone on for long, the patient begins to experience physiologic changes associated with starvation, including cardiovascular changes, bradycardia, and low blood pressure. Acrocyanosis and arrhythmias can occur, especially exercise-related ones. Reduced heart size may lead to mitral valve prolapse. There can be metabolic changes. Most have hypothyroidism, which should not be treated except with food. Laboratory findings are often normal except for the thyroid-stimulating hormone (TSH) level. Often there are gastrointestinal disturbances such as motility abnormalities. Nearly all of these imbalances are reversible, although osteoporosis can be a long-term problem if amenorrhea persists.

Behaviorally, these patients sometimes have unusual eating patterns (e.g., eating only carrots or keeping foods separated on the plate). They sometimes exercise excessively. There are also psychological features common in patients with anorexia nervosa, including high levels of performance in work and athletics along with a perfectionist approach to nearly all activities. There is also an eagerness to please others, anger inhibition, and low self-esteem despite a great deal of success. Normal adolescent rebellion is often lacking, inhibiting movement toward independence. The avoidance of an adult sexual identity is frequently problematic. For example, amenorrhea is viewed positively by anorectic patients.

There are commonalties in family features as well, including overenmeshment, a lack of generational boundaries, overprotection, lack of conflict resolution or perhaps even conflict avoidance, rigidity or difficulty during times of change. It is important to keep these features in mind because in addition to weight gain overall resolution of the problem entails at least some alteration in these features by the individual and the family. In fact, movement toward normal independence from parents is a nearly universal requirement for cure.

Assessment

Anorexia nervosa is most commonly presented to the family physician because parents have demanded that their child go to the doctor. Sometimes it is someone else who refers, such as a coach or a schoolteacher. Usually the teenager is resistant to any kind of evaluation and denies any problem; the parents are therefore the primary source of the history.

When assessing any eating disorder the history should include a detailed description of eating habits including any bulimic behavior. It should also include how patients describe their body image; history of weight fluctuations; their desired weight; history of their menstrual pattern; laxative, diuretic, or diet pill usage; their exercise and athletic participation; substance abuse; and mood and anxiety problems including suicidal ideation. The family members' response to the problems and attempted solutions should also be explored. It is helpful to include parents in the evaluation process. The patient, of course, should undergo a complete physical examination.

Laboratory tests might include a complete blood count; assays for electrolytes, blood urea, nitrogen, creatinine, calcium, magnesium, phosphate, cholesterol, lipids, amylase, total protein, and albumin; liver function tests; thyroid function tests; urinalysis; and in the case of the highly emaciated patient an electrocardiogram (bradycardia and low voltage are expected) as well as the usual vital signs. Weight should be measured with the patient gowned, as some patients alter their weight by putting lead weights in their pockets.

Treatment

The first treatment decision is whether to hospitalize. Patients must be hospitalized if they have acute complications of starvation or bulimic behaviors such as profound hypokalemia. At 30% below ideal weight, hospitalization is almost always required. At 25% below ideal weight, often other factors can be considered, including fulminant weight loss, patients' motivation to keep their weight above dangerous levels, or their motivation to stay out of the hospital by avoiding weight loss. The family's willingness to accept responsibility to make sure the patient stays engaged in treatment is also an important consideration.

If hospitalization is necessary for the anorectic patient, weight gain should be the primary initial treatment goal (new learning cannot occur in the face of starvation). This nearly always requires a behavioral reinforcement program based on weight. It is usually not useful to base these programs on food intake, as manipulative behavior ensues and makes it counterproductive.

A typical example of a behavioral program is shown in Table 20.1. The program entails weighing the gowned patient each morning (same time and scale) and having their activity level for that day be based on whether they have lost, maintained, or gained weight.

In extreme circumstances tube feeding may be necessary along with restraints. This usually requires an involuntary commitment for the patient over 18 years of age.

Patients can order any diet they want so long as it is balanced. This program is usually best instituted on a pediatric or medical floor rather than a psychiatric unit in the hospital. A target weight should be set soon after admission that is usually 15–20% below ideal weight. When patients reach this weight they are allowed to be discharged with the agreement that they will continue to gain. Incentives can be built into this program in that patients who adhere to the treatment program more rapidly is allowed to be discharged at a slightly lower weight with the understanding that they will gain more of weight as an outpatient. Those who are more treatment-resistant initially therefore spend more days in the hospital. When recovery of weight has begun to be successful, the focus of treatment can then include other issues common to anorectic patients.

For the patient with anorexia nervosa who does not require hospitalization, or even after hospitalization, the treatment plan still must focus on weight. At the initial appointment patients should be weighed while gowned and a minimum weight set at which they know they would be hospitalized. A target weight should be agreed upon, with realistic goals for the weight gain. A realistic goal is enough weight to begin menstruation, which is usu-

TABLE 20.1. Behavior Protocol During Hospitalization of Anorectic Patients

Weight gain of 200 g or more—is allowed activity ad libitum

    May walk around unit, go into hall to make phone calls, go to first floor with parents or nurse

    May go out of the hospital for lunch only when weight gain is progressive and patient seems stable

Weight gain of 100 g—bed rest with bathroom privileges (bedpan)

    May answer phone when someone calls but may not go out to make phone calls
    May have visitors
    May watch television, receive mail, bathe in bed

No weight gain or loss—bed rest, no bathroom privileges

    No phone calls but may know who called
    May have visitors
    May watch television, receive mail, bathe in bed

Weight loss of 100 g—bed rest, no bathroom privileges

    No phone calls but may know who called
    No visitors
    May watch television, receive mail, bathe in bed

Weight loss of 200 g—bed rest, no bathroom privileges

    No phone calls
    No visitors
    No television
    May receive mail, bathe in bed

Weight loss of 300 g—strict bed rest

    No phone calls
    No visitors
    No television, mail, bathing
    May only eat

ally about 10% below ideal weight. Patients should be warned that for the first few days they may gain weight rather rapidly as their body adjusts to not starving. Initially it is best to see them once a week.

The family should be discouraged from monitoring their weight, letting them know that they can feel secure that if the patient gets into a dangerous situation the doctor will inform them. Parents should be discouraged from pushing the youth to eat and in fact should be encouraged to focus their attention on other aspects of the child's life. Some reward should be developed for achieving weight goals, with the doctor's office reporting to the family when goals have been reached. Patients are the best source of deciding what rewards they would like for achieving certain weight milestones. For example, if they like to exercise, initially they might not be allowed to exercise at home; once they have gained weight, though, there can be a gradual increase in the amount of exercise they are allowed.

Nutritional counseling may be of use to patients if their eating disorder is of recent onset. However, if they have been highly interested in diet and nutritional issues in the past, it can be counterproductive to then send them to a dietitian or nutritionist, as they may use it for manipulative purposes. Greater attention to other areas of their life is a more important change in the long run.

They should not be given a special diet but should be expected to share the foods everyone else in the family is eating. They should be allowed access to the kitchen at home in a way considered "normal" for their family.

Altering the sequence of events around eating is also important. Often parents and others push food too much. Food can be made unappetizing for anyone when it is pushed on them. It is not useful for the doctor or anyone else to argue with a patient over body image. As they come to accept themselves as an adult this attitude alters on its own.

Once the weight gain program has been initiated, other issues should be addressed. Such issues as overdependence and difficulty moving toward the normal independence of adolescence, being involved comfortably and socially with peers, and accepting imperfections in one's performance are critical to long-term successful treatment. Seeing issues as all good or all bad should be addressed as well. For example, the patient might be asked to make a list of good and bad features of friends or family. The next step would be to scale them on a Lickert scale from 1 to 10 (1 being bad, 10 being good).

A useful way to frame the problems of anorexia for the patient and family is to tell them that people with anorexia nervosa are sometimes uncomfortable giving up the look of a child and taking on the look of an adult. Getting involved in normal teenage activity then aids the process. For example, encouraging the patient to start a new activity that allows age-appropriate interaction is helpful. Being involved with peers in unstructured, noncompetitive activity is helpful (e.g., going to a dance with a friend.

To address perfectionism and independence, finding some new activity at which they can work just for fun and accepting a mediocre performance from themselves would be useful. Parents getting less involved in some of these activities (e.g., sports) also supports more independence.

In the case of athletes, having the doctor and parent work with the coach to set a minimum weight at which the youngster can compete can also be useful. For example, many female athletes involved in sports such as gymnastics, cross-country, or dance or figure skating should know that there is a minimum weight at which they can compete or even go to practices. If the eating disorder is specifically targeted at performance in a sport, setting the weight standard can be curative alone and not require a comprehensive program. Working on issues of perfectionism in tandem may prove beneficial.

An eating disorder support group can be helpful for the isolated patient. It is not always useful, however, because at times the eating disorder peer group becomes a forum for its members to compete over how much weight they can lose.

Medications

In general, psychotropic medications have not been found useful for anorexia nervosa. Hormone therapy for prolonged amenorrhea may be important for preventing osteoporosis. Patients who have been starving themselves may initially feel nauseous when eating fuller meals. Usually eating small, frequent meals ultimately leads them to tolerate larger meals. Sometimes, however, metoclopramide helps avoid the nausea while they are getting used to the larger intake.

Bulimia

Patients with bulimia are preoccupied with food intake and use desperate means to control weight. They get caught up in binge/purge cycles. Their fear of being out of control of their eating leads them to control their weight by inappropriate means, such as fasting, self-induced vomiting, excessive exercise, and abuse of laxatives and diuretics. Bulimic patients do not become extremely thin; in fact usually their weight is within 10% of ideal. They become secretive and guilt-ridden about eating habits, which often leads to dysphoria or depressive symptoms including suicidal ideation. There is a high rate of substance abuse as well. A dual diagnosis of bulimia and personality disorder is common. They also tend to have unintended pregnancies if they are not amenorrheic. Patients with anorexia nervosa often have bulimia as well. In this case, anorexia nervosa is the diagnosis.

On the whole, bulimic patients do not have medical findings. Rarely they have parotid enlargement. Some have calluses or scars on the back of their hands. They can have dental erosion and gastrointestinal symptoms (e.g., motility problems, bloating, heartburn).

They usually have a troubled background, which sometimes includes substance abuse or depression in their families. Almost always there is some form of authority and control problems within the family. Issues of control appear to be central to the problem of bulimia and therefore are usually the primary focus of treatment. When the patients experience that they have better self-control in all areas of their lives, symptoms diminish or disappear.

Assessment

These patients most commonly present during their late teens or early twenties for a physical problem, at which time the question of bulimia comes up.

However, this occurs only if the physician develops some suspicion and asks probing question about the patient's eating habits.

The evaluation for bulimia is similar to that for anorexia nervosa. The history should include a detailed description of eating habits and of a typical bulimic event. It should also include a description of how patients view their body image; a history of their weight fluctuations; their desired weight; their menstrual pattern; laxative, diuretic, or diet pill usage; their exercise pattern and athletic participation; history of substance abuse; and mood and anxiety problems including suicidal ideation. It is useful to include at least one family member or significant other in the evaluation to have their description of the problem and attempted solutions. The patient, of course, requires a careful physical examination. Laboratory tests might include a complete blood count; assays for electrolytes, blood urea, nitrogen, creatinine, calcium, magnesium, phosphate, cholesterol, lipids, amylase, total protein, and albumin; liver function tests; thyroid function tests; and urinalysis. The weight should be determined with the patient gowned.

Plan

Hospitalization of the patient with bulimia is rarely necessary. Aside from profound hypokalemia, psychological factors are a concern. Suicide risk is probably the most important consideration. Although suicidal ideation is common among bulimia patients, they rarely have a plan. Outpatient treatment is therefore usually preferred. (If suicidal ideation is present, evaluate the same as for any suicidal patient; see Chapters 15 and 16.)

To begin treatment it is useful to frame the bulimia as being caused by a general sense of being out of control and looking for ways to be in control, with much of the focus on food intake. The "self-observational task" (see Chapter 1), which is helpful for many out-of-control behaviors, is a good way to initiate treatment. Begin by asking the patient to maintain a diary of all food intake and to document closely all actions and thoughts surrounding the binge/purge cycle in great detail. Any other related behaviors, such as laxative use, should also be described in the diary. The more detailed the description, the better.

At this point it is important to avoid asking patients to change, as they perceive it as the doctor trying to control them. The explanation for keeping the diary that appears to be most acceptable to most bulimic patients is that the first step in gaining control over one's food intake is to better understand it and keeping the diary is aimed at this goal. The act of being self-observant of the eating behaviors alters the sequence of events toward making these actions less spontaneous and impulsive and more controlled by the patient. This often has the effect of attenuating the behavior. It is not useful, however, to discuss this common outcome with the patient.

At the next appointment, patients who have already significantly reduced their bulimic behavior are told that changing too fast can be uncomfortable and so to continue to keep the diary and put off making any other improvements. This helps them feel in even more control and maintains the improvement.

If they have kept the diary but not improved, a small alteration in the sequence of events is requested. It is explained that it is aimed at helping them to gain more control, but slowly. Patients are asked to maintain their level of bulimic activity but plan the episodes each morning in detail. For example, if patients average two bulimic episodes per day, they are told each morning to write down what time they will be, how much will be eaten, how long this eating will go on, how long after the eating episode the purge will occur, how long the purge will take, and what the patient will do following the purge episode. This is again described as a small step toward gaining more control over the binge/purge cycle without being overwhelmed by moving too fast. This task often leads to improvement because it makes the bulimic behavior less spontaneous.

If the patient has improved, at the third meeting the patient is requested to not make any more changes for a while but to do more of the same. They can be told they have already made significant changes, and moving too fast may make them feel uncomfortable. It is safest to do more of the same about planning their binge/purge cycles and keeping a diary.

If they have kept to the plan but not yet reduced their binge/purge behavior, some small decrease in their behavior might be recommended. For example, there may be a small reduction in the amount of calories or food consumed, a greater length of time may be planned between the binge and purge episode, or just one binge/purge cycle per week may be eliminated while otherwise maintaining the rest of the plan. A detailed diary should continue to be kept throughout the treatment process.

At subsequent appointments, a gradual decrease in bulimic activity can be requested each week. Otherwise the plan remains the same. If no improvement has occurred by this point, it is probably time for a referral.

Because bulimic patients often are relieved of their anxiety through the binge/purge cycle, it is useful to substitute some other way to reduce anxiety. Relaxation exercises, biofeedback, or meditation may be suggested. If the patient has an ongoing substance abuse problem, treatment is likely needed before improvement in other areas can occur (see Chapter 12).

If patients live with their parents, at least a few sessions of family therapy are indicated. The goals of family therapy are to shift the focus of conflict (control) away from food and onto normal independence issues youths have with parents. Conflict between youths and parents is not abnormal, but the focus on eating behaviors is. Helping patients and their families deal with issues of control in other areas of their lives is of prime importance for long-term improvement of bulimic patients. Parents who are overly controlling are encouraged to turn control over gradually to their youngsters.

For the patient no longer living at home, family therapy may not be crucial, particularly if there is not a great deal of parental influence. If there is a controlling significant other, conjoint therapy can be helpful. Whatever in patients' lives leads them to feel out of control must be addressed so they believe they are more in control of their everyday problems.

Medication

Antidepressants have been found helpful for some bulimic patients who are depressed. However, it is important to keep in mind that often it is the dysphoria that motivates a patient to seek treatment. If their mood improves after taking medicine, they may lose all motivation to continue treatment for the bulimia. Selective serotonin reuptake inhibitors (SSRIs) sometimes cause nausea. Some antidepressants (those that are anxiolytic) cause weight gain. Appetite-suppressing antidepressants (e.g., SSRI's, bupropoin) are potentially anxiogenic and often have gastrointestinal side effects. Therefore prescribing antidepressants for bulimic patients must be done with caution. Adolescents have a low response rate to antidepressants in general beyond a placebo effect.

Case Report

F.E. was a 15-year-old girl well known to her family physician. She had suffered childhood asthma, which resolved spontaneously to a great degree when she reached puberty. Her mother now brought her to the office with concerns about extreme loss of weight. F.E. had excelled in gymnastics during the last 2 years, participating in the floor exercise, balance beam, and unequal bars. Her mother complained that the teenager had lost 7 pounds before the season began this year and was continuing to lose weight, "eating like a bird." In addition to twice-daily gymnastic practices, she was exercising evenings by bicycling long distances and skipping rope in the garage.

At this visit Mrs. E and her daughter were then separated, ostensibly for the nurse to weigh, determine vital signs, and prepare the patient for the physician's examination. Mrs. E was questioned regarding significant life events or family crises, and there were none. She was asked if her daughter left the table at the end of the meal and went into the bathroom or if she suspected her daughter of self-induced vomiting or laxative abuse. There was no history of these problems. The physician asked Mrs. E if this behavior had been going on the prior year and she reported that it had begun just before this gymnastic season. Mrs. E volunteered that her daughter ate only small amounts of salad without dressing and some fruit especially grapes. She drank either water, diet soda, or small glasses of skim milk. Mrs. E gave no history suggesting features of a dysfunctional family (e.g., enmeshment, overprotection, conflict avoidance, loss of generational boundaries, rigidity). She did describe her child as "a perfectionist" and" overachiever." Even as she said this she seemed to beam with pride. At the same time she appeared concerned about her daughter's health.

On examination F.E. was painfully thin but sinewy and strong. Her hair and skin lacked luster, and the skin appeared almost dirty. The thyroid was palpable normal. The chest was clear, and the heart had regular rhythm without number or gallop but at a rate of 45 beats/min at rest. The abdomen was scaphoid without mass, organomegaly, tenderness, surgical scar, or hernia. When questioned, the teenager reported she had begun menstruating at age 13 but had not had "a period" for 3 months. She was not sexually active. The physician expressed concern that she might be overtraining and reducing her body weight to a level below the point where she would have optimum performance. He was careful not to be critical or controlling but to offer advice as if he were a trainer or a coach. He expressed that his goal was the same as hers, to improve her athletic performance. He asked permission to discuss these matters with the coach.

When the office visit was completed the physician telephoned the gymnastics coach and made her aware of F.E.'s amenorrhea and weight loss. The coach was aware of this syndrome in young women athletes but expressed that she had not recognized it in this girl. She was quite willing to work with the physician to correct the problem. Together, a normal body weight for height was established, and the coach agreed to tell F.E. that she would not be allowed to perform until she had achieved this weight using the same rationale as the physician's about optimizing her performance. She agreed to provide "training table" advice to F.E. and her mother, as she was also the health teacher.

F.E. and her mother were given a plan to shop together and to buy nutritionally correct foods for the athlete. The coach also told the teenager that she was not to exercise to a great extent outside of supervised practice to prevent overtraining or "putting muscles out of balance." The coach reminded F.E. that she was the trainer and F.E. the athlete, and that she needed to stay with the coach's training program exclusively. The plan met with little resistance; and at the follow-up visit 1 month later F.E. had gained 4.5 pounds and had curtailed her solitary exercise. By the second month she had reached her goal weight and was allowed to participate again in gymnastics competition. The physician planned at some future date to address the perfectionism by encouraging F.E. to become involved in a noncompetitive activity as well.

References

Becker AE, Grinspoon SK, Klibanski A, Herzog DB (1999) Eating disorders. N Engl J Med 340:1092–1098.
Beumont P, Russell J, Touyz W (1993) Treatment of anorexia nervosa. Lancet 341:1635–1640.

Brownell KD, Foreyt JP (1986) Handbook of Eating Disorders: Physiology, Psychology, and Treatment of Obesity, Anorexia, and Bulimia. New York: Basic Books.

Carek P, Futreel M (1999) Athletes' view of the preparticipation physical examination: attitudes towards certain health screening questions. Arch Fam Med 8:307–312.

Hobbs W, Johnson C (1996) Anorexia nervosa: an overview. Am Fam Physician 54:1273–1279.

McGilley B, Pryor T (1998) Assessment and treatment of bulimia nervosa. Am Fam Physician 57:2743–2750.

Minuchin S, Rosman BL, Baker L (1978) Psychosomatic Families: Anorexia Nervosa in Context. Cambridge: Harvard University Press.

Sargent J, Liebman R (1985) Eating disorders. In Henao S, Grose NP (eds) Principles of Family Systems in Family Medicine. New York: Brunner/Mazel.

Slaughter J, Sun A (1999) In pursuit of perfection: a primary care physician's guide to body dysmorphic disorder. Am Fam Physician 60:1738–1742.

21

Adolescent Substance Abuse

RISK FACTORS

1. The adolescent with substance abuse is highly rebellious with poor impulse control.
2. Parental authority is either overly lax or overly rigid.
3. There is a high level of social anxiety that is ameliorated with alcohol usage or other drugs.
4. Teenagers who have difficulty fitting in, who are novelty seekers with little that is challenging in their lives, who are in poor social environments such as highly disrupted family situations, who are having little success with school or extracurricular activities, who have few family activities, and who have low self-esteem are candidates for substance abuse.
5. There is a history of family substance abuse.

ASSESSMENT

1. Red flags
   a. Parental suspicion of substance abuse by the teenager.
   b. Significant changes in the teenager's life style, such as less accomplishment in school and several other activities.
   c. Marked increase in rebellious activity.
   d. Change in peer group to a highly rebellious group.
   e. Unexplained health problems, especially if serious with altered mental status.
2. Screening questions
   a. Ask adolescents when they last consumed alcohol or other substances.
   b. If they admit to consumption, ask when they last consumed something before that time, and what and how much they consumed on each occasion.

3. History
   a. Specific example of drinking or substance abuse including social interaction leading up to usage and afterward, including parental response.
   b. When most and least likely to use substances.
   c. What the teenager likes about usage.
   d. What the teenager wants to change.
   e. The parents' perception of the problem and attempted solutions.
4. Indicators of pathology
   a. Onset of substance abuse prior to age 16.
   b. Any regular use by a 16 to 18-year-old.
   c. In post-high school adolescents, any substance use other than the weekend or if the use interferes with usual activity.

TREATMENT

1. For teenagers still living at home, parents must increase and maintain a highly structured environment with clear discipline.
2. For adolescents over age 18 or who have moved away from home, suggest a trial period of 1 month of abstinence to test their ability to control their substance use.
3. Suggest alternative activities that assert the adolescents' individuality and autonomy.
4. For adolescents who treat social anxiety with alcohol, seek alternative ways to become more socially comfortable.
5. For adolescents with low self-esteem, seek alternative ways to be successful.
6. For the high novelty-seeking teenager, seek activities directed at highly challenging activities (e.g., rock climbing).
7. For the teenager using substances to treat dysphoria related to major life conflicts, institute individual or family therapy.
8. For adolescents in whom substance usage is beyond their control, a substance abuse treatment program may be necessary. For those doing well in school or work, an outpatient program can be sought. When substance abuse is interfering with their ability to perform required tasks, an inpatient program is likely necessary.

Family physicians can make a real difference with teenagers who suffer from substance abuse, but it can be a challenge. In fact, the challenge starts with defining the problem. Studies show that there has been at least some alcohol consumption by more than 50% of high school seniors, and up to one-third have tried marijuana; 90% of college sophomores report the use of alcohol during their freshman year of college, with approximately 40% bingeing on the weekends with some regularity. After about the age of 22, there is a gradual but significant decline in the use of alcohol and other substances by most young people. About 10% of the population continue to have a substance abuse problem at some time in their lives (excluding nicotine). Nearly all who do started substance usage during their teens.

Although adolescents may not know the specifics of the statistics, they have a general sense of this reality; that is, although many teenagers use alcohol, for most it does not lead to long-term abuse. This makes the issue a complex one for physicians who treat teenagers. If they tell all teenagers that alcohol is dangerous for them, adolescents dismiss it as erroneous information and in some ways validly so. Yet there are serious risks involved that should be addressed by the family physician.

Certain risk factors are known to identify teenagers who are more likely to develop a substance abuse problem. Most youths who drink alcohol are motivated by rebelliousness, experimentation with adult identity, and novelty seeking along with some risk taking, sensation seeking, limit testing, and curiosity. In some respects what they do for risk taking is a matter of opportunity. Some teenagers define themselves through pole vaulting and others through driving 100 miles an hour, sexual activity, or drinking. To say that a certain degree of experimentation with alcohol and other substances is normal is not to say that it should be overlooked.

Because the primary motivations for most teenagers falls into the category of rebelliousness toward authority and movement toward adult identity, parents are in a position to make the greatest difference; and the family doctor's most frequent role is to support the parents. By the time teenagers finish high school, they have been exposed to an average of more than 50 hours of education on substances. Although the physician might be in a position to reinforce this education, additional information is likely to accomplish little. For most teenagers who do not have the risk factors discussed below, a parent providing firm limits regarding the use of substances is probably the most valuable and effective response. Teenagers who are grounded for a week because parents become aware the youngsters have consumed alcohol are probably not going to increase usage and perhaps will decrease it. Punishment has an impact because it hurts; but it also clearly communicates that the parents are opposed to their teenager's use of substances. It teaches them also that their parents are in a position to set firm limits.

For the at-risk adolescent, it is necessary for the family physician to take a larger role in treatment. Risk factors include serious rebelliousness and poor impulse control. Often this situation is seen in a family with either overly lax or extremely rigid rules. Sometimes it represents extreme disagreement between the two parents on rules, regardless of whether they are married, which may make the parents vacillate between being overly lax and overly rigid.

Sometimes teenagers find that alcohol or other drugs distract them from certain psychological or interpersonal problems. For example, they may self-treat a high level of anxiety, particularly social anxiety, with alcohol, making them feel more at ease in the social context. Some teenagers who have been ostracized by peers find their niche in a rebellious group characterized by the usage of alcohol and other drugs. Some teenagers have an extreme desire to seek novelty and excitement, especially if they find themselves bored and unchallenged in most areas of their lives. Some are depressed because of perceived failures, or they are in a poor social situation, such as having parents going through a divorce and using alcohol and other drugs to avoid their own problems and to treat their dysphoria. Some have never learned to control impulses adequately. Having parents who role-model substance abuse increases the risk considerably.

On the other hand, there are certain protective factors that, even in the presence of risk factors, may help youths avoid substance abuse. They include having parents who provide "tough love" (i.e., firm, caring discipline along with positive attention for success). They provide family togetherness, regularly having dinner together, going to church together, or participating in other activities as a family. Successes in organized activities, particularly for the student not doing well at school, can lead to increased self-esteem (e.g., the student who excels in athletics, music, 4H, a church group, or scouting). Teenagers do better if they see their future as important enough to delay immediate gratification in favor of future success. Teenagers who feel good about themselves are less likely to do things that are injurious, such as using substances beyond the norm.

Assessment

The most common red flag that presents to a physician pointing to adolescent substance abuse is the expression of parental concern. Usually if a parent suspects substance abuse, it is occurring. Another red flag is a significant change in teenagers' life style, such as a significant lessening of accomplishment in school or other activities: the greater the changes, the more concerning they are. A loss of interest in one sport or activity such as music is common, but teenagers rarely withdraw from multiple activities without significant reason. A marked increase in rebellious activity or changing their peer group to a highly rebellious or antisocial one is common. Any unexplained health problem, especially when the teenager is hospitalized with a serious unexplained condition, should raise consideration of substance abuse. This is especially true if there is a change in mental status.

Often a screening question (see Chapter 2) such as, "Have there been any major changes in your life over the past year?" during a routine examination can bring these issues to light. It is especially important to ask adolescents when they last consumed alcohol or other substances. This question could be asked in a slightly different way for at-risk teenagers: "Have you consumed any alcohol or other substances during the past month?" If the answer is yes, they should be asked when they last consumed alcohol or other substances and how much they consumed at the time. They should then be asked when their last drink or consumption of other substances occurred prior to that.

For adolescents who admit that substance usage is a problem, a thorough history of such use should be obtained. The history should include an example of a typical episode, including events leading up to and following usage; when usage is most and least likely; what is desirable about the substance; and what the teenager wants to change. Parents should be asked for their perception of the problem and attempted solutions.

Early age of onset is considered a strong risk factor for later problems. In an individual younger than age 16, any alcohol or substance abuse should be considered pathologic. In the 16- to 18-year-old, any regular usage of alcohol or other substances is considered pathologic.

Binge drinking on the weekend is common in post-high school adolescents. Drinking that occurs regularly other than on the weekend is considered pathologic. Substance usage that causes interference with activities is considered pathologic. Regular binge drinking on the weekend warrants close observation and counseling the individual with regard to risks.

The use of a urine drug screen to identify illicit substances can be helpful. However, if done without the knowledge and approval of the teenager it can do more harm than good. It should be considered only in specific circumstances. For example, a drug screen should nearly always be done in teenagers who are hospitalized with a life-threatening illness that might be secondary to drug usage or who have a severely altered state of consciousness. Another instance in which it can be useful is for the teenager who knows that a drug screen is required to compete in sports or to have a particular job.

On the other hand, if the teenager is in the office and the parents are requesting a drug screen because they suspect substance abuse, there are better alternatives. Ask the parents for the specific observations that led them to believe the teenager is using substances. If they are normal adolescent rebellious behaviors, such as temper outbursts at parents, define them as such. If they represent overly rebellious or limit-testing behavior (e.g., a drop in grades or spending time with the wrong crowd), substance abuse may be part of the picture. These problems should motivate parents to increase discipline regardless of whether substance abuse is discovered. If there are specific consequences for this behavior, teenagers are likely to decide that substance usage is not worth it. Often parents want the screening test to prove to the teenager that their increased control is justified. Although teenagers believe such control is never justified, the increased adverse consequences of their misbehavior provide external limits, making it easier for the teenager to stop the substance usage.

If the parents have observed their adolescent to have an altered mental status, they should operate on the assumption that the youth was a user and not have to prove it. Rather than performing the test without the teenager's approval, the parents can explain to their adolescent that they are concerned about the behavioral problems and they therefore are providing more structure. This should include a strict curfew and more requirements to inform the parents where the teenager is going. Teenagers often respond to these measures by saying that they are not being trusted. Usually at this point the teenager has broken rules such as coming in late for curfews, so the parents can simply respond that because of repeated rule violations they do *not* trust the teenager. The teenager must act trustworthy for a given period of time (e.g., a couple of months) before he or she can be trusted again. Ultimately in this situation the goal of the doctor is to place responsibility for providing structure on the parents if possible. If teenagers want a drug screen to prove they are not using, it can be useful but does not exonerate the teenager from responsibility for other rule violations.

Drug screens are highly reliable. Under most circumstances they can detect cannabis weeks after usage. The collection of urine should be observed by an adult if the teen had prior knowledge of the screen. There are a few false-positive results, which can be ruled out with a history of medication. Being at a party where marijuana was smoked is not an excuse for a positive result.

Treatment

Adolescents are rarely cooperative with attempted substance treatment unless it is to avoid a consequence such as losing their driver's license or grounding. Some adolescents agree to the challenge of not drinking for a month just to prove they have that much control. Even if they are not fully honest with the physician about the results of this test, they at least have a heightened sensitivity to their own behavior, which may lead them to change their substance usage.

For the overly rebellious teenager, more structured limit setting may be all that is necessary to reverse the course of substance abuse. For others who are having more needs met by substance usage, additional interventions may be necessary. It is important to identify the primary motivation for use and the benefits that result from the substance abuse. A less pathologic means of having these needs met can then be sought. For example, overly rebellious teenagers might be guided to alternative behaviors that assert their individuality and autonomy without the use of illicit substances. Specifically asking them what activities they would enjoy (even if it would make their parents uncomfortable) can provide this information. Developing a compromise with the parents then may help the teenager feel more autonomous. For example, the parents may reluctantly agree to let their teenager take a white water rafting trip if he or she remains free of drugs for a month.

For teenagers treating their social anxiety with alcohol or other substances, suggestions on how they can learn to become more comfortable socially may provide a useful alternative to the substance abuse. For example, guiding a shy person to a small group that shares a similar interest could be helpful. They might join a small computer club, rodeo club, or car club. Directing high novelty-seeking teenagers to activities that fill this need can provide an alternative to their substance usage. For example, joining a rock climbing club or taking up sky diving or sail boarding may give them the thrill seeking they might otherwise get from amphetamine, cocaine, or hallucinogens. Cost need not be an excuse, as drugs are also expensive. For the teenager using substances to treat depression relative to major conflicts going on in their lives (e.g., a divorce in the family) family or individual therapy may provide the best alternative for treatment.

Teenagers are concerned about having the support of their peer group, and they usually choose a set of peers because they reinforce their own viewpoints on what is desirable behavior. For example, a nonrebellious teenager is unlikely to choose a group of highly rebellious peers for friends. If parents provide their teenager with highly structured rules, it will likely eventually alter their friendship pattern. Adolescents then sooner or later discover that they have little freedom and no fun if they are always in trouble with their peers. This opens the door for them to become involved with a new group of friends. Encouraging the teenager to join a group that shares a mutual interest with them and is not extremely rebellious can be helpful.

The doctor and parents must be patient. A change in peer group often takes months. Usually it takes repeated episodes of rule breaking and consequences (e.g., grounding for a week or two) before a real change occurs. It is easy to become frustrated. Success usually comes by not overreacting, not giving up, and consistently providing structure and other alternatives for having needs met.

For teenagers who have markedly altered their life style and made the use of substances a central part of it, a structured substance abuse treatment program may be necessary to break the pattern. For the teenager who is still for the most part involved in school or work, it can be an outpatient program. If this fails or if the teenager has dropped out of many or most activities, an inpatient program is likely the optimal referral. However, once the treatment program has ended, the struggle remains. The parents must still provide a highly structured environment and other alternatives for meeting the teenager's needs before a long-lasting change is secure.

Case Report

H.H. was a 17-year-old high school student in his junior year. He was seen initially along with his mother, father, and stepfather after he had been caught a third time for substance abuse. On this occasion the police officer assigned to the high school had noticed rowdy boys at a basketball game; he had given them a breathalyzer test and found H.H. to be at the 0.02 level.

He had been caught similarly drinking about a month before. A year before he had been required to go to a diversion program after having been caught in a car with marijuana. His mother had made this appointment because she thought that the previous diversion program, which had consisted of watching movies about drug abuse, was of little value. She was hoping for something more substantial, thinking that a family meeting might help.

H.H. lived with his mother and stepfather, but his father had joint custody and he spent a lot of time with him. The father was first asked to describe his view of the problem. He thought his son's use was experimentation, not atypical for youths. He said his son's only problem was getting caught. Subtly he intimated that he had used substances as a youth and now he was a successful professional. He was concerned that his son, because of being caught, could lose eligibility on the tennis team. In all other areas including school, peers, activities, and family relations he though he was doing fine.

His mother's view of the problem was primarily that it was the peer group that caused him to get into trouble. She thought that his peers were troublemakers. She had told him on several occasions that he was likely to get into trouble again if he continued to hang out with them. Other than that she thought he was doing well in all areas.

The stepfather obviously liked H.H. and thought like he got along with him well. His view, however, was that H.H. was pretty lax about following rules. The stepfather thought it was not his place to lay down rules, but that H.H. needed stricter discipline. In other areas he thought he was doing fine.

H.H. went last in the discussion. In his view, the peer group was not a strong influence on him; in fact, he thought that he was a leader among his peers. Before the basketball game, he had secured beer from an older friend and supplied his two friends. He freely admitted to drinking an average of twice a month and using cannabis occasionally. He stated that he began alcohol use at the age of 14 and occasionally smoked cigarettes. When asked what rules he had at home, he said his parents were pretty slack. Academically, he was an A student. He was ranked in about the middle for tennis but thought he could move up this year. He was planning on going to college and was beginning to look at options. He liked his peer group. In general, he saw no problem but bad luck in getting caught again.

At the conclusion of the evaluation, the doctor told the family that he was quite concerned about some red flags for substance abuse. H.H.'s initiation of substances at the age of 14, his present regular use, hanging out with a group who regularly used alcohol, and the fact that he had gotten into trouble on several occasions with the substances were concerning. It was suggested to the parents that he was not ready for the freedom he had, that it was getting him into trouble. If things did not change he could at the very least make himself ineligible for tennis for the year and find himself with significant legal difficulties.

The family was told he needed more guidance at present in the form of structured rules. The parents agreed to work on that and in fact wanted to set that up at this meeting because the parents were otherwise rarely together. They developed a set of rules starting with his being grounded from all activities outside of school for 1 week and loss of use of the car for 2 weeks; and if there was even the slightest infraction of the rules during the next 2 weeks the grounding would be extended to a month. H.H. initially protested, but the parents stood firm. In the future if the parents even suspected substance usage, he would be grounded again with loss of car privileges. The father agreed to this regimen.

A follow-up appointment for 2 weeks with H.H. alone was set up. At that appointment H.H. stated that he had followed the rules—that he did not like them but understood them. Although he protested the increased discipline, his antagonism lacked enthusiasm. He stated that he had not used substances for the previous 2 weeks and that he had not found this to be much of a challenge. He thought that even when he started doing things with his friends again abstinence would not be a problem. He then had questions about searching for colleges. Follow-up consisted of calls to the parents, who stated that they had been keeping to the rules and that H.H. had been responding well. They promised they would be in contact if problems again developed. They were told it was likely he would challenge the rules at least once.

References

Beman DS (1995) Risk factors leading to adolescent substance abuse. Adolescence 30:201–207.

Botvin GJ, Baker E, Dunsenbury L, Botvin EM, Diaz T (1995) Long-term follow-up results of a randomized drug abuse prevention trial in a white middle-class population. JAMA 273: 1106–1112.

Fishman HC, Stanton MD, Rosman BL (1982) Treating families of adolescent drug abusers. In Stanton MD (ed) The Family Therapy of Drug Abuse and Addiction. New York: Guilford.

Heyman RB, Adger H (1997) Office approach to drug abuse prevention. Pediatri Clin North Am. 44:1447–1455.

Kaufman P (1979) Family therapy with adolescent substance abusers. In Kaufman E, Kaufman P (eds) Family Therapy of Drug and Alcohol Abuser. New York: Gardner.

Werner MJ (1995). Principles of brief interventions for adolescent alcohol, tobacco and other drug use. Pediatr Clin North Am 42:335–349.

Sloboda Z, David SL (1997) Preventing Drug Use Among Children and Adolescents: A Research-based Guide. NIH 97–4212. Bethesda: National Institute on Drug Abuse.

Trepper TS, Piercy FP, Lewis RA, Volk R.J, Sprenkle DH (1993) Family therapy for adolescent alcohol abuse. In O'Farrell TJ (ed) Treating Alcohol Problems. New York: Guilford.

22

Marital Problems

ASSESSMENT

Although it is helpful to have both members of a couple present for marital counseling, it can be done with only one member present so long as the plan is aimed at altering the interaction between the couple.

1. Obtain each person's description of the problem without interruption from the other partner.
2. Explore power and control in the relationship. Have them describe a recent decision they made together in detail from start to finish.
3. Obtain a description of how they modulate closeness and distance. Ask them specifically what they enjoy doing together and obtain a description of a recent time they have spent as a couple.
4. Investigate how anger is expressed in the relationship. Ask for one or two recent examples of when they had feelings of anger and how they responded. (Remember that silence and withdrawal is as much a response as more outward expressions.)
5. Investigate romantic and sexual expression between the couple. Obtain detailed descriptions of the sequence of events surrounding any sexual problems.
6. Investigate the possibility of jealousy and marital affairs. It is frequently useful to see each member of a couple individually for a least a brief period to investigate anything he or she may feel uncomfortable saying conjointly.
7. Investigate their commitment to continuing the relationship.

PLAN

1. Negotiate realistic goals for treatment. Both members of the couple must have at least some commitment to maintaining the relationship despite ambivalence. If ambivalent, they must agree to continue the relationship for a negotiated time to see how things work out. One or two changes can be worked on at a time.

2. If power and control is a significant problem:
   a. Begin with a self-observational task where each closely watches how they make decisions and writes the steps down in detail.
   b. After they have completed a self-observational task they should set up a structured time to negotiate a decision in which the goal is compromise. Specific ways in which they will alter their usual sequence of events surrounding decision making should be negotiated. They should then practice this new way of making decisions, keeping up the self-observational task.
   c. If successful, they can go on to more difficult issues. If unsuccessful, the physician should help them negotiate a compromise. Then go back to item b.
3. If closeness/distance issues are a problem:
   a. Have them negotiate a specific time for mutually enjoyable activity.
   b. If they have a pattern of avoiding this time, discuss with them that this resistance likely represents some underlying conflict that has not been resolved and attempt to resolve it.
   c. Give the assignment of having them surprise the other person once or twice a week with something unexpected that pleases the other person. Challenge their sense of creativity to promote positive results.
   d. Once they have had some positive recreational interactions, have them set up a regular schedule.
4. If anger expression is a problem:
   a. Begin with a self-observational task, writing down all angry feelings and interactions with the significant other.
   b. The following week have them set aside 20 minutes twice a week where each has a 10-minute period to tell the other what angered them that week without the other responding. Over time, allow increasing amounts of response but keep to timed periods to promote structure and control.
   c. Once they have found a way to make this work, have them make this exercise a structured part of their week.
5. If sexual problems are significant, once they have resolved other problems in their relationship address the sexual problems as described in Chapter 23.
6. If jealousy is a problem attempt to disallow any discussion of jealousy. If this does not work, assign it to a specific period of time. For example, once a week for 5 minutes the partner describes all of his or her feelings of jealousy without the other responding. It is important to ascertain that there is no flirtatious or other activity such as an affair going on that is promoting the jealousy.
7. If a marital affair has taken place but the couple still wants the relationship to continue the first step is make sure the affair has

stopped. Once it has stopped, it is best to make a referral for marital counseling.

Although patients rarely request marital therapy from their physician directly, it is not uncommon for marital problems to be brought up indirectly or in relation to other problems. They may be presented to the physician following a general health care visit or perhaps at the completion of a visit for another acute problem. For example, a woman in response to a question regarding birth control responds, "Why bother?" then complains about her husband's distance. Another common presentation is when patients come in for a psychological problem such as depression or anxiety and relate most of the problems they are having to their marital relationship. Although a referral for marital counseling is often most efficacious, many patients prefer to receive help from their family doctor.

Assessment

Although it is not impossible to perform marital counseling with just one partner, it is easier and usually more effective to have both present. Frequently when the initial patient brings up the problem, he or she expects the partner to balk at therapy. In this case it is useful for the physician to contact and invite the other member to participate directly. An effective approach is to ask the spouse for help in treating the other spouse's problem, avoiding anything that sounds like blaming them for the problem.

It is important that the physician not take sides and even avoid the appearance of taking sides. Therefore it is usually a good strategy to begin a conjoint marital session by directing questions to the party who is least known to the physician. It is important to obtain each person's description of the problem without interruption from the partner. When there is a great deal of distance in a marriage or one spouse is domineering at some point, each should be seen briefly alone by the physician. The main purpose is to ask about abuse or affairs, but other issues such as substance abuse, jealousy, or sexual problems are commonly brought up as well.

When each member of the couple describes the problems to the physician, there is sometimes a specific problem such as a disagreement over the way a child should be disciplined. However, much more often their complaints reflect broader relational patterns. They are often vague such as "We are having communication problems" or "We seem to argue a lot." It is useful under these circumstances to explore four common areas of marital problems so the presenting problem is clarified.

1. How are *power and control* handled within the relationship? How are decisions made? Does one person come across as domineering? Does the

other invoke guilt or manipulative behavior to get their way? The most useful way to explore power and control conflicts is to have the couple describe a recent decision they made together, including the specific sequences of interaction.

2. A second area of possible trouble is *closeness and distance*. All couples vacillate between too much closeness and too much distant, and they have various mechanisms to correct for either extreme. The most common problem occurs when a couple has an underlying conflict they are afraid to address and therefore spend more and more time avoiding each other. When you ask what they do together for recreation or enjoyment you find they spend little time together. The other extreme is less common but also occurs occasionally. The couple, after marriage, gets into the habit of spending all of their time together and feel rejected when one wants to spend time apart. Jealousy is often a co-problem here. When obtaining a description of how they modulate closeness and distance, it is useful to determine what they enjoy doing together recreationally and at what frequency. A description of a recent joint event is useful.

3. The third common area that sometimes leads to problems is *how anger is expressed*. It is easy to become judgmental regarding this area, depending on one's own views; but in general most ways of expressing anger are acceptable unless they become extreme. For example, if somebody yells loudly for 10 minutes and then cools down and is ready to discuss a problem in a more level-headed way, it may not be a problem. On the other hand, if it escalates into hours of yelling including name-calling and destructive threats or abuse, it is harmful. Alternatively, sometimes a member expresses anger by withdrawing and closing off communication. This may work if such expression of anger lasts a few hours and then the person is ready to discuss the issue. However, if it is an attempt to punish the mate by days of withdrawal, perhaps even weeks, it obviously can lead to a harmful effect on the relationship. To investigate anger it is useful to have each describe a recent anger interaction in detail.

4. Finally, *sexual issues* can obviously be a problem in a marriage, but it is also not unusual for sexual problems to be used as a disguise for one of the first three problems noted. That is, one member complains about sexual problems when really he or she is avoiding sex because of conflicts over power, closeness or expression of anger. Therefore if sexual issues are the presenting problems, it is useful to explore the other three areas and make sure there are no major problems in those areas before addressing the sexual issues. If there are sexual problems, obtaining a detailed description of the sequence of events surrounding the sexual problem is important.

Attempted solutions already tried should be explored. The most common attempted solution is avoiding arguments, which usually leads to the couple growing uncomfortably distant. Another common response to asking about attempts to make things better is trying to determine who is to blame for the problem. This usually leads to defensiveness and less openness to change. It is important to address the issue of blame if it comes up by immediately making clear that finding blame is not useful for finding solutions.

Plan

Before a plan can be developed it is important to negotiate realistic goals for treatment. The first step is assessing each of the partners' commitment to continuing the marriage. It is possible to treat a couple when only one member is interested in working toward change, but it is not possible to be successful at marital therapy when one member of the couple clearly does not wish the marriage to continue. An attitude of disgust toward one's spouse is more predictive of eventual disillusionment than anger. Once a person has absolutely decided to leave the marriage, it is highly unlikely that this decision can be altered. Ambivalence toward the marriage, however, does not contraindicate marital therapy. If ambivalence is strong, it is best first to develop a contract whereby they act as though the marriage will continue for a specified period (e.g., 4 months). They should be informed that sometimes things get worse before they get better.

Goals of therapy must be realistic, and usually only one or two changes can be worked on at a time. If the two spouses have different goals, it is important that they believe their needs for change are included in the treatment plan. It is often helpful to address the specific problems in the broader context of the four topics previously described. Start with small changes to have successes before larger changes are tackled. The following are interventions found useful when addressing the four common problem areas.

If *power and control* are problems, a useful way to begin is with a self-observational task. The couple is asked during the next week to twice set aside a half-hour to make a decision about some issue that is intermediate between the most conflicted issue and the least conflicted issue. They are to try to come to some compromise regarding this conflict in their usual way with one exception. That is, they are to observe the process of their decision-making and keep a diary of it upon completion of their task and bring it to the next meeting. Simple self-observation often alters the process enough that they have a much better experience with the decision-making. If they show improvement, asking them to continue the self-observation process twice weekly with more difficult decisions often solidifies the improvement. If they continue to have difficulty, the doctor can make suggestions on alterating the sequence of decision-making enough that a compromise can be reached. Problems are often associated with the belief that decision-making is a zero sum game (mathematic game theory, i.e., $x + y = 0$); that is, they cannot both be winners. One suggestion for altering the sequence is for each to suggest a compromise that gives the other an advantage; in other words, try to throw the game and see what happens. After a half dozen trials nearly all couples are able to demonstrate an improvement in their decision-making process.

It may be tempting for the physician to take sides in these conflicts, but unless both parties in the relationship feel empowered by the decision it is unlikely to succeed long term. The physician, on the other hand, need not be an expert at the decision-making process; simply being an outside observer who is not emotionally involved can give enough perspective to make suggestions that lead to a different process for the decision-making. The decision made is not important: It is the process on which they should focus. When the couple achieves some success, they can proceed to tougher decisions.

If *closeness–distance* conflicts are serious they can be addressed in several ways. Often the couple describes the problem as having no time or a lack of opportunity. Having them negotiate a specific time for a mutually enjoyable activity is the first step. It is sometimes useful to warn the couple that if they never find the opportunity to spend time with each other or if it leads to an argument it usually represents some underlying conflict that has not been resolved sufficiently. Facing the conflict directly usually leads to improvement.

A playful way to address closeness issues is to suggest that each member of the couple surprise the other once or twice during the week with something unexpected that would please the other person. This promotes the couple's sense of challenge and creativity in the relationship, often leading to positive results.

When *anger expression* is the problem, the intervention can begin with a self-observation activity. The couple can be requested to set aside 20 minutes twice a week when they can each tell their spouse for 10 minutes what angered them (however slightly) the previous week. Neither is to respond to the other's statement, and the time is to be adhered to strictly. They are then to write down the sequence of events of this session in some detail and bring it to the next therapy session. If the couple typically argues frequently, this session can take place three or more times a week. This exercise almost immediately creates a much more controlled atmosphere for the anger and alters the way the interaction occurs. Often this is all that is necessary for the couple to have a much different and more positive experience with expression of anger and one they can use as a model for future confrontation.

If this exercise does not lead to sufficient change, the next step is to make it an even more structured experience. The next week's assignment entails first one and then the other partner expressing anger for 10 minutes without either answering. They are then to take a 1-hour break and return with a 5-minute rebuttal to the other person's expressed anger. A diary is kept and the results reported. If no change has occurred, the next week they can add to the process an additional rebuttal; but each time there is a rebuttal there must be at least a 1-hour break before another response can occur. This slows the sequence of events to a point where they are much more likely to express their anger in a controlled, more productive atmosphere. With this approach eventually they are likely to find their own style of anger expression, which is likely to be different from the problematic one.

Sexual problems are sometimes related to avoidance of intimacy because of distance and conflict in the relationship. If so, the above interventions are helpful as a start. Issues covered with a specific problem with sexuality, are addressed in Chapter 23. Sometimes the reverse is true: When sexual problems improve, other marital problems resolve.

When a productive change has been realized in even one area of marital interaction, it is often useful to wait to see if it has a snowball effect on other problems. After making positive change the best approach may be to tell the couple to make further changes slowly and wait a month or two for a return appointment. After a month's time the doctor may find that other positive change has occurred, which makes further treatment unnecessary. If not, another of the problems can be addressed.

Two specific problems, jealousy and marital affairs, do warrant some specific discussion. In regard to jealousy, a pattern often develops wherein one person makes accusations and the accused denies them. The denier then attempts to prove innocence with all kinds of evidence, which leads to the accuser finding holes in the defense, and the pattern thus escalates. If the jealousy is of recent onset it often reflects some change in the relationship. Perhaps there really is an affair, but as commonly happens there has been some recent distancing within the relationship. The accuser senses the distance and fears an affair. If the jealousy is ongoing the accuser may be insecure, which is enhanced by the partner's distance, put-downs, or flirtations. Jealousy also can play a role in a relationship in the form of flattery. Being jealous is saying their partner is desirable. In this situation, unconsciously encouraging jealousy may reassure desirability.

One way to overcome jealousy begins with interfering with the sequence of events surrounding it. The doctor can simply state that discussion of this issue is not allowed until the other issues in the marriage are addressed. Often once the couple is feeling closer and more secure the issue of jealousy simply dissipates. Another technique is to encapsulate the discussion of jealousy. For example, give the jealous partner permission to express concerns but only at a specified time (e.g., 10 minutes once a week) and have the other person not respond to it. This alteration in the sequence frequently leads to resolution. Another approach is to alter the denier's behavior. Rather than attempt to deny the accusation by countering with the facts, the response might be to state that either the person trusts them or they do not, and that if they wanted to have an affair they could not be stopped. After stating this once they simply ignore the accusations. Once the sequence of events is altered, other issues (e.g., closeness and conflict) must be dealt with so there is less insecurity in the relationship.

If the physician becomes aware of an affair, it must be addressed before other issues can be confronted. If an affair has gone on long term it should be assumed that it is not a secret but may not be openly acknowledged. On the other hand, it is not always necessary to divulge an affair to the other party; it depends on the expected outcome of such a discussion. For example, if one is denying the affair, it may be because if they acknowledge it they will be forced to divorce the partner to save face when they may not otherwise wish to take this action. It is necessary, however, to have the affair end before marital counseling can proceed successfully. The physician must confront the offending party with the explanation that if the goal is to improve the relationship the affair must stop. Most often when an affair has occurred there are long-standing problems within the marriage. Referral to a therapist may be useful but only if the affair is to be stopped and if both members of the couple wish the marriage to continue.

Case Report

G.L. is a 35-year-old woman who was encouraged to see her family doctor by her sister, who had been counseled by the doctor previously. Mrs. L brought her reluctant husband to the session. She described the problem as being that her husband showing no feelings toward her. His emotional withdrawal worsened after she suffered three consecutive miscarriages over the past year. He also yelled at her for spending money on a number of occasions. She said the one thing they enjoyed together was taking care of their 3-year-old child.

Mr. L was frightened by his wife's threat to end the marriage and overall thought there was nothing wrong with their union. He was concerned at this time of great financial stress that his wife spent too much money. They were in danger of losing their farm.

Evaluating the marital problem, the physician thought that the husband's lack of emotional support was a problem but also concerning was their power struggle, which centered on finances. This had led to increasing distance in other areas of their marriage. They spent little time together and sexually had become relatively inactive. At the conclusion of the first session, the doctor gave the homework assignment that they make one small financial decision together and each keep a diary of this process to be brought to the next appointment. They were also to go out to dinner.

At the next appointment they had come up with a decision regarding buying a dishwasher together, which apparently was much needed. They both felt good about how they had decided to do it. They had not gone out to dinner together, however, making many excuses why they did not. Because their mutual decision-making had gone better than expected, at this appointment they received an assignment to devise an overall financial plan together. The doctor, reflecting on their avoidance of the assigned dinner together, said that perhaps her request was too fast for their ability to be close with each other. They were requested to just spend 1 hour taking a walk together some evening the next week. Mr. L was requested to write a letter to his wife in which he was to describe how he would have liked to support her at the time of the miscarriages. He was not to give her the letter until the next appointment. He responded that he felt that there was something wrong with him because he did not have feelings toward the fetus, so when the miscarriages occurred it did not feel real to him. The doctor suggested that this may be a natural difference between some men and women early in pregnancy but that he cared about his wife. He was asked what it was like to see her suffering, which should be the focus when he wrote the letter.

At the next appointment it was learned the couple had gone to the bank as part of the financial planning. On the way home Mr. L had broken down and cried because it was apparent that they would lose the farm. He had worked part time as a diesel mechanic. His wife pointed out that he was considered by his boss to be a naturally outstanding mechanic, and they would be more than happy to hire him full time. Mrs. L came across as extremely supportive. They both agreed to give the farm one last year to turn around.

Mr. L had not yet written the letter because he said he had no idea what to say. He was asked how his wife had treated him when he expressed his sad feelings about the farm and he had been quite pleased by how she showed him sympathy. It was suggested that perhaps she wanted the same. He seemed to understand. They had spent an hour together that week walking, which had gone quite well.

At the next appointment, Mr. L did bring in a letter to his wife, which in fact he had already shared with her. She was quite pleased by it. In fact, she had made arrangements for a sister to take care of their child for a weekend, while the two of them got a motel room. They thought that the compromises they had made on their financial plan were acceptable to both. On the other hand, they had gotten into a heated argument over how to spend time with the in-laws over the holidays. They were again requested to try to find a compromise and keep a diary.

They came back the following week, pleased with how they had made some compromises regarding the in-laws and had very much enjoyed their weekend. There was obviously much more closeness and much less hostility between them, and therapy was concluded.

References

Doherty WJ, Baird MA (1983) Family Therapy and Family Medicine. New York: Guilford.

McDaniel SH, Campbell TL, Seaburn DB (1990) Recognizing the signs of strain: counseling couples in primary care. In Family-oriented Primary Care: A Manual for Medical Providers. New York: Springer-Verlag.

Starling BP, Martin AC (1992) Improving martial relationships: strategies for the family physician. J Am Board Fam Pract 5:511–516.

23

Sexual Problems

ASSESSMENT

1. Assess overall marital functioning. If there are serious problems in the marriage address them prior to sexual counseling.
2. Consider physiologic contributions to sexual problems including medications that commonly cause sexual disorders (see Tables 23.1 and 23.2, below).
3. Obtain a detailed description of sexual activity beginning with how a couple shows desire for sexual interaction through conclusion of the sexual activity.
4. With both members of a couple present, determine their understanding of the other's sexual needs.

PLAN

1. Consider *sensate focus* exercises for many problems.
   a. The couple is told they should not have intercourse for the next month or two to lessen performance anxiety. They begin with twice weekly nondemanding caressing, excluding breasts and genital area. Good communication should be part of the process, and criticism and overcontrol should not be allowed.
   b. Continuation of step a but including the entire body, including breasts and genital area but not focused on these areas and not aimed at sexual arousal but simply enjoying touch.
   c. Maintain all qualities of the first two steps, focusing on exploring the sense of touch but adding the use of massage oils. If they have cheated and had intercourse, suggest that they are going too fast and that they slow down and keep to the sensate focus exercises.
   d. Again continuation of all the qualities of earlier step c but now doing mutual touching rather than your turn/my turn touching.
   e. Include intercourse, but the focus is still not on orgasm but enjoying the immediate feelings of touch.

2. *Female arousal disorder* symptoms include vaginal dryness, lack of genital swelling despite interest in sex and responsiveness to partner.
   a. If estrogen deficiency, treat with estrogen replacement therapy.
   b. If inadequate foreplay, provide education if necessary or refer the couple to a book.
   c. If lubrication is inadequate despite adequate foreplay and response in the postmenopausal woman, prescribe appropriate lubricant.
   d. If the above steps do not work, offer sensate focus exercises.
3. *Female orgasmic disorder.*
   a. Evaluate whether it is a primary or secondary orgasmic disorder.
   b. Evaluate whether there is sufficient foreplay or clitoral stimulation. If not, provide education for the couple or refer to a book.
   c. If secondary anorgasmia is the problem and is of relatively recent onset, sensate focus exercises are often effective.
   d. If the woman has primary anorgasmia and negative feelings toward sexuality, consider referral to a psychotherapist. If they have a positive attitude toward sexuality and do not wish a referral, a self-help book along with regularly scheduled appointments for both the patient and the partner may help.
4. *Sexual pain, dyspareunia, and vaginismus.*
   a. Evaluate if there is any specific reason for anxiety related to intercourse and any physiologic contributions to pain on intercourse including adequate lubrication. Provide estrogen for deficiency. Provide education for insufficient foreplay.
   b. If anxiety is related to intercourse, treat with a desensitization program
      i. Good vaginal muscle control can be developed by the use of Kegel exercises.
      ii. Once the above has been learned, vaginal self-dilatation with finger or graduated cylinders can be used while practicing overall relaxation exercises prior to penetration.
      iii. Once the above has been successfully achieved penetration by the partner should occur under the control of the woman.
5. *Hypoactive sexual desire.* Evaluate if fantasies are present. If recent changes in sexual interest are present, evaluate physiologic contributions, such as hormonal changes, iatrogenic causes, or psychological contributions such as a high level of recent stress or depression.
   a. If the problem is long-standing, referral is likely indicated.
   b. More commonly the problem is related to a discrepancy between the couple's desire for sex. It is important to have a detailed history of how sexual encounters are initiated and how the couple tried to resolve discrepancies.

  i.   Treatment should be directed at trying to develop a suitable compromise between the couple regarding frequency.
  ii. Alter the sequence of events. For example, have the partner with the least desire initiate sexual encounters at a frequency that is a compromise.
  iii. Another alternative is to have the partner with the greater desire initiate contact in the usual way but have a specified number of refusals by the less interested partner.
  iv. Alter sequences, such as altering time of day or using sensate focus exercises to initiate some encounters.

6. *Male erectile disorder.*
   a. Evaluate physiologic contributions to the erectile disorder, although distinguishing the physiologic and psychological contributions is often not possible. A comprehensive approach is usually best.
   b. If performance anxiety is a contributor or sole cause, use sensate focus exercises. Request no intercourse for at least 2 months. This removes performance anxiety.
   c. Medications such as sildenafil (Viagra) can be considered so long as the patient experiences arousal.

7. *Premature ejaculation.* Rule out other problems, such as lack of sufficient foreplay of the woman.
   a. Educate if necessary.
   b. Use stop/start technique.
      i.   Masturbate to a level before orgasm would occur, stop, repeat this process three or four times.
      ii. When the above has led to increased confidence in control, repeat step 1 start-stop technique except using a lubricant.
      iii. Once confidence is built, rather than stopping use a slow-down technique while relaxing the muscles in the buttocks.
      iv. When confident, practice with a partner. Begin with foreplay in the usual way; then, using a prearranged signal, stop rhythmic thrusting in the way that had been previously done during steps 1–3 (start-stop technique); begin again using the stop/start technique learned previously.
      v.   When confidence in step iv has been developed, repeat it; but rather than coming to a complete stop, use a slow-down technique as learned in step iii.
      vi. Pharmacologic agents, such as selective serotonin reuptake inhibitors (SSRIs) can be used to delay ejaculation to build confidence. Sildenafil can be used to maintain an erection for a longer period after orgasm has occurred to build confidence.

Many people turn to their physician for help when they have problems related to sexual concerns. Sexual problems not only can cause lessening of overall quality of life but also can, over time, erode otherwise good marital relationships. The most common factors related to sexual problems are misinformation, performance anxiety, and boredom, issues that family physicians are in an ideal position to address. Sometimes a sexual problem is the symptom of broader marital problems. The physician should rule this out by asking some screening questions. As discussed in Chapter 22, a four-question screen can usual detect serious marital problems: How are decisions made by the couple? How does the couple experience closeness with each other and allow independent activities? How is anger expressed? Is sexuality satisfactory for both partners?

Usually if there are serious problems in the first three of these areas it is best to address them before problems in sexuality are addressed, as it is difficult for the couple to work enthusiastically on their sexual problems when they are angry with each other over other issues.

Assessment

As with other assessments for brief therapy treatment, after a general description of the problem it is important to obtain a detailed description of the sequence of events surrounding the problem, including attempted solutions. The description should begin with a discussion of how the couple signals sexual interest to each other before the intimate behavior even starts. It should go though the sexual encounter and include how they act after sex, as this can either reinforce or discourage subsequent intimacy. In addition, it is useful to obtain a good medical history, including medications that could cause sexual disorders (Table 23.1). Iatrogenic causes of sexual disorders are

TABLE 23.1. Drug Categories Commonly Associated with Sexual Disorders

Anticancer drugs and hormones
Anticonvulsants
Antihypertensives
Carbonic anhydrase inhibitors
Cytotoxic drugs
Digitalis family
Diuretics
H_2-receptor antagonists
Pain medications
Psychiatric medications (selective serotonin reuptake inhibitors are the most
    common)
Recreational drugs (e.g., tobacco, alcohol)
Sleep medications

not uncommon. Without a history suggesting a physiologic cause (Table 23.2) an extensive workup is rarely indicated.

Plan

As with brief therapy for other problems, reframing (i.e., altering the way patients think about the problem or altering the sequence of events surrounding the problem) often leads to significant improvement. There are many misconceptions regarding sexuality, so often simple education can lead to marked improvement in sexual adjustment. For example, if the patient's description of the sexual encounter indicates that there is little foreplay or little clitoral stimulation, giving the couple information regarding this issue or directing them to a good book where it is discussed (e.g., Masters et al., 1994) can be quite helpful.

Anxiety related to sexual performance or expectations, such as performance anxiety, is a factor in a number of sexual disorders, such as arousal disorders, erectile disorder, premature ejaculation, and orgasmic disorders. Sensate focus exercises (Masters et al., 1994) can provide a foundation for many of the problem-specific treatments we discuss later. Masters and Johnson's development of sensate focus exercises evolved from the observation that couples enjoyed sexual activity less and had more problems if they focused on the goal of having a mutual orgasm, so intercourse became overly goal-directed. Couples with this focus lost their sensitivity to the joy of touching and caressing each other. Once the pleasure of this activity is lost, the whole sexual encounter can be less pleasurable and ultimately lead to a lack of satisfaction. This in turn leads some to lose confidence in being a good lover.

With *sensate focus* exercises the couples concentrate on the pleasure of touching without the goal of orgasm. The process can be divided into five steps. It can be varied for the needs of each couple.

Step 1. To lessen performance anxiety, the couple is told that they should not have intercourse for the next month or two while they are performing

TABLE 23.2. Medical Conditions Commonly Associated with Sexual Disorders

All degenerative diseases
Endocrine disorders including diabetes
Liver or renal failure
Depression
Pain disorders
Peripheral neuropathy
Respiratory disorders (e.g., chronic obstructive pulmonary disease)
Vascular disease

these exercises. They are then told that twice a week they should engage in "nondemanding caressing," excluding the breasts and genital area. Each partner should caress the other one for a period of time. Although no specific time should be specified, 10–20 minutes is a reasonable range. During this exercise, first one partner and then the other should caress every part of the body except breasts and genitalia, using different motions, different pressures, and different parts of the hand. A spirit of experimentation is key. Each partner should simply focus on touching and being touched. The person receiving the touch should occasionally give some kind of feedback on what they are feeling. It is important for them not to be critical in doing so and to allow themselves to experience each of the touching processes for a while before they comment on it so that they can be aware of how it is affecting them. This increases communication between the couple.

Step 2. The next stage is a continuation of the first. It should begin after the couple has had at least four sessions of the first step occurring over an approximately 2-week period. They should feel comfortable with step 1 before proceeding to step 2. The primary difference between the first stage and the second stage is that caressing the body can now include the breasts and genitalia. It is important to reiterate that the focus should not be on sexual arousal and should not lead to intercourse or orgasm; the focus should be on the pleasure experienced from touching the body for its own sake. In fact, it is a good idea to caution the couple not to overemphasize genital touching but to make it part of overall exploring as in the first step. In addition, hand-on-hand communication can be added. That is, the recipient of the touching can put his or her hands on top of the giver's hands and with subtle pressure can guide the hand toward what feels good. There should be some caution regarding this also: that the receiver does not try to control the touching and provides minimal guidance, allowing the giver a good deal of latitude. The one doing the touching should, while pleasuring the receiver, also explore the sensations in his or her own hands and fingers. This exercise should be done approximately twice a week for a couple of weeks with each partner taking turns being the receiver and the giver.

Step 3. At this point the couple has often "cheated" (i.e., had intercourse), which can be a positive sign that passion in the relationship is heating up; but it is best to caution against proceeding too fast to prevent the reemergence of performance expectations, which can be problematic. Therefore if they have had intercourse in the interim it is best to warn them that they may be moving too quickly. The third step entails maintaining all of the qualities of the first two steps with the focus on exploring the sense of touch but adding the use of massage oils. For those inexperienced with massage oils or lotions, educate them to warm them and to apply them to their hands first. The goal in this step is again to add to the variance of touch. Otherwise this step is the same as step 2.

Step 4. This is a continuation of step 3. It should not lead to orgasm or intercourse. The primarily change is mutual touching rather than your turn/

my turn touching. The couple can sit facing each other with their legs wrapped around the other person. They should experiment with different positions.

Step 5. This stage includes intercourse, but the focus is still on the immediate feelings of touch involved and not on the orgasm. Instruct the couple to start with the nongenital sensate focus exercises in the same way all the previous sensate focus encounters have occurred, with each exploring the other's body and sense of touch. Gradually continue with mutual touch including genital caressing. For some, maintaining the hand-riding technique as previously described, may be helpful but without being a "traffic cop". When both are comfortable, move so the woman is astride the man. Slowly continue with the sensate focus exercises; but the woman uses the man's penis around her vaginal opening to explore what the feelings are but does not rush toward intercourse. When penetration is desired, the woman should slowly insert the penis but only a short distance and again move slowly, concentrating on the feeling of touch involved and the different sensations. A period of quiet containment where the two lie together in this position with perhaps the woman squeezing her thighs and contracting her vaginal muscle can add to the experience. As this goes on, the couple may want to move toward quicker and deeper thrusting; but maintaining a slow rhythmic movement as long as possible leads to a quite different experience and allows new learning about love-making.

With those who have difficulty with step 5 it may be useful to have a number of sessions where orgasm is specifically avoided so the couple can learn to work on simply experiencing the pleasure of touch during intercourse. This again avoids performance anxiety.

The sensate focus exercises have been found helpful for altering the way a couple thinks about their sexuality and the sequence of events that lead to problems. These sensate focus exercises can be useful for a number of problems related to sexuality.

We now turn to specific disorders and how this exercise and other interventions can be useful. The most common sexual problems seen by family doctors are, for women, arousal disorder, orgasmic disorder, dyspareunia, and vaginismus. For both men and women, hypoactive sexual desire is a common problem. Men commonly suffer from erectile disorders and premature ejaculation.

Female Arousal Disorder

The primary symptoms of female sexual arousal disorder are vaginal dryness and a lack of genital swelling. Although interested in sex, the woman is not responsive to her partner's stimulation. Painful intercourse is sometimes associated. In the postmenopausal woman estrogen deficiency and related medical concerns should be ruled out. A description of the usual pattern of the sexual encounter should include how the couple communicates with each other their interest in sexual activity. There are specific concerns here: Are the signals understood by both partners so one does not feel pushed into it? For young couples and sometimes even older couples, inadequate foreplay can be the problem. Is the woman trying too hard to become aroused? If the issue is specifically one of technique or the need for greater lubrication, specific suggestions can be made. If the woman is trying too hard to be aroused or frustrated that she is not aroused, often the sensate focus exercises as previously described lead to good results. The physician can either go through the steps; or for some couples simply prescribing one of the many books that describe the sensate focus exercises can be suggested. The physician should, however, see the couple for follow-up every 2–3 weeks at least several times, as usually couples do best when they have a chance to talk over their new experiences with a physician. The important thing to emphasize is that the exercises should be done with the goal of learning how to feel good, not making sure orgasm is achieved by either partner.

Female Orgasmic Disorder

It is useful to divide woman who have difficulty with orgasm into two groups: one with primary anorgasmia and one with secondary anorgasmia. Primary anorgasmia includes women who have never or rarely achieved orgasm. Women who have secondary anorgasmic disorder are those who have previously reached orgasm on some regular basis but are no longer able to do so.

For newly married or sexually active women the problem may be an educational deficit regarding technique. Usually the problem is a lack of foreplay or clitoral stimulation, which becomes apparent when the doctor obtains a description of the sexual encounter. The physician can provide education or refer the patient to a self-help book.

Women who have secondary anorgasmic disorder (new onset) can be viewed similarly to those who have arousal disorder, and they are treated similarly. Often there is anxiety because the person is trying too hard to have an orgasm. Here sensate focus exercises as previously described can be quite helpful (see Female Arousal Disorder, above).

For women who have primary anorgasmia, it is important to evaluate their attitude toward sexual expression. If there are significant negative feelings toward sexuality as a result of their upbringing or if there has been sexual trauma in the past, referral to a psychotherapist is likely indicated. If there are positive attitudes toward sexuality, specific behavioral programs can be followed with good results. One such program was described by Barbach (1975) in her self-help book, *For Yourself*, which can be recommended to the patient.

A brief summary of her approach is that she helps the woman get in touch with her sensuality through gradual steps, initially alone and then with her partner. It is a much lengthier process than the sensate focus exercises. It is not necessarily a complicated process, and many people can follow Barbach's steps without help. However, it may be useful to have some scheduled appointments with the doctor to discuss any anxiety or questions the patient may have regarding the process. As this is a long-term problem, it also falls within the category of those that family doctors often refer to counselors or therapists when available.

Sexual Pain, Dyspareunia, Vaginismus

Painful intercourse, which in the case of vaginismus includes involuntary spasm of the muscles surrounding the vagina, is not an uncommon complaint. If there are overall negative feelings toward intercourse that cause the woman to become highly anxious, this problem must be addressed first. However if the woman has positive feelings toward sex, the problem often begins because of physiologic pain; perhaps she is newly initiating intercourse, and the vagina is not accustomed to penetration; or perhaps she has an infection. Often what maintains the problem is fear of the pain itself. It is first important to be certain that adequate lubrication is present during intercourse. Lack of estrogen, insufficient foreplay, and other physiologic causes should be eliminated. Following this stage, a gradual approach to help ameliorate the patient's fear of pain is usually successful.

The couple should agree on a gradual stepwise approach to the problem. The woman should feel in control of the sexual encounter, especially that she can stop if it is painful. Instructions on the development of good vaginal muscle control by use of Kegel exercises should be the first step. Vaginal self-dilatation with the finger or lubricated graduated cylinders can be used to help the patient gain confidence about accommodating the penis. Practicing overall relaxation exercises prior to penetration initially with masturbation and later with intercourse can also help relieve the problem. The couple should be educated to have sufficient foreplay to stimulate lubrication. Artificial lubricants may also be of some benefit initially if lubrication does not occur spontaneously in sufficient amounts. Usually if the above process is followed in a gradual way, where the woman feels in control of the sexual encounter good resolution should occur.

Hypoactive Sexual Desire

Hypoactive sexual desire is often difficult to assess because what is normal is often more subjective than objective. Sexual fantasy being absent provides strong support for this diagnosis. If there has been a recent change in sexual interest, hormonal (e.g., testosterone deficiency) and iatrogenic (e.g., antidepressant medication) causes should be investigated. High levels of recent stress should also be ruled out along with depression. In the situation where there is true sexual aversion by the patient, it often represents long-term guilt about sex or past psychological trauma related to sexuality. Referral is usually indicated.

If the situation is to improve, both members of the couple must desire a better sex life. If only one member feels pushed into seeking help, it usually does not work. It may represent a great deal of hostility in the relationship, which must be addressed first. In this case, more general marital therapy is needed before sex therapy has a chance for success. More commonly what is described to the family physician as hyposexual desire is really a problem of discrepancy between a couple's desire for sex. A certain degree of discrepancy can be considered normal. Most couples work this out without a problem. However, when it leads to significant unhappiness in a couple or conflict, therapeutic intervention should be attempted.

If people feel obliged to be more sexually interested they paradoxically lose interest. It is therefore important to investigate in detail the history of how sexual encounters are initiated, including how the couple subtly communicates they are interested in sex. Sometimes the problem is that one or both members of the couple misread the other's subtle messages as to whether they are interested. Specifically having the couple understand each other's signals in some cases resolves the problem.

When conflict has occurred around frequency, the conflict itself can exacerbate the problem. In this situation an approach similar to that described in Chapter 22 regarding marital counseling for dealing with power struggles can be helpful. Once a couple agrees that one or the other is not at fault but that it is an issue of compromise, they can work it out. Sometimes a useful exercise can be suggested: "Over the next 2 weeks sex is to be initiated three times a week by the more interested partner. The other partner is to refuse the sexual encounter twice, so the couple has a sexual encounter once." This alters the sequence of events in such a way that the doctor is blamed for the refusals and allows the couple to explore how they initiate and stop their sexual activity from a new perspective, often with a different outcome. Usually couples who can work out compromises related to other issues can also work them out when related to sexuality. If they cannot it might be a sign that they have power struggles in other areas as well.

Sometimes it is helpful to alter the sequence of events totally to help the couple take a different perspective of their sexuality, such as having them go on a vacation together, try altering the time of day when they have sex, or making some other change that alters their whole view of the problem. Another approach that frequently works is to treat the problem as an arousal disorder with the sensate focus exercises.

Male Erectile Disorder

Distinguishing the psychological and physiologic contributions to erectile disorder is often difficult if not impossible. Often both are involved. For example, as a man ages the erectile response may become less vigorous. If the man then worries about his performance as he is becoming aroused he may lose his erection entirely. After this he may worry more, compounding the problem. Diabetes, depression, alcohol abuse, and medication side effects are also common factors.

Even for the physiologic factors involved in erectile disorders, the history is most diagnostic. It should include investigation of the symptoms and medications listed in Tables 23.1 and 23.2. If the man has successfully masturbated recently, it is a strong indicator of a major psychological contribution. If the sequence of events includes his achieving an erection as he becomes aroused but soon losing it, it usually indicates a strong psychogenic component. The most important laboratory test is a fasting glucose assay. Prolactin, luteinizing hormone, follicle-stimulating hormone and testosterone assays may also be helpful. The neurologic examination includes evaluation of sensory and motor function in the genital area, including the bulbocavernous reflex, cremasteric reflex, and presence of an "anal wink." Checking for nocturnal penile tumescence can also be useful. If an erection is not achieved during rapid-eye-movement (REM) sleep a physiologic etiology should be strongly suspected. It can be checked easily using a snap gauge available from the pharmacist.

If the erectile disorder is significantly associated with anxiety, sensate focus exercises can be useful. The exercises can also be helpful diagnostically. If the patient achieves an erection during the exercises, anxiety had to have played at least some part in the problem. An important part of initiating the sensate focus exercises for erectile disorders is the direction that no intercourse should take place for a considerable period of time (e.g., 2 months) while doing the exercises. This is to remove the performance anxiety aspect of the problem. Usually what does occur during the course of the sensate focus exercises is that the couple on one or more occasions "cheat" (i.e., have intercourse). Because there is less fear of failure things go much better. Once this occurs it leads to more confidence, and improvement follows. Furthermore, the sensate focuses can lead to needed changes in behavior; for example, when men age, more and longer direct stimulation of the penis is sometimes necessary for sexual response.

Sildenafil (or similar drugs soon to be introduced) can be helpful. It helps overcome some of the physiologic contributions to erectile disorder. Taking medicine is easy and can help rebuild confidence in the man. However, when not necessary overreliance can occur. Like Dumbo's feather the man might believe that he absolutely needs it or he cannot fly.

Premature Ejaculation

Rapid or premature ejaculation is a common problem. Its etiology is not well understood, although some believe it is caused by habituation during adolescence. They surmise that teenagers attempting to achieve orgasm rapidly through masturbation become habituated to the pattern, and it continues during intercourse. Others see it as an anxiety disorder where the more the person worries about it the more they lose control, which leads to a recurring pattern. In any case, effective behavioral interventions have been developed, such as the stop/start technique.

The physician can recommend a self-help book on this technique such as one by Helen Singer Kaplan (1997) or briefly describe the process such as the steps outlined below. Often part of the sequence that needs to be altered is the patient's attempt to use distracting thoughts in the hope that it will prolong intromission time because it does not work. What they need to learn is to be able to stay at a higher level of arousal for a longer period of time. That is what the stop/start method addresses.

Step 1. The patient should begin by masturbating slowly, focusing on the sensations without trying to hold back. When he reaches a level of arousal before orgasm, he stops for a time: not long enough to lose the erection but long enough for arousal to diminish. This process is repeated three or four times, finally allowing the ejaculation to occur. This exercise should be repeated five or six times over a 2-week period.

Step 2. Again go through the process in step 1 but more closely approximate the feeling of intercourse by using a lubricant. This exercise should be repeated a number of times over a 2-week period.

Step 3. This process is similar, but rather than totally stop just before the point of orgasm slow down to slow stroking until the likelihood of ejaculation subsides, and then pick up the pace again. There should be no attempt to try to hold back but simply to enjoy the sensation while altering the rhythm to gain greater control. For some patients, doing relaxation exercises during this process is helpful such as relaxing the muscles in the buttocks.

Step 4. The next step requires a willing intimate partner. Begin with foreplay, which can be whatever is usually enjoyable for both partners. At the time of intercourse the woman should take the superior position, above the man. At a prearranged signal, the rhythmic thrusting is stopped just as it had been during the masturbation process prior to urgency to ejaculate; once the likelihood of ejaculation has subsided, the rhythmic thrusting should resume. It should be repeated, just as it had been during the masturbation process, three or four times before ejaculation is allowed to occur. The patient and partner should be warned that if at any point ejaculation does occur prematurely, there is nothing to be worried about, and an attempt should be made again in a few days, which is likely to be more successful. If the woman has not had orgasm, other means could be used to bring her to orgasm.

If problems persist, an intermediate step between steps 3 and 4 can be used. This entails using the same procedure as in step 3 but with the partner stroking the penis and using the signal for the stop/start technique.

Step 5. After five or six practice sessions of the previous step, the couple should try, rather than coming to a complete stop prior to orgasm, to slow down again, using some prearranged signal and then speeding up once the likelihood of orgasm has subsided.

Pharmacologic agents can be of some help. Paroxetine, for example, and other SSRIs have been shown to delay the ejaculatory response in men. Sildenafil, which although it does not delay orgasm, prolongs the erection following orgasm. This allows men to feel more confident in their ability to help the woman achieve orgasm, and this confidence can lead to less anxiety, which ultimately helps avoid premature ejaculation.

Case Report

Several presenters have reported the following case at different conferences. It is difficult to know who to credit, but it is an excellent demonstration of how even small alteration in the sequence of events during sexual activity can lead to problems and to their resolution.

A man calls the doctor asking to be seen for sexual counseling. He states that he and his wife have grown more and more distant and have not been sexually active for several months. He does not know the reason for it. His wife is agreeable to sexual counseling. He is going away on a business trip the following week, so they make the appointment for 2 weeks hence.

Two weeks later the patient calls again saying that the appointment is no longer needed. The doctor, curious as to what occurred, asks the patient if it would be okay to explain what happened. The patient stated that they had gone to a retreat for his corporation and the first evening there was a social gathering in which drinks were served. The retreat took place at a beautiful resort with small rustic cabins, but the cabins were so small their queen-size bed had to be pushed against the wall on one side. He slept on that side, with his wife on the open side. Not surprisingly sometime during the night he developed urinary urgency, and because he could not evacuate the bed on his side the only way to the bathroom was over his wife. While attempting to climb over her, she totally mistook his intention. One thing led to another and both were pleased with the results. Apparently he eventually got an opportunity to void.

Afterward they finally talked, and the following is a summary of their discussion. His wife recognized that he was stressed by work and thought that nicest thing she could do was give him some space. He was frequently up late at night, so the opportunity for sexual interaction arose less frequently anyway. He, however, thought that she was mad at him for not giving her much attention and so was withdrawing sexually. Because he felt for the next several weeks he could not give her the usual amount of attention, he accepted this and did not make any attempts to approach her sexually. Her response was to think that he was even more burned out and the best thing she could do was not put any more pressure on him. After a while each thought the other had become more distant and was fearful that they cared less about the marriage. In fact, his request for marital counseling with the doctor was the first indication to her that their distance troubled him.

The phone call to the doctor may have gone a long way to allow what occurred at the retreat to happen. This demonstrates how sometimes even a small change in the sequence of events surrounding a problem can alter everything.

References

Barbach LG (1975) For Yourself. New York: Doubleday.

Charlton RS, Yalom ID (1997) Treating Sexual Disorders. San Francisco: Jossey-Bass.

Kaplan HS (1989) How to Overcome Premature Ejaculation. New York: Brunner/Mazel.

Levine SB (1997) Solving Common Sexual Problems. New York: Jason Aronson.

Masters WH, Johnson VE, Kolodny RC (1994) Heterosexuality. New York: HarperCollins.

Rosen RC, Leiblum SR (1995) Treatment of sexual disorders in the 19990s: an integrated approach. J Consult Clin Psychol 63:877–890.

24

Domestic Abuse

PARTNER ABUSE

Assessment

1. Routine screen for domestic abuse is to ask if the patient has been kicked, hit, threatened, or forced into sexual behavior by anyone during the past year.
2. If the answer is yes, obtain a detailed description of the sequence of events that led to the abuse.
3. If the abuse has occurred more than once, explore if it has an escalating, cyclic pattern.
4. Obtain a detailed description of how decisions are made.

Plan

1. If the history includes serious threats of harm or past injury, recommend at least a temporary separation. If the patient refuses separation, an emergency escape plan is discussed in detail including knowing the location of a safe house and how to get there.
2. If substance abuse is a problem it should be the first target of treatment.
3. Address power struggles and codependency in the relationship. Treatment should proceed in gradual steps.
4. Recommend outside activities such as Al-Anon, getting a job, taking a course at school, joining a church group, getting involved in sporting activities. The patient can explain to perpetrators that this new activity is for their good, fulfilling their needs (e.g., a job reduces the financial burden or an outside activity makes the partner less demanding).
5. Lessening power struggles is best approached by teaching one or both of the partners to attempt to make decisions in a more compromising way. Moving toward this goal in small steps works best.

6. Inform patients that even if they do not follow the plan well, they still do not deserve to be abused in any way.
7. To maintain momentum in making changes, short weekly appointments work best.

CHILD ABUSE

If the child abuser is an antisocial personality, incapable of emotional responsiveness to others, the physician should be an advocate for removal of parental rights. In most situations, however, other alternatives should be sought. Table 24.1 lists the clinical indicators of child abuse, including neglect, physical abuse, and sexual abuse.

Physical abuse

ASSESSMENT

1. Determine the specific sequence of events surrounding a child's misbehavior, including what precedes it and what occurs afterward.
2. Ask the parents if they ever think they use too much force to control their child, become too angry or frustrated with their child, or fear loss of self-control.
3. The physical examination should include looking for bruising, burns, fractures, subdural hematoma, and retinal hemorrhage. Consider total body radiography.
4. Determine if there is a significant emotional relationship between the parent and child.

PLAN

1. If there is significant suspicion of abuse, report as required by law in all 50 states. Document according to the guidelines in Table 24.2.
2. Maintain a stance of therapeutic helpfulness toward the patient and the family.
3. Hospitalize if necessary to protect the child or if further investigation is needed.
4. If substance abuse is a problem it should be addressed first.
5. Help parents develop a discipline program that allows them to feel in control of their child without the use of corporal punishment.
6. Address highly stressful periods. It is important here to not make the parents feel inadequate or incapable. Help the parents feel like good problem-solvers.
7. If financial stress is significant, referral to financial counselors or other social service agencies may be helpful.

Sexual abuse

ASSESSMENT

1. How do family members show affection? How is privacy maintained for the child? How are household rules enforced? Specifically, are the parents in the role of being parents, and are children in the role of being children? Is the family highly secretive?
2. Adolescents should be seen alone for at least a brief period during health care maintenance visits. Preadolescents should be seen alone if suspicion is significant.

PLAN

1. If there is reasonable suspicion, a report must be made to authorities with proper documentation.
2. It is usually best to remove the perpetrator from the home if the child can be assured safety.
3. For nonantisocial parents, reuniting the family after a period of separation is the ultimate goal.
4. If substance abuse is present, it should be the first target of treatment.
5. Family structure (i.e., parents assuming adult responsibility and children behaving like children) should start with counseling the two parents.
   a. Parents should develop and put into effect a joint discipline program.
   b. Promote activities that clearly put parents in the adult role as protector.
   c. Encourage good marital interaction. Apply marital counseling for problems of marital intimacy.
6. Family secretiveness can be addressed by promoting peer group activities.
7. Counseling for the abused child is important initially.
   a. It should address any belief the child has that he or she is responsible for the abuse.
   b. Open lines of communication lessen secrecy.
   c. Guide the child to an appropriate child's role.
8. The perpetrator should be required to ask the abused child for forgiveness. The other parent should also seek forgiveness for not providing protection. This requires significant preparatory counseling.

CHILD NEGLECT

Assessment

1. Note any red flags (see Table 24.1 for a complete list).
2. The most common red flag is parents who express numerous complaints over the burden of raising their children.

3. If neglect is suspected, the physician asks the parents what makes the child unhappy and happy.
4. Obtain a description of a typical day for the child.
5. If children have signs of neglect they should be evaluated for other physical abuse as well.

Plan

1. In the rare circumstance where there is no attachment between parents and child, the physician should recommend placing the child outside the family.
2. If parental skill is a problem, providing proper education and perhaps referral to a nurse educator or parenting class would be helpful.
3. For the parent who competes with the child for need fulfillment, create a situation wherein parental need fulfillment is contingent on their fulfilling the child's needs; for example, the parents can have a clinic visit after they perform a required task for the child.
4. Substance abuse, if present, must be addressed before other interventions.
5. If poverty is present, make an appropriate referral to a social services agency.

Elder abuse

Assessment

1. It is important for the physician to maintain a level of suspicion for signs of elder abuse, including physical abuse, sexual abuse, overcontrol, nonbenevolent decision-making, financial abuse, and the most common form, neglect.
2. Red flags include isolating the victim from the health care team, an unexplained or unusual injury, overcontrol by the caretaker, unexplained poor health or unusually poor hygiene, lack of amenities that can be afforded, or alcohol or substance abuse by anyone connected with the caretaking or by the patients themselves.
3. Risk factors include a family or patient feeling overwhelmed by the patient's needs, burnout, being financially burdened, and social isolation.
4. Ask the family what it is like to take care of the patient. If their descriptions are laced with blame or a sense of powerlessness, frustration, or hopelessness, abuse or neglect is more likely. Asking what a typical day is like can be illuminating.

Plan

1. Confronting the sense of powerlessness and frustration in the caretakers while empowering everyone is the primary goal.
2. Reduce financial stress by social service referral.

3. Referral for respite care can reduce burnout.
4. Reduce social isolation by making specific recommendations and referrals for daily activities.
5. In unusual circumstances it is necessary to report to Social Services that assault or neglect is occurring.
6. Patient autonomy regarding reporting must be respected.
7. Scheduling frequent visits breaks down the isolation and therefore makes abuse or neglect less likely.

For physicians who work with patients in abusive relationships, a normal reaction to the abuse is to become angry, wanting to see the perpetrator punished and to rescue the person who is the object of the abuse. Although an entirely normal reaction, acting out these feelings is usually not the most helpful approach. First, it is important for the physician to keep in mind that, as with most problem areas, doctors are part of a team. Being judgmental and punitive may be an appropriate response to abuse, but police and the judicial system are responsible for these approaches. It is the responsibility of the doctor to report abuse in some cases, but beyond that the help a physician can offer requires a therapeutic mindset. We discuss therapeutic interventions for partner abuse, child abuse (including child sexual abuse), and elder abuse.

Partner Abuse

Partner abuse includes physical injury, sexual assault, and emotional mistreatment, such as threats and other forms of inappropriate control. Women are the most common victims of domestic abuse. Risk factors for women include low socioeconomic status, teenage to early twenties relationships, pregnancy, chemical dependence in either partner, and lack of support from the extended family. The risk factors are additive. Certainly abuse can occur when none of these risk factors is present, but those who have risk factors call for extra vigilance.

Some understanding of characteristics common to abusers and the abused is helpful. These characteristics are not universal, but when evident they guide treatment planning to some extent.

Men who abuse women often have feelings of inadequacy, helplessness, and perhaps most important to the problem a sense of powerlessness. They have low self-esteem, feeling as though others take advantage of them if they are not on guard. They often have a basic belief that "might makes right." They are egocentric and have a difficult time empathizing with others. They are frequently dysphoric or at least have anhedonia. Often they attempt to treat their chronic problems with alcohol or other substances. Although they may put up a front of independence, they are usually highly dependent on the persons they abuse. Outside stressors tend to exacerbate their sense of powerlessness, so they are most likely to abuse when they are having global difficulties. In response to the feelings of powerlessness, they tend to put up a front of invulnerability.

They feel they must control others or they might be controlled by them. This reaction is most pronounced in their most intimate relationships. The woman who is abused is most likely to be abused when there is a power struggle, and the abuser believes he is losing. He then asserts himself physically to regain control. These individuals are less likely to be abusive when they have a sense of being in control of their environment, when they successfully accomplish things important to them, and when they see others as subservient to them. When the patient describes the sequence of events surrounding the abuse, often these characteristics become clear.

It can be helpful during treatment to understand the characteristics commonly associated with chronically abused women as well. These women are often used to being submissive in relationships. They look for men who appear superficially strong and protective of them and take this protective quality as a sign of love and caring. The women often have low self-esteem, which is driven even lower by their highly critical counterpart. Although dependence is a part of all relationships, these women often become highly dependent on the abuser before they know them well. They sometimes have a history of substance abuse. Like abusers, the abused often have a history of abuse during childhood.

There is frequently a cyclic nature to abuse. The relationship starts with the man coming across as powerful and protective of the woman, and the woman responds by being attentive and grateful. As time goes on, however, the woman becomes more open about her needs. The man, having low self-esteem and low tolerance for power struggles, perceives this as criticism and controlling, which leads to tension building in the relationship. During this phase the man attempts to establish the woman's submissiveness by being verbally aggressive and dominating. The situation escalates if the woman does not accept the man's authority, and this escalation can lead to violence. Following the violence, the woman often reaccepts the submissive role, and the man is again solicitous. Outside stress leads to this exacerbation occurring more readily. Frequently one or both members of the relationship use substances that inhibit self-control. The abuser may resort to physical violence more quickly and with less self-restraint under the influence of drugs or alcohol. Most abusive situations involve substance abuse. Because both partners have low self-esteem, jealousy is often the trigger for conflict.

Assessment

Abused women often present to the physician with injuries for which the explanation does not quite fit. They present with psychological problems, with a description of the stresses in their lives being vague. Other red flags include a patient describing her significant other in terms such as jealous, controlling, domineering, prone to anger, or extremely frustrated by stress. These significant red flags should lead the physician to explore potential abuse. The most sensitive screening tools are written questionnaires, although few family physicians use them because of time limitations. It has been shown that if the physician simply asks whether the patient has been kicked, hit, threatened, or forced into sexual behavior by anyone during the past year often leads to disclosure (El-Bayoumi et al., 1998).

A detailed description of the sequence of events that led to the abuse should be obtained. Because abuse is often cyclic in nature, a broader description of the relationship's ups and downs over time should be discussed as well. The doctor might ask, for example, "All relationships have up periods and down periods. What have those been like in your relationship?" Particularly within this context, an evaluation can be made as to whether the abusive cycle has included an escalation of harm. The most dangerous abusive circumstances usually include an escalating level of violence over time.

A detailed description of how decisions are made should be obtained, including a recent example. Past attempts to improve the situation should be explored. It is also useful to have the patient describe the relationship when it is at its best.

Plan

In situations where the abuse has escalated to injury or serious threats of harm, urging the patient to leave at least temporarily is likely the best option. Some states have reporting laws regarding harm with weapons or in some cases threatening with weapons. Obviously these laws must be observed in all cases. On the other hand, it is important for the patient to have trust in the doctor's confidentiality. Involving the police can be helpful; but if the patient is highly resistant or if the situation does not appear headed to physical harm, other options should be explored.

A plan should be developed so if the situation does reach dangerous levels the person would be ready. This should include having useful items available to them if they leave and how to contact authorities, find safe shelters, and obtain legal advice. Restraining orders are only partially effective; if the risk of injury is high, a shelter is safer.

In most cases the patient does not want to break off the relationship but simply wants the abuse to stop. Although separation is safest and therapy is more likely to succeed if the couple separates at least briefly, if the patient is resistant to separation it can be counterproductive to press the issue. Being controlled by another person, even a doctor, does not teach independence; and at this stage that is one of the therapeutic goals for the victim. If substance abuse is present, treating this problem first greatly increases the chances of overall successful therapy (see Chapter 12).

Although it is important for these women to *not* feel responsible for the abuse, it is also important to help them feel empowered to do something about it. Often they present to the doctor with a sense of helplessness, wanting the doctor to rescue them, transferring the full responsibility of solving the problem to the physician. Once the crisis has subsided, they may fail to follow through, frustrating the doctor. There are approaches the physician can take to avoid this scenario. Two dynamics often lead to increased violence: a power struggle and the woman's high level of co-dependence.

Changing the level of independence the woman has in the relationship often catalyzes the fastest changes. In general, the men involved in these relationships are highly dependent on the women, but they cover it up because they must cover up any sense of vulnerability. Whereas fear of losing the relationship totally can move these men to desperate acts, small steps toward independence on the woman's part can have a salutary effect. The man resists even these small steps initially; but if the woman persists while professing her commitment to the relationship, the man's fear of losing the woman inhibits his overdemanding behavior and ultimately his abusive behavior. The more he senses the woman is under his control, the bolder he can be. Therefore, helping the woman move toward greater independence psychologically and in other ways (e.g., financially) creates more balance in the relationship and lessens abuse. The most likely way this can occur is for the woman to gain psychological and emotional support outside the relationship, which is probably why support groups are effective. Certainly one of the recommendations to these women should be that they find a way to attend a support group (e.g., those provided through women's shelters or Al-Anon.) The principles taught and the support system found in Al-Anon closely align with the therapeutic needs of the abuse victim.

Becoming involved in activities that allow women to gain outside connections also helps. Taking an outside job, taking a course at a school, joining a church group, and getting involved in a sporting activity are likely to help the woman gain access to emotional support. A job is often best, as it can provide greater emotional and financial independence. The insecure perpetrator may sense the new activities as a threat to his control. It may be helpful to guide the woman to reframe the activity as being "for the abuser." That is, a new job takes financial pressure off him, and a new physical activity can help the woman be physically fit for the significant other. Some women attempt too rapidly to prove their independence to the significant other by going to a bar without him. Although the attempt to prove their independence in this way is understandable, it is misguided. It does not usually provide the woman with genuine support and inflames jealousy, leading to an escalation of violence. A gradual approach is best.

Attempting to lessen power struggles can be slow but helpful. It entails changing the way the couple makes decisions together. In abusive relationships both the man and the woman see the result of their decisions as either he is the winner or she is the winner. In mathematic thinking this is called a zero sum game. With $A + B = 0$, if A increases in value B must decrease to keep the constant 0. Because these men are extraordinarily sensitive to feeling out of control, they use whatever means, including violence, to win. Having the woman alter the usual sequence of events around decision-making (i.e., making a compromise about the goal) can deescalate the problem. For example, when the couple is making a decision about a rule for their child, the man says the woman is wrong, and the woman says the man is wrong. Each then tries to prove that the other one is incorrect. At this point the woman is instructed to think of a compromise between their positions. She should suggest to the man that if he accepts some middle ground she would back up the mutual decision, emphasizing how much he is winning from the compromise. Often this solution prevents the usual escalation. It is important to keep in mind that this is often as much of a change for the woman as it is for the man. However, the woman should also understand that even if she does not promote compromise, *she does not deserve to be hit or abused in any way.*

To induce patients to make any change initially, the physician may have to provide support for the patient by having regular frequent short appointments (e.g., weekly). The frequency of appointments should be reduced as they move ahead to other activities so the woman does not become overly dependent on the doctor.

These approaches have little effect in highly violent escalating relationships. However, when the woman does not want to leave the relationship and the relationship for the most part is nonviolent, this approach can be beneficial. It is common in family practice. Once the patient has benefited from this approach she may be more open to marital counseling as well.

Case Report

S.B. is a 42-year-old woman who was in her third marriage of 5 years' duration. She had three grown children and worked regularly at a technical job. She was seeing her family physician for her regular annual examination. As part of the routine history she had mentioned dysphoria. Upon further history and review of systems, the only positive finding on her examination was dysphoria without vegetative signs. After she received some patient education on general health care maintenance, the doctor asked her more about her unhappiness. She related it to distance in her marriage that had been increasing over time. The doctor recommended a follow-up appointment to discuss this further, including the suggestion that she bring her husband. She said there was no way he would come to the follow-up appointment, so she was encouraged to come alone.

A week later, while getting the history, it became very clear that issues of control were most prominent in the relationship. He had been controlling early in their relationship but had become more controlling over time. His control had gotten to the point where he would become hostile toward her if she did not walk the right distance from him. He would not let her go to the store alone, he said, because she would spend too much money. She was not allowed to see any of her friends. Recently he had tried to control how often she saw her family. He had not become physically violent until recently when she had argued with him over a farm chore, and he had shoved her several times. She was not physically hurt but was frightened.

When discussing the problem it became apparent that he was extremely dependent on her, and we discussed how she could use her withdrawal from him as a way to motivate him to give her back some control. In fact, she acted as if she was a child and he an adult. We began by focusing on the television (TV) remote control, which he totally controlled. The specific recommendation was that over the next week she offer to compromise with him regarding programming on the TV. If he did not compromise she would leave the room, read a book, and not talk with him at all until the next morning.

We also discussed an escape plan, calling the police and so on, if he escalated his violence in response to any of her behaviors. This plan fit with her goal to make the relationship better, not to leave it.

At the follow-up visit a week later she stated that little had changed. She had argued more about TV programming but had not left the scene as we had discussed. She was highly resistant to any of our suggestions, so we suggested that our request was probably too difficult for her and that for the next week we simply wanted her to keep a detailed diary of their interaction including her feelings so we could figure out a smaller step in the future. We also congratulated her for not allowing us to control her.

At the next appointment a week later, she stated that she had not prepared the diary but had in fact followed through on the TV plan on several occasions. When he would not compromise on the TV programming she had left. She was amazed at the results. Later on a number of occasions when she had requested a compromise with the TV he had become angry but gave her the remote control and become silent. She had done a good job of requesting input regarding the TV but was surprised in a positive way about the results of this encounter. Our next suggestion related to her family. We suggested she tell her husband she was going to visit them at a certain time the following week and then, without requesting permission as she had done in the past, she should just get in the car and go. The next week she followed through on this plan, and when she returned he yelled at her. As we requested, rather than getting into an argument with him she just ignored the yelling and went to be alone in the house.

Our next suggestion related to church, which he would not attend with her. We said she should offer to go with him but if he did not go she should simply go herself. At the next appointment 2 weeks later, she stated she had not gone to church. He had argued that they had to do things around the farm, and she had given in. A month later she returned, stating that although she had not yet followed through on the church going she felt much more freedom related to visiting her family. On several occasions when he became angry with her while doing chores on the farm, she had just gone into the house and ignored him the rest of the day. He then yelled at her, and she had responded very little. That weekend he asked her to go with him on a vacation for the weekend, and they went. She enjoyed this, as they had done it early in their relationship but had not gone for more than a year.

We suggested some other steps regarding visiting friends. She was rather defensive in coming up with excuses why she would not carry out this step. She thought that things were enough better that she wanted to stop therapy at least temporarily. Although the doctor was not in agreement that she was ready, they compromised: If things got back to the way they were she would return. The most important thing the patient had learned was that withdrawal was a much more powerful tool for change than confrontation.

Child Abuse

Child abuse, including neglect, physical abuse, and sexual abuse, is usually propagated by parents or other family members. Child abuse presents a number of challenges for the family physician. First, identifying abuse is often not easy, and neglect is even more difficult to identify. When abuse is suspected, the best course of action is not always clear either. It is, of course, the first duty of the physician to provide physical protection for the child. However, reflexively removing children from their parents can do more harm than good. Intervention for an abused child must be thoughtfully provided.

Some abusers are antisocial personalities with little in the way of conscience. These circumstances, although painful to observe, are simple to address, as advocating removal of parental rights is clearly the correct action. Other abusers care about their children but have a sense of powerlessness, low self-esteem, and a belief that "might makes right." They view children as equal in their thought processes, essentially regarding them as little adults, and therefore are unable to empathize with the needs of children. They are frequently immature to the point that they see their children as responsible for nurturing them rather than the other way around. Sometimes they are substance abusers and impulsively act out, later regretting their actions. A large percentage of violent and sexual acts occur under the influence of a substance. Many of these abusers can improve with treatment. This makes the course of action much more complicated for the doctor.

A large number of the individuals characterized above in fact never abuse their children. They may have the tendency but are lucky to never be so stressed by life circumstances to feel powerless. Physicians along with other professionals and nonprofessionals may help them through tough periods, providing a safety net for risky times. Family doctors are in a position to apply preventive interventions that make abuse significantly less likely. Although there is a considerable overlap of the characteristics associated with various forms of abuse, there are also differences. Therefore we take up, in turn, physical abuse, sexual abuse, and neglect, discussing the identification, evaluation, and treatment for each.

Physical Abuse

Characteristics of the vulnerable child include premature birth, birth of a child to an adolescent, a child who is often ill, and hospitalization of a neonate—all high stress situations that challenge bonding. It has been recognized that not infrequently one child is singled out for abuse in a family, and that this child has the lowest level of attachment to the parents. In fact, the lack of a good bond between parent and child adds significantly to the likelihood of abuse.

One early preventive intervention is to facilitate the biologic propensity for bonding during the first day and weeks of life. For example, encouraging close parental contact with the neonate is most important to those at risk and those least likely to aggressively pursue it, such as teenage mothers. Skin-to-skin contact and close eye contact are important cues to early biologic bonding.

Assessment

When the history of an injury does not match the physical finding, physical abuse should be considered. The indicators listed in Table 24.1 are those most often seen. Asking the parents to describe what they do when the child misbehaves frequently brings out many of the characteristics commonly associated with abuse, such as the parent who fears loss of control and sees force as the only way to maintain control over the child. Asking parents if they ever think they use too much force to control their child can be useful. Similarly, asking if they ever become too angry or frustrated with their children can be revealing. Determining the specific sequence of events around a child's misbehavior can be helpful.

If there is a strong suspicion of abuse, other investigation should be considered, including a complete view of the child's body looking for bruises and burns in different stages of healing; a radiographic series to look for fractures in different stages of healing; examination for subdural hematoma; and a thorough examination of the retinas for hemorrhage (shaken baby syndrome).

Plan

If there is significant reason to believe that abuse has taken place, it must be reported. All 50 states require that suspected abuse be reported. The word "suspected" requires judgment. Although there is some controversy, the re-

TABLE 24.1. Clinical Indicators of Various Types of Child Abuse

Neglect
  History of untreated medical conditions
  Inadequate immunization
  Absence of necessary health aids (eyeglasses, hearing aids)
  Malnutrition
  Developmental delays
  Poor hygiene
  Rampant dental caries
Physical abuse
  Bruises or welts resembling shape of article used to inflict injury
  Burns (cigarette, immersion, patterned)
  Lacerations, rope burns, facial injuries
  Fractures
  Abdominal injuries
  Central nervous system injuries (reflective of shaking)
  Chemical abuse
  Symptoms of suffocation
  Munchausen syndrome by proxy (caregiver makes up symptoms or induces
    illness)
Sexual abuse
  Abrasions or bruises on labia, penis, anus, inner thighs
  Distortion of hymen
  Abnormal anorectal tone
  Sexually transmissible disease
  Pregnancy
  Chronic abdominal or anal pain
  Recurrent urinary tract infections
  Precocious sexual activity
Behavioral findings for any type of abuse
  Depression or suicidal tendencies
  Anxiety
  Enuresis
  Sleep disturbances
  Excessive masturbation
  Poor interpersonal relations or withdrawal
  Aggressive behavior
  Poor school performance
  Role reversal (child becomes caregiver)
  Child is overly compliant during the office visit

Adapted from American Medical Association (1994a)

porting of questionable abuse is not always helpful and in some cases has caused harm to a child who it turns out was not abused. For example, children are often separated from their parents for periods of time during the investigation. Similar types of separation have been found to be harmful to children, so the likelihood of benefit must exceed the probability of harm. As in all areas of medicine, judgments must be made.

If abuse is reported to authorities, it does not necessarily terminate a good doctor/patient relationship. Although in some instances alienation does occur, it is not inevitable if the doctor openly discusses the findings with the parents. The physician should maintain a stance of being there to help the family, not to judge it, but letting them know that there is an obligation to report. Often the doctor/family relationship can be salvaged to the family's benefit, particularly if it has been strong. Sometimes, in fact, the parents have felt guilty about losing their tempers and hurting their child, and they are relieved that something can be done to help. It may be helpful to reassure the caring but abusive parent that the physician's goal is to solve the problem, not separate the family.

If an abuse is reported, it should be done according to the guidelines for documentation of abuse as shown in Table 24.2. Sometimes to protect a child immediately during the investigation and to provide a chance to evaluate further, hospitalization is necessary. Often there is a physical finding that can be used as a rationale for the hospitalization and further investigation. Foster families or safe houses are available in most communities to

---

TABLE 24.2. Guidelines for Documentation of Abuse

1. Perform standard health assessment, including medical history taking and notation of relevant social factors.
2. Record chief complaints and describe abusive event or neglectful situation using the patient's own words when possible rather than the physician's assessment.
3. Give detailed description of injuries, including type, number, size, location, stages of healing, color, resolution, possible causes, and explanations given for their presence. When applicable, record location and nature of injuries on a body chart or drawing.
4. Describe observed behavior.
5. Give results of all pertinent laboratory or other diagnostic procedures.
6. Offer opinion on whether injuries were adequately explained.
7. For child abuse, give location of alleged abusive events, if known.
8. Supply photographs and imaging studies, whenever applicable.
9. Report any other significant facts that address the who, what, where, why, and when of injuries.
10. If incident is reported, give name of agency and person investigating, and list actions taken.

Adapted from American Medical Association (1994a)

provide refuge on an outpatient basis. Removing the perpetrator from the home is often better than removing the victim so long as safety can be ensured.

Beyond reporting the suspected abuse, the physician can offer important guidance to the family. This is especially true for the at-risk family where parental behavior has not yet reached the point of requiring a report.

Two factors associated with potential abuse are amenable to family practice intervention: parental stress and discipline problems. Avoiding issues of blame and thus avoiding parental defensiveness increases the likelihood of change. Helping the parents feel empowered rather than helpless is critical for change to occur.

It is important to avoid making the parents believe they are inadequate or evil. Because the goal is to help them believe they can be good parents, supporting their appropriate interactions with their children while at the same time finding better ways for them to provide discipline is the central theme. This must be done with some finesse, as these parents are prone to low self-esteem. A statement such as the following can help. "Your child is very trying at times. He [or she] is a real limit tester. I understand how you can become angry and frustrated, so to stay in control you must do some special things. In the past you resorted to corporal punishment to maintain control. Although resorting to physical punishment can control the child for a short time, over the long run the power of this action diminishes until it has little value. Children learn to take their spanking and soon afterward go back to their bad behavior. On the other hand, children want their parents' attention so much that by denying attention when they are bad or giving them extra attention when they are good parents can gain a great deal of power over their children's behavior." Although studies have not definitively shown corporal punishment to be a poor child-rearing technique, it is best to guide parents at risk for abuse away from this form of discipline.

If the parents accept the need for alternatives to corporal punishment, a discipline program such as one contained in Chapter 17 can be used. Feeling more empowered in this way, parents are less likely to resort to abusive punishment to control their children.

Helping parents cope with the stress that contributes to child abuse often requires referral. For example, if financial problems are prominent, referral to a financial counselor may be helpful. Interventions for substance abuse (see Chapter 12) and marital counseling (see Chapter 22) can be helpful for avoiding stress that leads to child abuse in at-risk families.

Child Sexual Abuse

For some family physicians, the identification of child sexual abuse, knowing the suffering it causes children, elicits the most hostile response of all. However, as with other areas of abuse, maintaining a therapeutic approach gives the physician the best opportunity to affect change positively for the benefit of all involved.

Sexual abuse may start at a young age, but more often it starts at pubescence. The perpetrator of sexual abuse is most often a family member or someone close to the family, such as the mother's boyfriend. Many characteristics of the perpetrator are similar to those described for physical abuse. Some additional characteristics, however, are commonly present.

Perpetrators, on the one hand, may appear to have an overly inflated ego, although within the family they view themselves in the role of another child, unable to control their impulses and not being responsible for their actions. Often the abuser has a difficult time separating his needs from the needs of others.

Often these families are secretive, and its members are highly insolated from people outside the family. Keeping family secrets is one of the family rules long before sexual abuse occurs.

Finkelhor (1984) identified four preconditions that are often present when child sexual abuse occurs.

1. *Offenders see their emotional and sexual needs as going unmet.*
2. *Offenders often lack internal inhibitions that would prevent them from sexually abusing a child.* This may be the result of substance abuse, mental illness, or a lack of protective feelings toward the child (which is inherently less in some stepparents compared to natural parents); or it may be the result of some other inability to bond, such as an abusive background.
3. *External inhibitions that would normally block abnormal behavior are overcome.* The propensity of these families to keep secrets and to maintain a high degree of isolation and the lack of normal psychological and physical boundaries between family members are often prevalent in families where sexual abuse occurs.
4. *The child's resistance to abuse is overcome.* Children might be so emotionally deprived they do almost anything to obtain some form of attention. They may themselves be desirous of protecting the perpetrators. That is, they have loving feelings toward the perpetrators and do not want to hurt them by holding them responsible for their actions. Even more likely, the mother may have long given a subtle warning that she would take sides with the father or stepfather, and the child would become a traitor to the family. The mother's defense is usually a result of her own guilt for sexual withdrawal and her extreme dependency needs.

Assessment

Identifying child sexual abuse is often difficult. The signs are frequently subtle and overlap problems in other areas. Evidence of trauma to anatomic locations such as the perineum or the presence of venereal disease in a young teenager or child is an obvious red flag. The presence of venereal disease in a teenager who denies sexual activity should make the physician suspicious, although obviously for the 17-year-old who denies a sexual encounter there could be other reasons. The physician may see the child come across sexually. In addition, the child often takes on an adult role precociously. The child or teenager who is overly sexually precocious or extremely uncomfortable in the presence of a man may indicate a red flag situation. Sometimes the dating behavior of a teenager who dates only members of ethnic groups other than that of their family can raise suspicion, as does the presence of physical abuse.

It is important to interview the teenager alone if there is any suspicion of abuse. In abusive families, interviewing the teenager alone is likely to be highly resisted by a parent; and it is another red flag that abuse might be occurring. When the teenager is interviewed alone, a good question to ask is if anyone is making them uncomfortable because of their sexual interest.

For the preteenager in whom abuse is suspected, it is better to explain the difference between good touch and bad touch with the mother present and ask the child if anyone has touched them in a bad way. For the preschool child, the interview can be quite time-consuming and requires significant expertise. If there is reason for suspicion, an appropriate expert should be consulted. When interviewing and examining a child for suspected sexual abuse, it is important to respect the child's boundaries. If children do not want to answer questions or be examined, they probably should not be unless there is a medical reason beyond establishing abuse. Violating them even if it is by a doctor does not help them gain a sense of control over their own bodies. It becomes just one more example of inappropriate control by others.

Reporting sexual abuse is required by law and is extremely helpful to the child. However, as stated previously, reporting also can cause some ill effects and so should be done thoughtfully and only for significant indications. Every attempt should be made to obtain a clear history from the parents as well as the child. Interviewing the parents should be done in a nonjudgmental, nonaccusatory way using primarily open-ended questions while maintaining a therapeutic rather than a punitive approach. Asking questions about how family members show affection and how privacy in the child's bedroom is established are useful entries into the discussion. A highly defensive response is common among abusers and their family members. The mother, in fact, may strongly defend the father or stepfather from a daughter's accusations. While being honest about the need to report, doctors should emphasize their desire to help the patient and family.

Plan

If it can be done safely, removing the perpetrator from the home is better for the child than removing the child. If it can be garnered, support from the family is most helpful during times of crisis. For many families treatment for sexual abuse can be highly effective in terms of reuniting the family after a period of separation from the perpetrator and preventing recurrence while achieving a better level of overall adjustment. This helps prevent the victim from feeling guilt or believing that she is responsible for destroying her family. Most abused children want to feel safe and in appropriate control but want to remain in the family. If possible, this should be the goal.

There is a wide range of treatment programs available. The effective ones achieve a better than 50% success rate. Success is defined as return of the child to the family without further incident. Factors associated with the likelihood of successful treatment include perpetrators having genuine remorse for their behavior, their having feelings of protectiveness for the child, their succeeding in overcoming alcohol and drug abuse if present, and a reduction in social isolation by family. It is also essential during the course of treatment for the spouse/significant other to hold the perpetrator responsible for his or her actions *before* forgiveness is offered.

During the treatment process it is helpful for the physician to maintain close contact with members of the therapy team. Although initial therapy may be directed primarily at the perpetrator and the victim separately, ultimately family therapy is an important part of the process. Victims often believe they are responsible and suffer much guilt. This problem should be addressed in preparation for the family therapy. An essential part of this process is the perpetrator apologizing to the victim during a family session. It is also helpful if other adult members in the household apologize to the victim for not being available to them to hear their secret and being trustworthy enough for the victim to share the secret. This process not only establishes that it is the adult's responsibility rather than the child's for what has happened, it also breaks down the secrecy in these families, allowing healing to occur and safety to be established.

Marital counseling helps the adults develop a better sexual adjustment with each other. It is important to encourage a family structure that supports adult roles for adults and children's roles for children. Children should become involved in age-appropriate activities, such as sports, church, or the school band. When these changes have been established in the family, the physician can be reassured that the likelihood of sexual abuse is significantly reduced.

The family physician is in the ideal position to institute a preventive intervention in families who present with red flags for child sexual abuse but in which sexual abuse has not yet occurred. Small changes in the way families interact can lead to large differences in the overall outcome regarding child sexual abuse. Giving specific recommendations for children to be involved in outside activities can markedly reduce the social isolation of the family. Recommendations regarding parenting that place the parents in the role of being in charge of the child and protector for the child rather than being seen as a "friend" or competitor of the child can be valuable in many areas including prevention of sexual abuse. Identifying and treating parental substance abuse, marital discord, or sexual problems can make the difference between sexual abuse and a normal interaction in many of these families.

Case Report

D.B. is a 15-year-old high school student who is brought to the clinic by her mother for evaluation of depression. Her mother was concerned about her skipping school and missing her job as a cashier because of dysphoria; she thought that medicine would help. Upon further investigation it was found that D.B. had no vegetative signs and in fact was quite active starting in the afternoon. She often went to her cousin's house where she stayed despite the fact that her mother forbid her to do so because they were known drug abusers. She came home late, although she stated that she had no curfew. Her mother said they were best friends, although she was frustrated that D.B. did not obey her.

D.B. related her dysphoria to an older brother who is married and living in the area but who had rejected her and the rest of their family. The doctor, however, believed the dysphoria was related to her having gotten significantly behind in school and in danger of failing. Helping the mother develop some structure was the primary goal of the first appointment.

At the second appointment D.B. was seen without her mother. She expressed a great deal of hostility toward her stepfather who had lived in the house with them for more than 10 years. Two years previously he had been referred to Social Services because he had watched her undress. On this occasion she stated that one of her brothers had caught him peeking through a crack in the bathroom door. After the appointment, Social Services was called.

We asked that D.B. return with her mother the following week, and we called the stepfather to meet with him as well. During the meeting he vehemently denied any voyeuristic behavior. He stated that 2 years before he had watched her undress and that had taught him a lesson, although he had an explanation for why he had watched her. At the request of Social Services, he had now moved out of the house but hoped to return soon. Social Services had decided not to pursue the investigation further so long as he was out of the house until the doctor stated he could return. The doctor told the stepfather that the goal was to have him return to the house ultimately but that before that occurred certain steps had to be taken.

The stepfather's view was that the biggest problem with D.B. was that she was out of control and had no rules. We therefore requested that he meet with D.B.'s mother outside the home and that they draw up a list of rules for D.B. The purpose of this was to clearly put the father in a parental position along with the mother, rather than their being like peers to the girl.

At the next appointment the stepfather said they had made up the rules. He said he also had sent both his wife and D.B. a dozen roses, and that D.B. had asked him to help search for a car for her. The physician discussed the inappropriateness of the roses for the daughter and talked about guidelines by which he could be clearly a parent to her, not a friend. The doctor asked him to come up with a list of things he had done in the past that could be misconstrued as being more her friend than her parent. She also asked him to write a letter to her in which he described ways he had made her uncomfortable and apologize. He was not to send it but return with it to the doctor at the next appointment.

At a separate appointment with D.B. D.B. said that things were going better, and she was attending school on a regular basis. At the next appointment, after her mother had given her the new set of rules, she got into a confrontation and threatened suicide, at which time the police were called and she was taken to the hospital. By the next morning she was no longer feeling suicidal. A meeting was held with her and her mother. She agreed that she would follow the rules even if she did not like them. The mother agreed to hold her to them, including the consequences. The physician (with the help of the hospital social worker) made arrangements for her to attend an alternative school. She was then discharged to home. At the next appointment with the stepfather it was agreed that he could help his stepdaughter look for a car so long as the mother was with them.

From this point on D.B. did well, liked her new school, followed the rules, and was no longer breaking curfew or going over to the drug house with her cousins. The mother felt much more empowered. The physician met with the stepfather, and overall his letter was appropriate. She made a number of suggestions and had him rewrite the letter before giving it to D.B. The process of reuniting the family began with the stepfather going to the house for dinner.

Child Neglect

Child neglect includes failure to provide for the medical, environmental, nutritional, educational, emotional, and supervision needs of the child. Because there is a broad range to these needs, neglect is often difficult to identify. From a legal standpoint, it is often difficult to prove unless the neglect is severe, which is rarely the case. Only when it is severe does it identify a parent who truly does not care about the child. More often when children are neglected, the parents do care but have difficulty maintaining the role of the protective caretaker.

This situation may arise for a number of reasons. Perhaps the parents have never learned to care for themselves. It is difficult to take care of a child when you do not take care of yourself. Perhaps the parent grew up in an atmosphere where there was always competition among members of the family to have their needs met. In this case, they may see the child as a competitor or may view the child as one who should nurture them. When the family is impoverished, it can have a profound effect on neglect. Despite the difficulty of identifying and treating neglected children, family doctors in many instances can make a difference.

Assessment

Probably the most easily assessable red flag for neglect is children who are behind in their immunizations. Although this is a highly sensitive finding, it is not specific for neglect. A parent who vehemently complains about the burden of caring for their child requires more suspicion. Falling behind on the expected growth curve is a more serious indicator. Weight, then height, then head circumference, respectively, increase concern. (See Table 24.1 for a more complete list.)

If there are red flags, the doctor should gather the following information. Asking parents what their child needs to be happy and what makes their child unhappy often brings out what needs of the child are going unmet. If the child gets into trouble or has frequent somatic symptoms, asking for the sequence of events around these occurrences can be illuminating. The common pattern of problem behavior emerging in response to the child who is being ignored is often seen. Care should be taken to avoid putting parents on the defensive as much as possible. Parents who respond to these questions by regarding their children as competitors rather than under their protection are most concerning. A medical evaluation for neglect should include a complete physical examination with attention paid to any signs of physical abuse (neglect is a risk factor for physical abuse), a developmental screen, and of course a close look at height, weight, and head circumference. Asking parents to describe their child's typical day can be an eye opener for the physician.

Plan

If children are not having their needs met in terms of food, shelter, or essential medical care, it must be reported. The same laws usually apply to neglect as to abuse. Often the doctor can maintain a good relationship with the parent and stay involved so long as the doctor expresses a desire to help and is not judgmental. The physician can explain to the parents that the family needs help with taking care of basic necessities, and by reporting this fact the physician wants to make sure that help is available to the family and the child. If the doctor is uncertain about the child's health status, sometimes admitting the child to the hospital allows enough time for the necessary evaluation. A neutral explanation for further evaluation can be given to the parents, such as: "Further workup is needed to explain a physical finding."

If a report to Social Services is needed, presenting this necessity to the parents often helps diagnostically in discovering those parents who really do not care about their child. Those who have no attachment to the child easily give up responsibility for the child to others. In this situation, encouraging

Social Services to find an alternative living situation for the child is likely best. In the more common circumstance where the parents have an ambivalent relationship toward the child or lack of parental skill, alternatives to removing the child should be sought.

In some situations it is simply ignorance that leads the parents to be inadequate caregivers especially in the case of infants. In this situation regular visits from a nurse educator can help. Along with providing education the nurse can role-model and give positive reinforcement for good parenting. When the child becomes a toddler, referral to parenting education classes can be helpful.

For most neglectful parents, many of whom are dependent themselves, the overall strategy is to help the parents have their needs met in ways that are not viewed as competitive with their children. A common pattern that develops in families where parents are not providing for their children's needs is that the children respond by becoming more demanding and manipulative in an attempt to have their needs met. This in turn leads the parents to find the children less enjoyable to be around and to view their children as bad. This leads the parent to give the children even less, which of course makes the children more needy and more demanding and manipulative.

One approach to reversing this cycle is to find a way to give the parents more attention for giving the child more attention. An example is a mother who had somatoform complaints that she used as an excuse for not taking appropriate care of her child. She was given several assignments and told the doctor wanted to see her again after she completed the assignments. This meant that the doctor would give her more attention for giving her child more attention. Other members of the treatment team, such as social workers and others, can become involved in similar reinforcements. In some situations the extended family can be called on to help. Perhaps a grandparent could be asked to provide babysitting once a week for a job well done by the parents.

The more creative the ways to meet parental needs by giving reinforcement when they provide care to their children, the more effectively can neglect be altered. The hope is that by helping parents develop a good relationship with their child they will ultimately enjoy the relationship and it will be self-reinforcing, requiring less outside input.

Substance abuse, if present, must be dealt with before any other intervention is likely to help (see Chapter 12). Poverty, leading to neglect, should result in referrals to social service agencies.

Elder Abuse

Elder abuse has been increasingly recognized as a problem. Many family physicians are surprised when elder abuse is uncovered. This is concerning, as lack of recognition is probably the greatest barrier to resolution of the problem.

Elder abuse is seen in a number of forms, including physical abuse, sexual abuse, overcontrol, nonbenevolent decision-making, financial abuse, and the most common form, neglect. In the case of physical abuse, the spouse is usually the perpetrator. Other family members are more commonly guilty of ignoring autonomy, stealing resources, and neglect. The most common source of neglect is the elders themselves. In situations where the family is not around to supervise or be involved on a regular basis, the perpetrator may be some other caretaker on whom the patient is dependent.

Assessment

It is critical that the physician maintain an index of suspicion for elder abuse so it does not go unrecognized. Red flags for the physician are in many ways similar to those noted with other forms of abuse. The most common red flag is an attempt to isolate the victim from the health care team. For example, the perpetrator may not want the patient to talk alone with the doctor. The victim may be hesitant to talk openly as well because of embarrassment, fear of retaliation, or wanting to protect the perpetrator (particularly a spouse). Other red flags include unexplained or unusual injury, overcontrol by the caretaker, unexplained poor health care or unusually poor hygiene, a lack of amenities they could easily afford, and alcohol or substance abuse by anyone connected with caretaking or by the elders themselves.

Probably the most important risk factor for abuse is when a family member feels overwhelmed by the needs of the patient. Extraordinary time responsibilities may lead to burnout and depression, which may ultimately lead to frustration, anger, and then abuse. Financial burden may lead to neglect or abuse. This can be especially important in the case where there is forced cohabitation with family members. Social isolation by the family can further exacerbate the problem. In the rural environment social isolation is almost inevitable unless the family takes active steps to avoid it. Although more services are offered in urban areas, proactive steps must occur there as well.

Psychological problems including substance abuse and mental or emotional disorders are common in the abuser. A history of violence in the family is a definite risk factor. Children who have been abused by their parents may, in turn, abuse their parents when the parents become elderly and dependent. A spouse who has always abused his wife is likely to continue to do so in old age. Dementia may disinhibit aggressive tendencies. As with all forms of abuse, people who have low self-esteem and often feel powerless are much more likely to become abusive under stress.

In general, if the physician suspects abuse based on the above red flags, the next step is to speak with the family and, if applicable, other caretakers. Without suggesting blame, asking the family members or other caretakers for their views on why the patient's health is less than expected is usually productive. If the description is heavily laced with blame, a sense of powerlessness, frustration, and hopelessness, abuse or neglect is likely. Asking family and caretakers if they ever get so frustrated with caretaking they find themselves getting overly rough with the patient or ignoring them for long periods can provide useful information. If abuse is suspected, the physician must find a way to see the patient alone. Patients can then be asked how they feel they are being cared for and if they have been hit or inappropriately touched. If the patient lives alone, asking how they get food, medicine, and social interaction provides information on self-care. Asking the patient to describe a typical day provides the best understanding of the patient's life style.

Plan

Most states do not have specific reporting laws regarding elder abuse, although many forms of abuse (e.g., physical assault or neglect) are illegal in and of themselves. Nearly all states have adult protective services. Often discussing the patient with them can help decide whether to make a formal referral. Without reporting laws, however, the decision to report is grayer, especially because abuse and neglect run along a continuum and the minor problems are the most frequent. Certainly in the case when there is immediate danger to a patient's life or serious compromise to their functional abilities, reporting is obvious. However, when the neglect or abuse of a more minor nature occurs, it may be better to approach it in other ways. In all cases when elderly persons have the mental status to provide informed consent, their autonomy must be respected. The doctor's disrespect for their autonomy in this case could be experienced by the patient as abusive itself.

Confronting the sense of powerlessness and frustration of caretakers in a supportive way is most often the best way to decrease elder abuse. The goal should be to empower everyone—patient, caretaker, family members—to help them feel involved and part of the solution. This avoids making people defensive while markedly reducing the likelihood of future neglect or abuse. Reducing stressors (e.g., financial stress and the burdens of the caregivers) in most cases works better than punishment for infractions. Because solutions may require efforts from several disciplines in addition to the family, the family physician often finds it useful to call a health care team meeting. In some cases it must be preceded by a family meeting to help prepare them to see the health care team meeting in the proper context, that is, as an attempt to get support for everyone involved, rather than as a desire to determine who is to blame. The overall goal should be to reduce the caretakers' burden and reduce social isolation. Often this means getting other organizations involved, such as the senior citizens center, visiting nurses, and social services. It can be framed to the caregiver as being for the patient's good. If the caregiver burns out they are no good to anyone.

When abuse or neglect is suspected or confirmed, it is important to schedule frequent appointments or visits from health care providers for ongoing evaluation. This practice not only leads to early detection of a deteriorating situation, it can have a profound effect on the problem behavior by decreasing the isolation. If nothing else, the potential perpetuator feels more restrained.

References

Domestic Abuse

American Medical Association (1994a) Diagnostic and Treatment Guidelines on Child Physical Abuse and Neglect. Chicago: American Medical Association.

American Medical Association (1994b) Diagnostic and Treatment Guidelines on Child Sexual Abuse. Chicago: American Medical Association.

American Medical Association (1994c) Diagnostic and Treatment Guidelines on Domestic Violence. Chicago: American Medical Association.

American Medical Association (1994d) Diagnostic and Treatment Guidelines on Elder Abuse and Neglect. Chicago: American Medical Association.

Baker N, Mersy D, Tuteur J, et al (1996) Family Violence Monograph, 205th ed. Kansas City, MO: American Academy of Family Physicians.

Reid S, Glasser M (1997) Primary care physicians' recognition of and attitudes toward domestic violence. Acad Med 72:51–53.

Steiner RP, VanSickle K, Lippmann SB (1996) Domestic violence: do you know when and how to intervene? Postgrad Med 100:103–116.

Partner Abuse

Ambuel B, Hamberger LK, Lahti J (1996) Partner violence: a systematic approach to identification and intervention in outpatient health care. Wis Med J 95:292–297.

El-Bayoumi G, Marum ML, Yolanda H (1998) Domestic violence in women. Med Clin North Am 82:391–401.

Holmes MM (1995) The primary health care provider's role in sexual assault prevention. Womens Health Issues 5:224–232.

Melvin SY (1995) Domestic violence: the physician's role. Hosp Prac 30:45–53.

Wilke WS (1996) Highlights from medical grand rounds. Cleve Clin J Med 63:199–202.

Child Abuse and Neglect

Bethea L (1999) Primary prevention of child abuse. Am Fam Physician 59:1577–1585.

Craissati J, McClurg G (1997) The challenge project: a treatment program evaluation for perpetrators of child sexual abuse. Child Abuse Neglect 21:637–648.

Dubowitz H, King H (1995) Family violence: a child-centered, family-focused approach. Pediatr Clin North Am 42:153–166.

Finkelhor D (1984) Child Sexual Abuse. New York: Free Press.

Guidry HM (1995) Childhood sexual abuse: role of the family physician. Am Fam Physician 51:407–414.

Jenny C, Sutherland SE, Sandahl BB (1986) Developmental approach to preventing the sexual abuse of children. Pediatrics 78:1034–1038.

Madanes C (1990) Sex, Love, Violence. New York: Norton.

Mayes A (1995) Twenty years in the evaluation of the sexually abused child: has medicine helped or hurt the child and the family? J Med Assoc Ga 84:244.

Elder Abuse

Krueger P, Patterson C (1997) Detecting and managing elder abuse: challenges in primary care. Can Med Assoc J 157:1095–1100.

25

Problems Associated with Chronic Illness in Adults

ASSESSMENT

1. After bad news about a chronic illness is presented to the patient and family, and education is repeated several times, evaluate the initial adjustment. How do they understand the illness and treatment process? Is guilt excessive? Is family cohesion leading to social support? Do they have concerns over pain management?
2. Two months after diagnosis the family should be reevaluated for overall adjustment to the illness. In addition to the questions in item 1, ask them to describe a typical day and how the illness has changed their day. Evaluate whether the grief process has led to excessive withdrawal or overdependence. Are they involved in as much normal activity as the illness will allows? If there are problems regarding adherence, evaluate how the patient and family are feeling about being in control of their care and the goals for treatment.

TREATMENT

1. If guilt is a problem, treat with:
   a. Education
   b. Forgiveness from close associates or those in authority (e.g., pastor)
   c. Penance
2. If denial is a problem, treat with education. If further education does not work, reframe the problem as accepting the illness as a sign of strength.
3. If adherence is a problem related to control issues, attempt to renegotiate goals and the treatment process. Look for acceptable compromise.
4. If withdrawal and social isolation are problems, prescribe specific new activities or a timeline for becoming involved in past activities. Use physical and occupational therapy if necessary.

5. If overdependence or learned helplessness is a problem, prescribe specific activities that would demonstrate more normal adjustment and some independence. Give specific tasks to the family that give more attention to the patient for normal behavior and less for sick behavior.
6. If the family has become overly distant, prescribe specific activities the family can do together.
7. If power struggles are a problem, discuss with the patient and family how decisions should be made.
8. If there are marital problems, evaluate couple activities as well as sexual activities and prescribe new ways to approach these problems.
9. If patients experience grief for an extended time, explore opportunities to engage in meaningful activity, which can bring new meaning to their lives.

Two families have a member diagnosed with diabetes. Both families initially are in pain and have difficulty adjusting. Months later one family has for the most part returned to a normal life style despite the need for adherence to treatment protocols. The other family remains centered on the disease, dropping out of many of their usual activities; they are overwhelmed and burdened by the treatment protocol. Prior to the illness both of these families were well adjusted. In fact, the family that had the most difficulty adjusting was the more educated and financially successful one.

There were precursors that, although subtle, could help the doctor identify the family at risk and could help guide them to a better adjustment. Turk and Kerns (1985) reported that most families, despite going through a painful adjustment period, ultimately return to normal functioning. However, a significant number of families have long-term adjustment problems. The most important factors are as follows. First, how significantly does the illness directly affect the functional status of the patient? The stage of life of the patient should be considered in this context. For example, as much as removal of a breast from a 70-year-old may alter one's body image, consider the impact it would have on a 25-year-old-woman. When the chronic illness disrupts a patient's ability to perform usual roles in the family (e.g., work, caretaking, self-care) and forces the younger generation to take care of the older one, it creates havoc throughout the family system. Sometimes learned helplessness develops in response to an illness. Because of their illness a patient cannot participate in the activities that brought them closer to their significant others. They also discover that being taken care of for their illness makes up for the lost attention and closeness. On the other hand, they learn that when they act more self-reliant they lose this attention. This process often unconsciously leads to learned helplessness.

The initial response to the diagnosis of a chronic illness has been defined by many as a grief reaction, with the commonly associated dynamics of denial, guilt, anger, mitigation, dysphoria, and adaptation. It is important not to view this reaction as pathologic depression. Defining this reaction as depression rather than grief places it in the category of an illness, whereas grief reactions are considered normal. The ultimate resolution of grief comes with redefining the meaning of one's life while accepting the loss. This goal does not come easily for anyone; it is achieved only through struggle.

Complicating factors when grieving for chronic illness are common. Many illnesses (e.g., multiple sclerosis and asthma) are characterized by periods of exacerbation and relapse. For the patient this has been defined as the Democles syndrome. In Greek mythology Democles was offered a great feast but was forced to partake of it while sitting under a heavy sword suspended by a single thread. The patient may enjoy their renewed health but not without feeling the constant fear of the illness hanging over them by a single thread. How the associated issues of grief (i.e., denial, anger, guilt, mitigation, dysphoria, adaptation) are confronted has a profound effect on adjustment. Those who cope best usually have broad areas of competence, giving them a good chance to find areas of competence despite disability. They are usually flexible. They can tolerate the need for dependence when they have to but strive for independence. The doctor should encourage these characteristics.

Families who do best are able to approximate their usual normal behavior as closely as the illness allows, particularly when the illness is in a steady state. This can be complicated, however, by even defining what is normal and what is abnormal. For example, a patient presenting with a chronic cough and an enlarged lymph node is diagnosed with lymphoma. The lymphoma is treated and is in full remission. The person develops a cough related to an allergen, yet the cough provokes significant anxiety, not only in the patient but in significant others. Although acting normally can be quite beneficial, it is important for the physician to be aware that *acting normally* is different from *being normal*.

Four family characteristics appear to have the most profound effect on family adjustment. The family's balance between cohesiveness and individuality is one characteristic. The families that most successfully cope with significant illness usually are good at pulling together during the initial acute phase and later return to a more normalized state of allowing some dependence while encouraging maximum independence. Families who have problems tend to remain at one extreme or the other.

Control issues can also interfere with adjustment. When a family member or the entire family has a sense of powerlessness, power struggles ensue. This can have a dramatic effect on adherence to the treatment protocol.

Rigidity versus flexibility is another determinant of adjustment. The family may adjust in creative ways and find solutions to problems or remain in old ruts even when they do not work anymore.

How families resolve conflict can have an important impact on family functioning as well. Marriages have a much higher rate of dissolution following the diagnosis of a chronic illness in the family. Highly stressful times, like illnesses, commonly lead to more conflict because they usually require more cooperative decision-making. Patterns of avoidance or overly hostile mechanisms of dealing with conflict can lead to distancing of family members to avoid the anger. This can begin a cycle devastating to the marriage and family (Minuchin, 1978).

Assessment

Initially it is difficult to assess whether a family is likely to make a good adjustment. It is best to assume that they will. Education about the illness and treatment is all that may be necessary during the initial adjustment. This should nearly always include the family as well as the patient. Because the time of initial diagnosis is emotionally charged, the patient and family find it difficult to focus and learn everything that needs to be learned. Therefore education must be undertaken small steps and repeated several times. The ensuing grief reaction should be described as normal, although the physician maintains vigilance for excessive guilt or destructive anger. Family cohesion should be heightened early; and if support is lacking for the patient or other family members the problem should be addressed, probably at a family meeting.

Fear of physical suffering is often described as the initial concern of patients and their families and most certainly should be discussed early. Giving them a plan for addressing concerns such as pain or at least letting them know it is a high priority for the doctor can be reassuring. For example, explain to them that chemotherapy has had a reputation for causing suffering, but it is now much improved.

By 2 months after the diagnosis most families are beginning to return to some semblance of normal. This is a good time to reevaluate the family's overall functioning. Are they returning to their usual activity as best they can? It is useful to ask the family again for their understanding of the illness. If despite repeated education there are still gross misconceptions about the illness, denial is likely. Denial is not necessarily pathologic unless it interferes with adjustment or adherence to treatment.

The best way to determine the more subtle adaptive changes is to ask them to describe a typical day and how it has changed since the illness had been diagnosed. The doctor should closely evaluate whether there has been excessive withdrawal from socialization or activities that used to be important. Whether there have been unnecessary changes in parenting roles, dependence, or overprotection should also be scrutinized. Hope and meaning in the patient and family's lives may take a while to be reformulated in light of the illness. By 6 months following the diagnosis, the doctor should ask patients if they are getting involved in meaningful activity. If the patient is married, it is useful to check on related issues of normalcy (e.g., sexual functioning) and how the disease has altered the marriage.

After a period of remission a flare-up of the disease can be a time of renewed grief, possibly turning into despair and depression. It is important to reevaluate patient and family function a couple of months after the first major flare occurs.

Treatment

For families who are having difficulty, intervention should be targeted at the specific problem. Guilt is one of the most common early causes of poor adjustment, and so it is the first issue to address if excessive. A number of approaches can be helpful: (1) education to clear up misconceptions on the illness; (2) forgiveness from a meaningful significant other or spiritual leader; (3) penance for a perceived contribution to the illness and a request for forgiveness. (See Chapter 28, section on guilt.)

If adherence to the treatment protocol is a problem, most likely denial or control issues are the primary concern. The first step is to attempt to renegotiate with the patient and family agreeable goals and the treatment process (see Chapter 10).

If denial is a problem after several months, reeducation should be attempted; but it is unlikely to be effective. In this circumstance, it may be useful to explain respectfully that their denial as understandable given the dysphoria of accepting the disease. Then give them the choice to not accept the disease until they are strong enough. This reframing of acceptance as strength often helps people past the denial stage (see Chapter 10).

If withdrawal and isolation are problems, the physician should prescribe a gradual return to normal activity. Because it is likely to meet with some resistance, the physician should negotiate what new activity the patient would attempt and try to gain family support in encouraging this. Follow-up should be regular (e.g., weekly) until some return to activity has been appreciated. If there is much resistance with a lot of "yes— but" responses, it may be worthwhile to involve physical and occupational therapists early, even if it is not physically necessary. Gaining confidence that the patient, despite the illness, can perform activities helps both the patient and family get back to their usual activities as quickly as possible.

If overdependence or learned helplessness has occurred and has not resolved after several months, the physician should specifically prescribe some activity that would demonstrate a more "normal" adjustment and some independence. For example, a 20-year-old returns home from college because of surgery for ulcerative colitis and is still at home despite having recovered from the surgery. The doctor should call a family conference to develop a specific plan for a return to school. Close follow-up should be maintained until this readjustment has occurred. If there is much resistance to this movement toward independence, a more gradual approach may be needed. One way to deal with the resistance is by requesting that the family undertake the difficult task of acting as though things were normal for a brief period (e.g., an hour a day). They are then to take note of how this exercise alters things. As they learn to tolerate a short period of normality, the experiment can proceed in gradually increasing increments. What is likely to occur is that needs are met in new ways, and the family members gradually desensitize the fears that led to overprotection.

If a family becomes overly distanced in response to illness onset, prescribing a family activity to bring them together can get them past this hurdle. It can be useful to set this up as a challenge in some cases. For example, "It is difficult for your family to let others see your pain, but it also robs you of supporting each other." If the family used to attend church or go to a restaurant together this activity can be suggested as a start. It is best to start slowly with these activities and gradually work to increase their frequency.

If power struggles become a problem, it is best to discuss specifically who in the family makes decisions and when and how it takes place. Often problems develop when people are overprotecting one another by not communicating painful information. For example, an elderly father's adult child may not want to confront his parents directly over the perception that they are not capable of driving or making decisions. The battles occur indirectly and therefore go unresolved. If mental status is compromised, as when brought on by a stroke, it is still best to address specifically how decisions can be made in the family. When the physician brings these issues up directly for discussion in a family conference, most families can resolve them quite well.

If the patient is married or involved in a romantic relationship, specific issues of sexuality should be addressed including, if necessary, an open discussion of how sexual interaction can take place with the couple despite disabilities. Often these discussions are avoided by the couple, but once they take place there is much relief. All that is needed in these instances is the physician's leadership in facilitating the discussion. In the case of a single person not involved in an intimate relationship, it is sometimes useful to discuss changes in body image with them and the best adaptation that could be made. Again, these issues are often of great concern to patients, yet they do not bring them up unless the physician initiates the discussion.

Sometimes, despite adaptation to the illness by the family and patient, problems develop because of a lack of opportunity to engage in meaningful activity. All too often, for example, it is easier for government administrators to put someone on total disability benefits than to give them vocational rehabilitation and work opportunity. Although laws such as the Americans with Disabilities Act may be helpful, often the physician needs to guide patients to pursue their rights assertively. It can have therapeutic and practical benefits.

The ultimate goal of the family physician should be that the chronically ill patient and family can maintain meaningful activity and relationships in their lives. Addressing the problem areas gives the best opportunity for this to occur. As Sir William Ostler said, "The way to live to a ripe old age is to develop a chronic disease and learn to accommodate to it."

Case Report

J.P. was a 63-year-old man who developed idiopathic cardiomyopathy. His work as foreman of a construction crew was seriously affected by symptoms of congestive heart failure. After a thorough cardiovascular workup confirming the diagnosis, the patient underwent treatment with furosemide (Lasix) and a series of antiarrhythmia medications, each of which caused side effects requiring discontinuation.

Previously healthy, the patient became fearful about this condition, which was worsened by a series of therapeutic failures with the antiarrhythmia drugs. J.P.'s marriage had been plagued by long-standing power struggles. With the advent of J.P.'s illness, his wife began to offer frequent advice regarding J.P.'s daily activities, food choices, and other matters out of appropriate concern for her husband's heart condition. J.P. interpreted this as a further bid for control, however. His rebellion was to the point of making choices that were detrimental to his condition.

Despite their struggles, this couple had enjoyed a healthy and active sex life. However, perhaps owing to the physical disability of the cardiomyopathy, a conditioned response to shortness of breath, the effects of medication, fear, or escalating marital discord from the control dynamic, J.P. developed impotence. His wife's reticence to have sexual activity because of fear for her husband may also have been contributing.

When J.P. was placed on a third antiarrhythmia drug his anxieties became so great that he undertook recklessly to mow a weeded vacant lot in hot weather with a push mower. He collapsed later that day in the home and was rushed to the hospital after successful treatment of a malignant arrhythmia by paramedics.

J.P.'s family physician recognized the problems with adjusting to chronic illness while the patient was in the intensive care unit. He met with J.P.'s wife and reframed J.P.'s obstinacy, lack of adherence to necessary life style changes, and his disregard of her good advice as a response to his fear. Mrs. P. was informed that J.P.'s behavior was as if he was trying to prove to himself or others that he was still okay. Mrs. P. was asked to refrain from making constructive reminders of what was or was not healthy behavior, as it was serving only to remind J.P. that he was ill. The physician promised to inquire frequently about these behaviors to ensure that these essential elements of care were not disregarded.

Near hospital discharge, the physician met with J.P. and his wife to discuss sexual matters. The possibility of temporary impotence perpetuated by performance anxiety or perhaps the effect of one of his previous medications was hypothesized. The couple was counseled that a few weeks after discharge they might return to normal sexual activity using the female superior position to reduce cardiac workload during intercourse. Mrs. P. was reassured that this was no more physically stressful for her husband than other everyday tasks he was able to perform. The physician predicted success but promised to be available to discuss the problem again if sexual dysfunction recurred.

Over the next several months J.P. became increasingly accommodated to his limitations, was compliant with taking the medications, and suffered no more side effects of prescribed drugs. In retrospect, the physician wondered whether the patient's prior problems with medications were true pharmacologic events, the results of a hyperadrenergic state due to the patient's stress and failure to accommodate to his disease, or a psychosomatic resistance to treatment. J.P.'s sexual dysfunction resolved. Marital dynamics seemed to improve for this couple, and certainly J.P.'s cardiac condition was no longer part of the "battleground." Thirteen months later J.P. died suddenly of an arrhythmia, a not unusual outcome of this disease. His wife told the family physician at the funeral that their last year together was perhaps their happiest.

References

Golden WL, Gersh WD, Robbins DM (1992) Psychological Treatment of Cancer Patients: A Cognitive-behavioral Approach. Needham Heights, MA: Allyn & Bacon.

McDaniel SH, Campbell TL, Seaburn DB (1990) The developmental challenges of chronic illness: helping families cope. In Family-oriented Primary Care: A Manual for Medical Providers. New York: Springer-Verlag.

McDaniel SH, Hepworth J, Doherty WJ (1992) Challenges in chronic illness. In Medical Family Therapy: A Biopsychosocial Approach to Families with Health Problems. New York: BasicBooks.

McDaniel SH, Hepworth J, Doherty WJ (1992) Childhood chronic illness. In Medical Family Therapy: A Biopsychosocial Approach to Families with Health Problems. New York: BasicBooks.

Minuchin S (1978) Psychosomatic Families. Cambridge, MA: President and Fellows of Harvard College.

Peteet JR, Abrams HE, Ross DM, Stearns NM (1991) Presenting a diagnosis of cancer: patients' view. J Fam Pract 32:577–581.

Rolland JS (1994) Families, Illness, and Disability: An Integrative Treatment Model. New York: BasicBooks.

Turk DC, Kerns RD (1985) Health, Illness, and Families. New York: Wiley.

26

Problems Associated with Chronic Illness in Children

ASSESSMENT

The following four questions should be asked of the parent of a child with a chronic illness. Starting at school age they are asked of the child as well. Reevaluation should take place after times of transition.

1. What activities interest the child, and at which of these activities are they good?
2. Do they have at least one good friend or, for preschoolers, are they beginning to learn to interact with peers?
3. How are they doing at preschool or school, including academic achievements, peer relations, and relations with teachers?
4. How are they getting along with family members, including how the parents maintain discipline and what parent/child activities are enjoyed outside of caretaking for the illness?

The following questions should be directed to the parents.

1. Describe any guilt feelings you have.
2. How are you receiving social support?
3. How do you balance the needs of family members?
4. How is the child's illness affecting your marriage or if unmarried your social life?
5. Are both parents in general agreement over health care issues?
6. How are you getting along with the health care team?

TREATMENT

1. If guilt is a problem:
   a. Provide education on the course of the illness and treatment process.
   b. If still a problem, recommend asking for forgiveness from significant others, clergy, or through worship and spirituality.
   c. If still a problem, recommend penance.

2. If social isolation is a problem, a specific plan for reconnecting with friends and family should be developed. A support group is helpful for some.
3. If the family has become illness-centered, recommend specific activities considered normal and non-illness-related. Normal discipline should be prescribed as much as possible.
4. Teaching the children self-care and helping them develop as much independence as possible is good preventive intervention as well as treatment for adolescent rebelliousness. At adolescence the doctor should begin to meet privately with the patient, keeping the parents informed of concerns when necessary.
5. Balancing needs in the family when problematic should entail developing a specific weekly schedule. This may require compromise by everyone.
6. If burnout is a problem, appropriate referral to Social Services may be of benefit. Once the child has reached school age, the stay-at-home mother should be encouraged to have outside activities or vocational interests.
7. If conflict between parents includes the child's health care program, schedule a meeting to work on compromises.
8. If adherence is a problem, discussing how decisions are made between the health care team and the patient and family should be discussed and compromises developed that allow the patient and family to feel empowered.
9. If there are poor relations between the health care team and the patient or family, a care conference should be requested to improve communication and compatibility.

"A good parent is not to lean on but to make leaning unnecessary." This aphorism highlights the goal of most parents. While achieving the goal of independence is filled with challenge for all parents, for those with children suffering chronic illness it is manyfold more difficult. For certain illnesses it is impossible, and different goals must be established. The stress of rearing a chronically ill child is enormous. Mental health problems in families who have children with chronic illnesses are reported to be two to three times higher than in families with healthy children. On the other hand, although this rate of psychopathology is high, it nonetheless represents only a small number of families with chronically ill children. Therefore a reasonable goal of the family physician is that the family with a chronically ill child remains psychologically healthy. There is much the family physician can do to facilitate this goal.

The time of the initial diagnosis and times of relapse are crisis points for nearly all families. For some, relapses have a greater potential to incur a pathologic response than the initial diagnosis. At the time of relapse the family is much more aware of its meaning, and naïve optimism is not possible. Grief is the universal response. Working through grief successfully has some common components. Guilt must be addressed. No matter how unreasonable, parents tend to believe there is something they should have done to prevent the illness or the relapse. The problem is especially difficult when an accident or mistake has been made (not egregious negligence), such as an automobile accident caused by a moment of human error. In such cases excessive guilt is nearly universal. To make matters worse in those cases, the other parent in some instances continues to blame the spouse overtly, subliminally, or even subconsciously. This can occur even when blame is questionable or erroneous, as in the case of a type I diabetic child who has an uncle with type I diabetes.

Social isolation must be confronted. The extended family and friends are initially supportive but usually drift away after sometime. Most people are so busy with their nuclear family there is only so much time to donate to the extended family. The resulting lowered social support for one or both parents can lead to problems and is often exacerbated when the parents are divorced or alienated from their families. Introverts prefer being solitary and so may not have well developed social networks, although at highly stressful times they too benefit from social support. Sometimes lack of support occurs when the two parents are out of sync with their grief, which is not uncommon. For example, sometimes the mother has a highly expressive grief response after a grave diagnosis, whereas the father is initially stoic. The mother interprets his reaction as uncaring or unfeeling. As time passes she starts to feel better, at which point the father may be feeling grief. Each might view the other as unsupportive in these circumstances.

Control issues occur with a small but significant number of patients. Some are seen because certain parents are prone to power struggles. In other circumstances, true disagreements can develop over goals or treatments. Compliance problems may be an issue, as patients or parents may view the doctor's interventions as being overcontrolling or overly burdensome. The doctor's style or approach can ameliorate or exacerbate this struggle (see Chapter 10). A sense of powerlessness may be especially pronounced in the child with a poor prognosis.

Another common problem is differentiating normal from abnormal. A compromise between appropriate vigilance of the child's health care status versus an overpreoccupation with the chronic illness is a difficult course to navigate. For example, all children are moody at times. On the other hand, it reflects an exacerbation of many illnesses (e.g., diabetes), or it can be a side effect of drugs (e.g., steroids). Underreaction could lead to physical morbidity; overreaction can reinforce a sick role with lower functional status than necessary.

Times of transition of either the child's developmental life cycle or the illness process usually present a significant exacerbation of stressors, increasing the risk of developing new problems. The transition of beginning school, entering adolescence, or moving out of the home to become an autonomous young adult can be stressful for all families but particularly for those with children who have a chronic illness. We discuss common problems of transition below.

The initial problem for children born with a serious illness is bonding. Bonding is related to physical proximity, including touch and eye contact. Most parents can negotiate the separations required by hospitalizations. Some parents, however, such as teenagers, are at risk for bonding problems, and the child can develop lifetime sequelae as a result. Important preventive interventions entail the physician attempting to facilitate a close bond between parents and child. Neonatal intensive care units are well aware of these dynamics and do everything possible to facilitate bonding. The family physician, often most trusted by the parents, is in a prime position to encourage this process.

The movement of the 2- or 3-year old toward autonomy can bring new problems. Sometimes it is difficult for the parent to provide firm limits when a child with a chronic illness throws a tantrum. Children use whatever means they find to have their way and can fall into a pattern of using their disease as a manipulative tool. For example, diabetic children may threaten not to eat if they are not given the foods they want.

School is a time for children to learn how to get along with their peers and explore their own abilities, which affects their self-esteem. These areas can lead to problems as well. Children rarely attempt to make friends with disabled children, who might look different or cannot play on the playground on a par with them. Children who recognize that they always are in last place can easily develop problems with self-esteem.

Adolescence presents another difficult transition when dealing with chronic illness. The primary issues of adolescence include, for example, dealing with altered body image, sexual development, and becoming more autonomous from parents; these factors can all be affected by illness. Adolescents' need to move away from primary parental support and toward their peers is frequently complicated by disease. Teenagers usually form their peer groups by being involved with those who act and look most similar to them, which often excludes children with chronic illness. Adolescent autonomy can be complicated. Care plans are usually experienced as overcontrolling by a teenager. Rebelliousness can center on adherence to a treatment protocol in these situations. It can be pronounced when the physician appears authoritarian or as "siding with the parents" by expecting high standards or technical outcomes of treatment (e.g., normal hemoglobin A1C level). The teenager is likely to be noncompliant in this circumstance. The alternative is a negotiated goal between doctor and teenager, as we discuss under Treatment, below.

Family adjustment is a significant variable. Balancing family needs is extremely difficult especially when the chronically ill child demands a great deal of time. In single parent families the demands can become impossible and lead to burnout. Siblings who do not get enough attention can develop manipulative, even pathologic ways to do so. Sometimes a cycle develops where the parent has an underlying resentment for the extreme demands of the sick child. The parent then feels guilty for these feelings and ameliorates this guilt by overindulgence, making the child even more difficult to handle and exacerbating the cycle.

Marriages have been found to be at higher risk in these families. If the child needs aides in their home, there is loss of privacy. At times there is sleep deprivation because the parents are vigilant about the monitors that are often required. Mothers sometimes have a difficult time sharing caretaking for the ill child, neglecting their own needs.

Sick children can become an easy excuse for parents to not confront the conflicts they have with each other. Sometimes children play into this by using their pathology as a distraction when the parents develop or express hostility toward each other. As a study of brittle diabetic children has shown, the symptoms in these children exacerbate at the time of heightened marital conflict. When a doctor sees a chronically ill child going through repeated periods of unexplained exacerbation, they should keep a sharp eye out for this possibility.

Despite the challenges, most families navigate chronic illness without developing mental health problems. Certain protective factors have been found to be important to this process. Families that do well develop an attitude that their child is normal with an illness rather than define their child by their illness: "I have a child with diabetes" versus "I have a diabetic child." These families adequately resolve their guilt feelings. They develop a balance between providing for the needs of the sick child, the needs of others in the family, and the needs of the marriage. Finally, it is protective when the parents can work well together to make decisions for their child even if other areas of the marriage are not good or they are divorced.

Assessment

Because families with chronically ill children are at high risk for mental health problems, it is important that the physician regularly assess risk factors so early intervention can prevent problems or they can be detected early when treatment is most effective. Because most problems develop at times of transition, the most efficient approach is to evaluate at these times (e.g., after the initial diagnosis, a serious relapse, or a developmental change such as entry into school, adolescence, or leaving home). Most children and adolescents with chronic disease are seen regularly for follow-up, so the family physician can easily include a few of the questions listed below during regularly scheduled visits.

The following four questions aimed at the child's adjustment and five aimed at the family comprise a brief but comprehensive evaluation. They are unlikely to make the child or parents uncomfortable when asked.

1. *The child and parents should be asked what activities they are interested in and at which of these activities they are good.* These questions reveal whether the child is involved in age-appropriate activities and thus is not being overprotected. It also examines self-esteem issues. Children should believe they are good at something (e.g., academics, art, sports, playing Nintendo, chess).
2. *Does the child have at least one good friend?* Even if there are problems with the peer group, if children or teenagers have at least one good friend with whom they regularly do things, it can be protective. It is critical to avoid social isolation. Pets can help, but they are not a total answer. The question for preschoolers is if they are learning to get along with peers.
3. *How are they doing at school or preschool?* This includes academic achievement, peer relations, and relations with teachers. The answer gives an idea of overall adjustment outside the family.
4. *How are they getting along with family members?* What do you enjoy doing with your child? When your child needs discipline, how do you provide it? It is important to evaluate if the child is overly indulged or is receiving age-appropriate guidance and discipline. On the other hand, does the child get non-illness-related attention from the parents? How do siblings interact?

The questions directed toward the parents include the following.

1. *Do you have guilt feelings?* If so, how do you handle these feelings? It is important to make it clear that most parents feel guilt, so it is not an abnormality. A desirable answer is something along the lines of, "Although I do have occasional guilt feelings, I also know that we are doing the best we can and it's not really our fault." An alternative that also reduces concern is, "Yes, I feel some guilt, but I'm working it through with the help of others."
2. *Who do you rely on for social support? Are you able to spend time with friends?* The answers help the physician understand if the family is overly enmeshed with each other as and if there is outside support.
3. *How do you balance the needs of family members?* Do the other children have time with the parents to spend in a normal way for their age? Do the parents have opportunities to pursue any of their interests, recreational as well as vocational?
4. *How is the child's illness affecting your marriage?* Are you usually in agreement regarding health care decisions? This question is no less important when a couple is separated or divorced. Do you enjoy a regular activity together? This answer gives an overall indication of whether there are any major conflicts between them, as highly conflicted couples tend to avoid each other even when the conflict is not overt.
5. *How do you think you are getting along with the health care team?* Issues of adherence to the treatment protocol is a good test of how the

relationship is going between the family and the medical community. If there are problems with adherence, the first issues to explore are the possibilities of a power struggle or conflicting goals. This is especially common when the patient is a teenager.

Treatment

Treatment should be aimed at the specific problems encountered. In the following section we address treatment approaches in the order they usually develop. Grief issues can often be handled through education by describing the common grief process. Normalizing the process often helps people feel more in control. This normalization should include a discussion of people's differing ways of confronting grief and differing timetables. When family members respect divergent grief processes they can more easily provide support for each other and resolve many problems.

When there is a problem with grief, excessive guilt is often the cause and must be confronted to avoid pathologic sequelae. To start, it is useful to explore the family's understanding of the disease, making sure there are no misconceptions that lead to guilt. It is important to determine if the family is socially isolated, as feedback from close associates helps ameliorate guilt. If social isolation is found, a specific plan for reconnection should be developed. Simply telling a family to socialize more rarely helps. Support groups or contacts with others who have dealt with the same disease can be helpful. If the family has good social contact and support, such groups are not always useful. Referral to a pastor can be helpful for some. (As with any referral, referral to a clergyman should be done with some knowledge of the referral source.) Guilt is sometimes alleviated when some meaning or value is found for the challenge posed by the illness. Having them write a letter expressing their feelings to someone close to them, God, or a religious authority sometimes helps even if the letter is never sent. When guilt is so pronounced it leads to depression, an approach to guilt resolution such as that described in Chapter 28 is sometimes necessary.

Because children with disabilities are better adjusted when they are treated as normally as possible, the doctor should intervene when the family becomes illness-centered. Educating the family as to all the ways the child is normal is a start. For example, "Although your child has below normal intelligence, he can compete in sports, which could benefit him." Second, normal discipline should be employed as much as possible. For example, "The steroids your daughter takes for asthma are not the cause of her tantrums, so she can be put in her room for a time-out like any other child." Third, having the child involved in as much normal activity as possible has long-term benefits. "Your child's diabetes should not prevent her from going to church camp."

Starting early to teach children self-care for their disease helps them develop normal independence. It also helps separate the child's treatment protocol from later adolescent rebelliousness. For example, the child who develops diabetes during preadolescence and has learned self-care is much less likely to manipulate diabetic control rebelliously toward parents during adolescence.

In fact, at adolescence, mirroring other development changes, it is time for the physician to manage the routine appointments differently. One of the authors refers to this transition as the "medical bar mitzvah." Parents are asked to give their teenager a measure of privacy, allowing the doctor and teenager to meet privately for their regular appointments. The parents can be told it is time for the adolescent to have an adult available to them to discuss their treatment and personal issues in private. Almost all parents allow it. In some instances they demand that issues such as birth control and substance abuse be open to them, which is not ideal but should initially be agreed to simply to open the door. This approach usually greatly reduces the likelihood of the teenager using medical adherence as a rebellious tool.

If the adolescent does become rebellious toward medical management, parents often become more vigilant, which makes the outcome worse. One approach is to take the parents out of the management loop. Start by telling the parents, "I will inform you if there is a serious problem, but otherwise I would like you to trust that your teenager and I are working things out together. Yes, there is some slight risk in your not being as involved, but there is more risk in your being involved and the teenager rebelling against you. I will meet with the teen regularly (once a week to start); your job is to treat your child as if he [or she] does not have an illness." It is useful to start by seeing the teenager frequently (even if not necessary for managing diabetes control) to reassure the parents. A similar approach to other high maintenance illnesses such as cystic fibrosis or asthma can also be employed.

Preventing social isolation for the more severely handicapped child can be a real challenge. However, even when disabilities significantly prevent them from competing athletically or academically, with some creativity an activity can be found to get them involved with a peer. Sometimes school-teachers can be asked to help. Playing chess, a computer game on the web, and billiards or playing in the band are examples of opportunities for the child to experience being on an equal basis with other children. Another option is certain formal groups. For example, a Scout or church group with a sensitive leader can sometimes be recruited to help guide and direct peer interaction to make sure the child feels included. In many areas summer camps are available for children with disabilities or chronic illnesses to help them develop socially as they move toward independence. Activities often include disease self-management and self-esteem building activities. They can be especially helpful for guiding a child toward independence from overly protective parents.

When balancing the needs of the various family members is a problem, it is useful to have a meeting with either the parents or the family to discuss specific ways to address this problem. In general, the more specific the plan the more likely it can lead to real change. For example, give them a homework assignment to develop a weekly schedule that considers the needs of all family members. It is important for the family physician to plan a return visit to discuss the outcome of the assignment. Not only does this help address any snags in the plan, it promotes completion of the assigned tasks. Social Services can sometimes be asked to help them obtain respite care services if required to accomplish these goals. If there is strong resistance to marriage time, the doctor should entertain the possibility that the illness is being used as an excuse to avoid a marital conflict or some other problem such as guilt. If burnout and significant mental health problems are not to develop, especially for the single parent, it is important that respite care somehow be attained. Once children have reached school age, it has also been found that the mother having outside activities or vocational interests can help prevent enmeshment with the child.

When decision-making about the child's medical care needs has become a source of conflict between parents, regardless of whether they are married, this issue must be addressed or serious problems will develop. Not infrequently the child's symptoms exacerbate during times of conflict between the two parents even when the parents believe the child is unaware. For married parents, meeting with the doctor conjointly to work out a solution usually resolves the problem unless it represents long-standing marital conflict. Whatever is decided it must appear to both parties as a compromise plan and not appear as if either has won a contest of who was "right." When the lack of conflict resolution represents a more general marriage problem, marital counseling may be beneficial if the couple agrees.

In the circumstance described earlier where the child's illness problems become a way to avoid focusing on marital conflict, the doctor's intervention is important and complex. Referral almost never works because the parents in these circumstances rarely admit to a problem. The doctor must keep the overt explanation for working on the problem focused on the child's difficulties. This explanation provides the physician with enough flexibility to make recommendations to the parents to help them deal with conflict in a way that does not exacerbate the child's symptoms.

For example, after hospitalizing a child several times for diabetic ketoacidosis the family physician suspects that problems at home are contributing to the brittle diabetes. Fueling this view is the observation that the child does well in the hospital but returns soon after discharge. In the hospital the mother is ever present, but the father seems distant. On the one occasion the physician spoke with the parents together the father seemed concerned about the child, but there was unexpressed tension between the couple. The doctor can only assume that the child is more sensitive to this "tension" than the physician can ever be. Because in somatizing families this "tension" is unlikely to be acknowledged, the physician must deal with it indirectly. The doctor does this by requesting that the couple work together on a plan for better diabetic control. It is important for the family doctor to spend time with the couple working on this plan lest the couple revert to avoidance patterns. Although the plan focuses on good diabetic control, the physician should require that the plan include a number of activities the couple performs cooperatively. The doctor can emphasize that the child's management is difficult and complicated and only with good coordination can it be successful. When there is "tension" between the couple it should be pointed out as normal but that a compromise must be found. Follow-up must be planned to include both parents. These sessions can take a half-hour to an hour but are time savers if it prevents further diabetic crisis. The same is true for other illnesses.

If the couple is separated or divorced with high conflict interfering with treatment, the physician may have to broker a compromise by meeting with each parent individually. It is often useful to "blame" the child for the problem to win the cooperation of the parents: "I'm concerned your child is manipulating both of you with his [or her] diabetic control. Only by working together can you help your child alter this behavior." Again, the resolution must seem to be a compromise to both parties not requiring either to "give in" if it is to be a lasting resolution. This is true even if the physician believes one or the other is a better solution. On rare occasions when parental discord seriously interferes with illness management, the physician may have to notify the Child Protective Services of neglect. In this situation, it is best for the doctor to describe the problem and let the agency explore culpability so the doctor can remain neutral. This wake-up call in some cases leads to improved cooperation between the warring parties.

When there is an adherence problem in the chronically ill family, it implies a power struggle or disagreement between the doctor and someone in the family. Although, as stated in the Assessment section, sometimes the power struggle is within the family and not between the health care team and the patient. When it is with the health care team, making sure the parents feel part of the decision-making process is essential. Sometimes when a number of consultants are involved this includes coaching the parents on how to be assertive with other health care professionals. When possible, this is a better choice than the physician being assertive on behalf of the patient, although sometimes this is necessary as well.

Occasionally as a result of grief, guilt, or personality nurses or other caregivers become targets of hostility. It is important for the family doctor to not be triangulated (take sides) here. Triangulation can occur only when one party gives "he/she said" or "he/she did" information to the physician. This cannot occur when both parties are with the physician. Usually the situation can be improved by calling a care conference and exploring alternative ways for needs to be met. Although logistically difficulty and emotionally taxing, it can help alleviate many problems.

Research studies and anecdotal reports have shown the benefits of the primary care doctor coordinating care. This is especially true when several subspecialists are involved. Family physicians, rather than withdrawing when pediatric subspecialists are involved, should maintain responsibility for the overall care of the child.

Case Reports

As a youngster, President Theodore Roosevelt suffered childhood asthma so severe his entire family feared for his life. His periodic bouts of asthma consumed the family's attention. His parents were said by all to have an idyllic marriage. When young Theodore left home for college his family worried greatly that without their attention at times of asthma exacerbations he would not survive. Surprisingly, Theodore did not experience another bout of asthma until he returned home at the Christmas break after his first semester.

Knowing the dynamics of chronic illness during childhood, one may speculate with fair assurance that Mr. and Mrs. Roosevelt likely had relationship problems. As their marital stress escalated and approached a point where there was likely to be some confrontation, little Theodore "learned" that if he were to experience an exacerbation of his asthma family attention would be diverted to him and marital confrontation would be avoided. Considering the effects of psychological stress on adrenergic function, acute-phase reactants, and the pulmonary system this "learning" need not have been conscious.

W.B. was a 7-year old type I diabetic who had been hospitalized four times in 1 year for ketoacidosis. None of these episodes was associated with noncompliance with insulin therapy, concomitant infections, or any other known precipitating factor. Once hospitalized, W.B.'s treatment and recovery were not particularly complicated. W.B.'s parents would stay at the child's bedside together for hours. They showed mutual concern and caring for their child. Recognizing this as a problem case, the managed care company responsible for this family authorized a comprehensive, interdisciplinary diabetes team evaluation. The social worker and psychologist on the team identified a troubled marital relationship as a possible factor in W.B.'s recurrent ketoacidosis.

The family physician and psychologist worked as co-therapists to W.B., his parents, and his three older siblings. At a family session they saw the nondiabetic children as close with their mother, whereas W.B. and his father appeared quite close. To test their hypothesis, the therapists asked the parents to develop a plan for how they would work together on monitoring W.B.'s blood sugar levels more closely. The doctors initially would not let the children join the discussion. Mrs. B soon complained that her husband was there to have fun with W.B. and would help when things got bad; but when it came to daily care of the illness it was all her responsibility. W.B. came to the rescue arguing on his father's behalf. This was followed by the other children joining the argument in defense of the mother. The two "camps" showed increasing discord until this reached a dramatic level, at which point W.B., the youngest, said that he was not feeling well, that his blood sugar was probably low, and that he needed some candy. The problem was forgotten, the family stress noticeably diminished, and attention was focused on W.B. Believing their suspicions confirmed, the therapists collaborated to involve W.B.'s parents in a series of visits designed to educate them about complicated diabetes and help them develop strategies to work together to prevent deterioration of W.B.'s condition. During the educational sessions the effect of stress, epinephrine (adrenaline), and norepinephrine on liver glycogen and gluconeogenesis was explained. Framed in this way the parents agreed to receive counseling aimed at working together for diabetic control. W.B. had another bout of ketoacidosis 1 month after this therapy began and then no episodes over the following 3 years.

Most couples who successfully use counseling for their children's health decline marital counseling. However, when the physician suggested counseling might help their marriage in areas other than the health of their children, this couple expressed openness. The family physician met several times with the parents, uncovering intimacy and control issues. These problems spilled over into the sexual arena. Using techniques described in Chapter 22, the family physician was able to help the couple.

References

Golden WL, Gersh WD, Robbins D M (1992) Psychological Treatment of Cancer Patients: A Cognitive-behavioral Approach. Needham Heights, MA: Allyn & Bacon.

McDaniel SH, Campbell TL, Seaburn DB (1990) The developmental challenges of chronic illness: helping families cope. In Family-oriented Primary Care: A Manual for Medical Providers. New York: Springer-Verlag.

McDaniel SH, Hepworth J, Doherty WJ (1992a) Challenges in chronic illness. In Medical Family Therapy: A Biopsychosocial Approach to Families with Health Problems. New York: BasicBooks.

McDaniel SH, Hepworth J, Doherty WJ (1992b) Childhood chronic illness. In Medical Family Therapy: A Biopsychosocial Approach to Families with Health Problems. New York: BasicBooks.

Minuchin S (1978) Psychosomatic Families. Cambridge, MA: President and Fellows of Harvard College.

Peteet JR, Abrams HE, Ross DM, Stearns NM (1991) Presenting a diagnosis of cancer: patients' view. J Fam Pract 32:577–581.

Rolland, JS (1994) Families, Illness, and Disability: An Integrative Treatment Model. New York: BasicBooks.

Turk DC, Kerns RD (1985) Health, Illness, and Families. New York: Wiley.

27

Problems in the Nursing Home

ASSESSMENT

1. For a reported problem in a nursing home, discuss the problem with a representative of the nursing staff. Explore with the staff how the problem occurs within the context of their typical day. Establish who is most bothered by the problem.
2. Evaluate patients in their room. If cognitively able, have the patients describe a typical day and their view of any problems or concerns during the course of their day. Explore how they get along with others, including nursing home staff, other residents, and family members during visits.
3. Evaluate what needs might be met by the problematic behavior (e.g., need for control, attention, emotional intimacy, avoiding a sense of purposelessness of life, boredom). If questionable, a mental status evaluation should be completed.

PLAN

1. In a few cases simply changing the way the patient's day is organized or adding an activity is all that is needed.
2. Usually a case conference is required to alleviate the problems. The conference should include nursing home staff, in some cases recreational or rehabilitation staff, a social worker, family, and if cognitively able the patient.
   a. If there are conflicts in the family over care of the patient, a family meeting should precede the care conference.
   b. The care conference should begin with each person defining his or her view of the problem within the patient's life context and solutions that have already been tried.
   c. Obtain a consensus of the group on realistic goals and expectations.
   d. Explore options that will have the patient's needs met in a new way.

> e. A behavioral program should be developed that reinforces pro-social ways of having needs met and extinguishes the problem behavior.

Thomas Jefferson wrote in the Preamble to the Constitution that there are certain inalienable rights: life, liberty and the pursuit of happiness. Sigmund Freud wrote that psychological health requires us "to love and to work."

Unfortunately, when patients are admitted to the nursing home, requirements for maintaining life are often so consuming that pronounced compromises must be made in the areas of liberty and the pursuit of happiness, particularly in the areas of maintaining meaningful relationships and meaningful activities. In response, patients often get into power struggles with the staff to the point of using manipulative or antisocial behavior. Other patients, when faced with the loss of control over their lives or insufficient social intimacy, respond by becoming withdrawn and inactive (learned helplessness).

The nursing home staff, sometimes overwhelmed with the task of keeping a large number of patients in the best possible physiologic condition with the inherent conflicts with other needs, often quickly resort to the use of medication. In recent years, however, more enlightened nursing home staffs have turned to other methods to deal with behavioral problems, using medications for behavior restraint only as a last resort—when nothing else succeeds and residents and staff are made uncomfortable.

Assessment

Dealing effectively with behavioral problems in the nursing home usually requires a team effort, with the health care team, the patient, and the family working together. Commonly, it is the family or nursing staff that brings a problem to the physician's attention.

It is often best to assess the problems in two parts. The initial action is a visit to the nursing home where the physician, prior to seeing the patient, discusses problems with a representative of the nursing staff. When getting the information from the nursing personnel it is useful to obtain a description of a typical day for the patient and of the problem behavior within the context of that day. It is important to establish who is most bothered by the problem.

It is usually best to evaluate patients in their own rooms rather than in an examination room, as it gives the physician more information about the context of the problems. Often patients do not recognize that there is a problem, or if they do they describe it as the nursing staff bothering them. Again, obtaining a description of a typical day from them and when the problems are most likely to occur along with the sequence of events surrounding the problem is useful information. By the end of the assessment, the physician should have some idea as to what needs are being met by the problematic behavior—whether more control, attention, or closeness, avoiding a sense of purposelessness in life, or boredom. Finally, the assessment should include a mental status examination unless the patient's cognition has been evaluated within a reasonable period of time.

Plan

After this evaluation simple changes in the way the patient's day is organized may make a difference in how his or her needs are met. For most patients a care conference is necessary that includes nursing care staff, preferably the charge nurse and at least one other member of the nursing staff who has regular contact with the patient. If the patient is in a rehabilitation program it is often useful to have a member of that treatment group present; the nursing home social worker is often valuable at the meeting as is at least one spokesperson for the family. If there is dissent within the family or poor family communication, it is often useful to have family members representing different viewpoints at the meeting. It is most often useful to have patients present also for the meeting, unless they are so cognitively compromised they are unable to really understand the proceedings of the meeting and become uncomfortable, disrupting the ongoing process. If family members are highly conflicted it may be of value to meet with them prior to meeting with the larger group.

The care conference should begin with each person, in turn, defining the problem, sequence of events, attempted solutions, and how they see the problem fitting into the context of the patient's life. Each person should have an opportunity to speak without interruption. If patients are cognitively competent, they should, depending on their wish, go either first or last. It is often useful to give the patient's family a special place also at the meeting so they can feel empowered, usually asking them to go first with a description of their concerns. The physician need not go into great detail with those who have already been interviewed.

Before a treatment plan is offered, it is important to define and obtain a consensus from the group on realistic goals and expectations. Sometimes a compromise must be reached between family members and nursing staff as to what the goals might be. It is usually important to find some middle ground regarding this to gain cooperation and make it less likely that someone will undermine the plan if they do not accept it. A physician's expertise on what goals are realistic is also a component. Because unrealistic goals lead to failure on everyone's part, it is better to set low goals and achieve them than to set too high goals and fail.

When strategizing a treatment plan, the physician should consider what needs were ultimately met by the problematic behavior. Problem behavior, as stated, can lead the resident to feel more in control, gain more attention, deal with boredom, or in the case of social withdrawal and inactivity avoid the uncomfortable process of facing the meaning of one's life. A successful plan alters interactions and the sequence of events in a direction that makes it less likely for the problematic behavior to meet these needs while at the same time provide alternative behaviors that are likely to meet the needs.

For example, a patient with good cognition may be causing trouble that leads to the family being called. The family may then argue with the staff, and the patient thus gets attention from the family for the problems he or she is causing. The patient is likely to change if the family is available more often when things are going well than when trouble occurs. This can be explained by saying, "Because your family will save time by not getting calls for problems, they will have extra time to spend with you, taking you to church or perhaps shopping on Saturdays, if you make the special effort to get along with the staff." Similar compromises can be worked out with control issues. "If you agree to take your meals in the dining room, rather than in your room, the staff will be able to spend less time on that so they can arrange to make sure you can choose whoever you want to help you with your bath; otherwise you will have to have whoever is available."

Regarding a patient who gets into difficulty when bored, along with those who are trying to find some value or meaning to their lives, it is sometimes useful to try new activities that fit into what used to give their life meaning in the past in a general way. For example, if residents have been "caretakers" (i.e., enjoyed taking care of other people either as a parent or in some other similar activity), finding ways they could help people in the nursing home can be useful. Initially it may take some kind of reward to entice them to do it until they discover that the activity is rewarding in itself. Although there may be laws that prevent patients from performing jobs in the nursing home, if the job is defined as therapy it is acceptable that the patient undertake some volunteer jobs. By giving them a sense of purpose, patients feeling much better about themselves.

For the patient whose mental status is compromised, programs based on "classic conditioning" are likely to be most effective; that is, immediate consistent rewards are given for good behavior, whereas extinguishing responses (i.e., no reward) or even uncomfortable experiences can be associated with problematic behavior. An extinguishing response must never be disrespectful or painful. An example might be every time patients spit at a staff member, that staff member (after making sure the patient is safe) leaves the room and ignores the patient for 20 minutes even if screaming ensues. This approach often alters the behavior even of patients who are highly compromised. Classic conditioning, however, takes time to be effective for the demented patient. It may take many repetitions of both the positive and extinguishing responses before behavioral change is seen. Inconsistency of staff response totally inhibits the success of the plan. Staff must be made aware that it is likely to take some time before the target goals are reached, but they must keep working at it or it will never happen. For example, a patient who enjoys being touched can expect frequent pats on the back when they are quiet versus being ignored when they scream.

It is important to gain consensus on this plan. Strong disagreement by nursing staff or family leads to recurring problems

Case Report

M.T. was an 82-year-old woman residing at the Shady Oaks Nursing Home. On monthly rounds the physician was approached by the nursing staff and asked to prescribe haloperidol or valproic acid for the patient's "unreasonable and demanding behavior." Although pressed for time, the family physician asked for an exact description of the behavior. He learned that the patient pushed the call light requesting the head of her bed be pulled up or down, the curtains be opened or closed, and to be helped to the bathroom (she needed no assistance and, when taken, might or might not urinate). The patient was usually verbally abusive to staff, criticizing everything they did. Requests for assistance were not concordant with the patient's true functional status; that is, she asked for things to be done for her that she was perfectly capable of doing for herself. These requests sometimes occurred many times an hour.

The physician asked what time of day was worst and the nurse replied that it was "all the time." He asked what preceded the behavior (e.g., what might trigger the behavior). There was no important information forthcoming. He asked what the staff did in response to these unnecessary requests for assistance and the nurse reported that staff regularly argued with the patient, pointing out her abilities and telling her that they were "too busy" for her to interrupt them needlessly. The nurse reported that M.T. was asking for her pain pills more often than they were ordered (hydrocodone/acetaminophen 5.5/500 qid as needed for pain) and would become verbally abusive when she did not receive them. She complained of severe pain the nurses believed was not real.

The physician reviewed the chart and was reminded that this patient suffered mild vascular dementia and was depressed. Her blood pressure control was adequate; she was on a lipid-lowering drug and two baby aspirin daily. She had received fluoxetine 40 mg daily for the past 4 months. A pretreatment Geriatric Depression Scale (short form) had scored 9, and a repeat test 1 month ago scored 4. These tests, then, indicated a high likelihood of major depression before treatment and significant improvement after treatment. On visiting with the resident the physician found her irritable and critical of the staff. She said she was lonesome for home and family. During her earlier life the resident had been a debutante and then a socialite, and the physician suspected some narcissistic personality traits. The resident was obviously lonely.

The physician later met with the Director of Nursing, the staff nurse, and the nurse's aide caring for the resident on this shift. He pointed out that the resident was showing some signs of learned helplessness and that her motivation for these behaviors was to "get a rise out of the staff" to receive attention. He reminded the staff that people may seek attention even if it is negative attention. He pointed out that the nursing care plan would have to be shared with the other shifts, as consistency would be critical to making behavioral changes. He suggested that the resident wanted to "get their goat," and it might be best if they did not give it to her. He recommended a reverse token system. The resident would receive five tokens at the start of each shift. If the patient made unreasonable demands or was verbally abusive, the staff would withdraw one token. They were not to show any emotion but simply withdraw a token and explain why to the patient. At the end of each shift if the resident had even one token remaining she could "spend it" for a 30-minute pleasant one-on-one activity of her choice with the staff person of her choice.

Regarding the patient's pain control, the physician accepted the patient's need for better control. He suggested that perhaps he had erred in prescribing the pain medication on an as-needed basis. He explained to the staff that she might feel obliged to escalate her symptoms to obtain effective medicine. The physician prescribed timed-release oxycodone scheduled each 12 hours and a rescue dose of her prior pain medicine up to twice daily as needed for breakthrough pain.

He assured the resident that he intended to increase the dose of the long-acting pain medication until it was strong enough to control the pain almost all the time. He told her about the token system, framing it as a way to provide time and attention fairly to the resident. She might use staff time for little services or save it for a pleasant activity. He also pointed out that many of her criticisms might be well taken, but she was making her complaints to the wrong people. He told her he had arranged for her to meet with the Director of Nursing each Tuesday morning for one-half hour, at which time she should list her complaints in a formal fashion.

These interventions were noted in the doctor's progress note and physician's orders. The staff incorporated them into the comprehensive nursing care plan, thereby avoiding any appearance of resident abuse but focusing on therapeutic intervention.

For a brief time the resident's behavior worsened. The physician had to reiterate the importance of the treatment plan and inform the staff that no medication was available to change this behavior unless it were designed simply to "snow the patient." He reminded staff of the clause in "OBRA 87" rules clearly disallowing physical or chemical restraints for the purpose of facility convenience. He asked them to increase their efforts and to be sure that the staff on the other shifts had "bought into" the plan and were following it consistently.

He received no further calls about this resident. When he visited the home the following month the nurse reported that the plan was beginning to work and that the patient almost always was able to retain at least one token and receive her reward. The physician directed staff to increase the "price" of the reward to two tokens and later to three and then four. His initial interventions for pain had also worked and required no further upward titration. The Director of Nursing reported that after two meetings on Tuesdays, at which the resident had made only a few feeble complaints, M.T. herself had declined to meet any longer.

These improvements were maintained over many months, and at the end of 1 year the fluoxetine was discontinued. Several nurse aides actually expressed a preference for caring for M.T. and continued to have one-on-one activities even after this option was deleted from the care plan. The physician dictated a quick memo to the Director of Nursing with a copy to the nursing home administrator expressing his appreciation to the home and its staff for a job well done on this case.

References

Carstensen LL, Edelstein BA (1987) Handbook of Clinical Gerontology. New York: Pergamon.

Christie-Seely J (1984) Working with the Family in Primary Care, a Systems Approach to Health and Illness. New York: Praeger.

Mace NL, Rabins P (1991) The 36-Hour Day. Baltimore: Johns Hopkins University Press.

Slama K, Smith D (1995) Sleep Disorders in Old Age Monograph. Providence RI: Manissess Communications Group.

Smith D (1995) Behavioral Intervention Monograph. Providence, RI: Manissess Communications Group.

Smith D (2000) Recognition and treatment of anxiety in long term care. Ann Long Term Care 8(3):88–89.

Smith D, Amundson L (1995) Psychotropic Medication Compliance by Elders Monograph. Providence, RI: Manissess Communications Group.

Stewart JT (1995) Management of behavior problems in the demented patient. Am Fam Physician 52:2311–2317.

28

Death: Dying and Grief

GIVING BAD NEWS

1. Bad news about diagnosis should be presented with a significant other present.
2. Diagnosis, treatment options, and a broad description of the prognosis should be short and, at first encounter, not detailed. Expect to repeat it on several occasions.
3. Always provide some form of hope, even if it is assurance that the patient can be comfortable.

ASSESSING PATIENT AND FAMILY ADAPTATION

Predictors of good adjustment include the following.
1. A supportive, well functioning family, which includes a balance between cohesion and independence.
2. Open communication among family members including positive feelings and anger.
3. A sense of control over one's destiny.
4. For families who offer good support, education and discussion of treatment options is usually all that is necessary.

PROBLEMATIC DENIAL

1. Denial can be beneficial unless it interferes with treatment.
2. For problematic denial, the doctor communicates with great empathy that the patients have good reasons for denial, explains the reasons in terms of protection against painful reality, and recommends that they maintain the denial until they are ready to accept the illness.

PATHOLOGIC GRIEF

1. Preventive intervention: After 3 months promote a return to some normal socialization and activity for the family and patient (as much as possible). Make sure guilt is being adequately addressed.

2. Significant signs of pathologic grief include excessive guilt, depressive symptomatology lasting longer than a year (should gradually diminish after 3 months), prolonged social isolation or withdrawal, emotional lability or numbing, denial interfering with one's life style, somatoform disorders, substance abuse, or marital or family problems.
3. If pathologic grief is a problem:
   a. Evaluate and treat unresolved guilt through the four-step process (see text).
   b. Develop a specific plan for returning to usual activities and overcoming social isolation. This may require the help of significant others to help the person become involved in new activities.
   c. If persons feel their lives are purposeless as a result of the loss, help them explore what used to give their life meaning and develop a plan for returning to meaningful activity.
   d. Learned helplessness: Family members should be directed to reinforce nonsick behavior rather than reinforce dependent behavior.

FAMILY PROBLEMS

1. If in response to a dying patient or grieving, the family is disengaging rather than pulling together during a crisis, it is often related to difficulties with anger, guilt, burnout, power struggles, or past jealousies.
2. Organize a family conference to discuss how the family can help the patient and each other through this difficult period.
3. Define anger as a normal reaction to guilt and give them specific ways to resolve it.
4. Power struggles: Discuss how the family can make decisions together.
5. Jealousy: Discuss how the family can be more supportive of each other.
6. Burnout leading to guilt and withdrawal: Develop realistic goals for treatment and realistic ways to meet them.
7. For patients who do not have good family support, refer to a support group.

The importance of the family physician to dying patients and their families has been demonstrated repeatedly. Unfolding events often lead the physician to develop an involved relationship with the patient and family, a relationship usually strongly valued by them. Although there is no correct way for a patient and family (family is meant to include significant others) to face this suffering, there are ways the doctor can help guide care toward the best adjustment possible and help reduce the likelihood of pathologic, psychological, or social sequelae. The family physician taking care of the patient and family is in an ideal position to assess the process and intervene when there appear to be problems.

Giving Bad News

The way bad news is presented to the patient and family, if done well, can lay the foundation for good communication throughout the course of the illness. Giving bad news is best done with a spouse (or significant other) present who shares the experience with the patient and can provide support. Giving bad news over the phone or indirectly through another, such as a nurse, is avoided if possible. The initial disclosure from the known, trusted family doctor is also usually superior to learning it from subspecialists or surgeons, even if they have more facts on the pathology or treatment.

To decrease anticipatory anxiety as much as possible when there is significant suspicion leading to a diagnostic procedure, the patient should be requested to have a spouse or family member with them at the follow-up appointment. The doctor might put it this way, "Whenever we do this kind of test just in case something is found that requires treatment, I prefer to have a spouse present to discuss the disease and treatment. So as a precaution, please bring someone with you for your appointment."

At the appointment, when the new diagnosis is discussed, with everyone including the doctor seated, the physician should start with a simple, short explanation of the diagnosis, treatment options, and some broad description of the prognosis. The doctor should begin with any positive signs, as little information is processed after the diagnosis is announced. In fact, the doctor should expect little to be understood beyond the diagnosis at this initial encounter. Patients should be encouraged to ask questions. The doctor should accept some silent moments while the family and patient gather their thoughts and feelings. In the case of terminal illness, the question "How much longer do I have?" sometimes comes up. Predictions by doctors have not been shown to be particularly accurate, so the question is best answered using broad parameters rather than a specific length of time. For example, the doctor might say, "Most people with your condition live 3 weeks to 18 months, a few live longer or shorter times." It is always important to give some kind of hope even if it is only reassurance that the patient can be kept comfortable. The physician should expect denial at times, as this is a way for people to deal with overwhelming grief. Denial should be accepted as normal so long as it does not interfere with required treatment. People acknowledge poor prognoses at a rate they can handle.

Assessing Patient and Family Adaptation

The emotional intensity during both anticipatory grieving and subsequent bereavement often leads families to pull together, but it can also lead to exacerbation of past disconnections. Although some individual characteristics (discussed below) lead to poor adjustment, support by a well functioning family is the single best predictor of adequate adjustment to death or dying.

Families who cope with a severe illness and grief the best are those who have a good balance between cohesion and independence among the individuals, openly communicate both positive feelings and anger, and have some sense of control over their destiny. For those who have problematic support, referral to a support group (e.g., cancer support group, church group) is helpful. For patients who have good family relationships, the family physician can focus primarily on keeping them well informed and giving them a sense of control over their care.

Problematic Denial

Denial initially is expected and helps the patient and family adjust to painful news at a rate that can be tolerated. It is only when it is excessive that it becomes a problem. The physician then must decide if the denial has become so troublesome an intervention is necessary. The treatment described below is usually effective, but it is likely to unleash a painful response.

When necessary, one way to help a family past troublesome denial is to use a restraining approach (as described in Chapter 1). The physician describes all of the reasons they do not want to accept the diagnosis. For example, the physician might say, "It is extremely painful to accept the diagnosis of this disease, which is likely to lead to premature death. In fact, it is so painful that some people don't have the strength to acknowledge it. They are afraid that the sadness will become so overwhelming they won't be able to function, or they are fearful their family will crumble. I can see your reason for not wanting to believe that you have this disease, but the denial now is causing problems regarding treatment that would be beneficial. However, you know what is best. If you are not yet ready to accept this diagnosis and the grief that goes along with it, I recommend that you avoid accepting it as long as you need to despite the repercussions."

Nearly always in the face of this restraining reframe, patients and families drop their denial at least in part and are more accepting. They also suffer more psychological pain, than if they maintained the denial.

Family Problems

Families commonly pull together in the face of bad news, motivated by the common problem of caring for a dying person and the feelings of camaraderie in mutual loss. For some families, however, facing tragedy leads to the opposite: conflict and alienation. Families who have difficulty dealing with anger or who have frequent power struggles or jealousy because of feelings of neglect are particularly prone to these difficulties. For these problems a family meeting to discuss how they can best help the dying patient can be helpful.

For families experiencing conflicts with each other over caretaking decisions, it is often useful to define the anger as a normal reaction to grief, particularly the frustration of dealing with painful feelings. This reframing of anger allows families to not push each other away. It may also be helpful to request that the family put long past conflicts on hold in order to be helpful in the immediate crisis situation. (Techniques discussed in Chapter 22 regarding the resolution of marital conflicts can also be employed if the simple request to ask them not to get into past problems does not turn things around.)

If family members have in the past had a sense of powerlessness, it can make them more sensitive to control issues with the doctors as well. It is important in this instance that the physician clearly communicates to the family that the family's and patient's decisions will guide the treatment and that the physician will develop a partnership with them as far as treatment decisions. It is sometimes useful to discuss specifically how the family would like decisions to be made, including the issue of advanced directives.

As time goes on with a terminal disease, other issues may become prominent. Burnout particularly can lead to guilt and withdrawal or to frustration and anger. The physician in this situation may need to sit down with the patient and family to talk about realistic goals and realistic ways to reach them. Opportunities for the family to obtain necessary relief from caregiving responsibility should also be discussed. When these issues are most troublesome, usually pronounced guilt feelings are at the root and must be discussed and dealt with directly.

Early Signs of Problems

Social withdrawal from everyone for more than a few weeks, dropping out of normal activity when unnecessary for more than a few weeks, guilt to the point of self-destructiveness, or any other symptoms that do not begin to resolve within a few months should be given some attention by the physician. Some short-term social withdrawal, anger, guilt, sadness, sleeplessness, general anxiety, loss of appetite, and lethargy are well known signs of normal grief. As stated, time plus family support for most is not only all that is needed, but it is usually the best remedy. It is not helpful to define symptoms of normal grief (e.g., depression) as pathology.

Pathologic Grief

To evaluate how a family is doing after loss of a loved one, it is useful to meet with them a month or two later to discuss the death. If there is an autopsy, it can be discussed as well. At this point, feelings of guilt can be assessed. A month or two after the loss the family should be making plans to get back to some normal activities if they have not already done so. Some may even be thinking about new activities that will give new meaning to their lives, although perhaps they do not yet have the energy to engage in them.

It can take a year before the bereaved parties are functioning at their normal level. Treatment should be considered if there is no improvement regarding guilt, withdrawal, isolation, and inactivity after 3 months. Intervention early for these problems can prevent a pathologic grief reaction from developing.

Signs of unresolved grief include the following.

1. Dysthymic symptoms (particularly a pervasive sense of worthlessness and self-blame) that have not diminished after several months
2. Prolonged social isolation, withdrawal, or alienation
3. Emotional numbing or flat emotional presentation
4. Inability to cry
5. Strong denial
6. Persistent compulsive overactivity without a sense of loss
7. Persistence of a variety of physical complaints, such as headaches, fatigue, dizziness, or multiple injuries
8. Profound identification with the deceased or prolonged acquisition of symptoms associated with the illness of the deceased
9. Extreme, persistent anger (may be directed at the physician)
10. Alcohol or drug abuse, persistent requests for sedative or narcotic medications (must be addressed immediately)
11. Marital or family problems (can be especially prominent after the death of a child and not uncommon after the death of an elderly parent)
12. Work or school problems

Addressing one of more of the following three primary issues usually leads to a significant improvement regarding unresolved grief.

1. Pathologic guilt
2. Isolation and inactivity
3. Loss in the meaning of life that cannot be redirected

When thinking about how to deal with pathologic guilt, it is useful to consider how guilt is dealt with normally by people. People commonly assuage guilt using four successive processes, usually proceeding to the next one only if the preceding one does not work. (1) They seek to discover if they are at fault. (2) If they believe they are at fault, they ask for forgiveness from the injured party. (3) They ask for forgiveness from a higher authority, such as their pastor, other respected person, or God. (4) They seek to pay penance and then again request forgiveness.

When guilt is overwhelming, the physician can help them through this process. First, give them information about the usual cause of the death and realistically what could have been done to prevent it. If this does not help, suggest that they discuss their guilt feelings with family members or significant others. A family meeting with the family physician might help. If this does not work, explore with the bereaved who they would look to as having enough authority to offer forgiveness. If this fails to relieve guilt, some plan for paying recompense adequate to relieve guilt can be planned.

For example, a woman who is convinced that she could have done more for her sister who died of end-stage complications of diabetes was seen for pathologic grief. Many people had tried to help her by educating her about the natural course of diabetes and offering reassurance. She had talked to her pastor previously without relief. This having failed, we decided penance was required. We requested she work for 1 year in a hospice program as a volunteer before she would be allowed to have any enjoyment. She initially reacted, stating this would be a most painful activity for her, to which we agreed. Six months later she returned stating that she thought that she had paid penance enough and she was ready to go on with her life. Her symptoms of pathologic grief were much improved, so her penance was concluded.

Withdrawal, isolation, and inactivity can maintain an unresolved grief reaction. Often people who are in this situation have in the past habitually withdrawn into a cocoon when under stress. It usually was time limited, and after a period of time they returned to their usual activities and functioned normally again. Faced with a serious loss, some are mired in their isolation. The common reaction is, "I'll get back to my usual activity when I feel better." This often leads to a downward spiral with the onset of many depressive symptoms. Usually the patient must discover that the opposite is the case: In fact, returning to their usual activities, including interpersonal activities, leads to the resolution of many of the symptoms of pathologic grief. Specifically discussing a plan to become reinvolved in activities in a stepwise fashion is required to motivate them to change. Sometimes the family must be mobilized to help the bereaved become involved in activities that are meaningful. For the person resistant to making any changes in regard to their withdrawal, isolation, and inactivity, it is sometimes useful to use an "as if" approach (described in Chapter 1). Specifically, the patient and family (or friends) are requested to, for a brief time perhaps starting with an hour a day, act "as if" they were feeling somewhat better; everyone is to treat them as though they were normal for the hour. The duration of "normality" is then gradually increased.

Sometimes when people are mired in pathologic grief secondary gain is involved. When exploring the sequence of events surrounding the withdrawal and social isolation, it may become evident that when the bereaved is morose, withdrawn, and inactive others attempt to "cheer them up." This happens not infrequently when the person who died has been a caretaker-type person. This leads to the survivor, usually not consciously aware, establishing a pattern of being sick to turn friends and family into caretakers (developing learned helplessness). If this is the case, it is helpful for the doctor to define "help" as ignoring the sadness and offering to do more normal activities, thus giving the sufferers more attention when they are "well" than when they exhibit symptoms.

The final stage of grief entails finding new meaning in one's life and finding new ways to have needs met that were once met by the person who died. The meaning of one's life is usually integrally tied in with family, so when someone dies some of the survivor's own value and purpose is lost and must be redefined. If the physician finds that there is unresolved grief that is not diminishing even many months after the death, it is time to inquire as to what brought meaning to their life prior to the loss and see what can be extracted from that past relationship and be incorporated in their future, giving their life new meaning. Specific activity directed at exploring these possibilities or beginning new activities to engage in this process of developing new life meaning should be the focus of the therapeutic interaction.

For example, the widow of a college president not only loses her husband but also her avocation. She has for many years coordinated the visits and served as hostess to the many dignitaries who visited the university. After her husband's death she became isolated and inactive. The physician asked the grown children to see if their church needed someone to organize the church's social events. Her pastor called her and asked for her help in setting up a social function at the church. Initially she was reluctant, saying she did not have the energy, but at the pastor's urging (after the doctor assured the pastor she was not ill) she agreed. She gradually found the energy to set up church functions regularly, and her symptoms disappeared.

Case Report

J.L. was a spry, mentally competent 82-year-old man, the patriarch of a large family-owned business. Mr. L had lost considerable weight and was mildly depressed. He continued to ignore these problems until he began to experience epigastric abdominal pain. He was hospitalized by his family physician; and after a workup in which newfound diabetes, elevated liver enzymes, and an elevated serum amylase were discovered he was scheduled for a computed tomography (CT) scan of the abdomen. The family physician then discussed his concerns about pancreatic cancer with the patient and his wife. The following morning on rounds the physician was met by Mrs. L and two of the patient's sons who implored the physician not to tell their father if cancer was discovered. They predicted that Mr. L would be greatly distressed by this news, and they preferred the physician to tell only them. The physician immediately expressed reluctance, but the family was emphatic.

The CT scan did indeed show evidence of cancer of the pancreas. The physician called a meeting of the family to discuss these findings. He began by suggesting that an oncologist might be consulted at this point as there are some treatments available that might help J.L. in terms of prolonging life or lessening his suffering. He then told the family that it was a malignancy that was almost certainly fatal.

The physician explained to the family that if they kept this news secret from J.L. it was likely that the patient would realize there was something terribly wrong but would be emotionally isolated from his family. He would likely know that they were keeping something from him, and it might cause him to be angry or feel alone in his time of greatest need. He, however, might not tell them to protect them from his distress. Having reframed this issue for the family in this way he went on to say that it would be a breach of his professional ethics to not share the diagnosis and prognosis with a competent patient. Having heard this reframing, the family reached a quick consensus to recant their insistence that the physician keep the diagnosis from their father. They appeared to grieve the prognosis. The physician then asked that they go to the bedside and that he would be along in a few moments after he finished charting.

When the physician came to J.L.'s room, the family was at the bedside. The physician asked permission to sit at the edge of the bed then proceeded to tell J.L. that he was there to discuss the results of his tests with him. He began by suggesting an oncology consultation to provide any helpful treatments that might be offered at this point. The physician told J.L., however, that he had a malignancy, which was severe and in most cases proved fatal.

He asked J.L. what he was thinking then. J.L. replied, "I thought it was something like that." The physician promised to supply more information the next day and encouraged J.L. and his family to be prepared with any questions they might have. He said he would write a consult order for an oncologist in whom he had great confidence but that he intended to remain on the case. He promised to interpret any recommendations the other physician might have in language that could be understood if that were necessary, to let J.L. and his family know what they can expect from any intervention suggested by the specialist, and to provide any necessary measures for comfort and relief of pain should that occur.

The physician reviewed J.L.'s already documented advance directive and asked if that was still the way he felt. J.L. replied that it was. He congratulated J.L. on his good judgment and courage .

References

Bloom-Feshbach J, Bloom-Feshbach S, (ed.) (1987) The Psychology of Separation and Loss. San Francisco: Jossey-Bass.

Davis G (1999) Anticipatory grief in patients of dying children. Am Fam Physician 59:2435.

Farber S, Egnew T, Stempel S, et al (2000) End of Life Care Monograph, 250/251th ed. Leawood, KS: American Academy of Family Physicians.

Marris P (1974) Loss and Change. New York: Pantheon.

McDaniel SH, Campbell TL, Seaburn DB (1990a) Anticipating loss. In Family-oriented Primary Care: A Manual for Medical Providers. New York: Springer-Verlag.

McDaniel SH, Campbell TL, Seaburn DB (1990b) Looking death in the eye. In Family-oriented Primary Care: A Manual for Medical Providers. New York: Springer-Verlag.

McDaniel SH, Hepworth J, Doherty WJ (1992) Caring for dying patients and grieving families. In Medical Family Therapy: A Biopsychosocial Approach to Families with Health Problems. New York: BasicBooks.

Prendes C (1997) Dying with dignity. Am Fam Physician 56:55–56.

Schneiderman L (1997) The family physician and end-of-life care. J Fam Pract 45:259–262.

Shapiro ER (1994) Grief as a Family Process: A Developmental Approach to Clinical Practice. New York: Guilford.

29

Resolving Problems of Advanced Directives and End-of-Life Decision-Making

1. Discuss advanced directives as part of health care maintenance visits for all patients over the age of 60. Discuss advanced directives with patients who have an illness that may result in premature death once they have accepted their illness.
2. Bring up the discussion of advanced directives in a way that emphasizes patients maintaining control over their care under all circumstances. Give them a handout to read and share with their families.
3. Document advanced directives in a way that ensures compliance. For example, make sure they are sent to the hospital or nursing home on admission.
4. Recognize red flags that indicate problems in end-of-life decision-making.
   a. High conflict families
   b. Excessive denial of terminal illness
   c. Excessive guilt
5. When end-of-life decision-making is a problem, call for a care conference. Make sure that all significant others who are likely to play a role in end-of-life decision-making are present, even if it requires teleconferencing.
6. Structure the care conference in the same way as a brief therapy session would be structured (see Chapter 1).
   a. Each person present expresses his or her concerns about the patient without interruption.
   b. The physician provides education, which includes a discussion of treatment alternatives such as cardiopulmonary resuscitation (CPR), respirators, dialysis, tube feedings, palliative care.
   c. Discussion should include the likely outcome of treatment and its effect on functional status.
   d. Discuss levels of functional status that may make a difference in their desire for treatment, such as permanent coma, irreversible loss of cognitive ability, whole body paralysis, terminal illness.

e. Allow patients to go first and describe their desires for advanced directives. This should include who they would like to speak for them in case they are unable to speak for themselves in the future.

7. If problems develop when patients are unable to speak for themselves, the doctor should call a family conference. The discussion should center on what the patient would want if they could speak for themselves. Control, denial, and guilt should be addressed as well.

8. For families in which problems persist, help of the clergy or a hospital ethics committee is sometimes helpful.

Ten years of experience on an ethics committee of a large hospital has demonstrated that most common problems related to end-of-life decision-making result from of a lack of timely discussion regarding advanced directives. Once the patient has a compromised mental status, without prior discussion there is often uncertainty as to what the patient wants. This leads to guilt and either a bias to do everything possible, no matter how burdensome or futile, or reluctance to make decisions at all. Chapters throughout this book have stressed early intervention as fundamentally important to prevent serious and chronic problems. In the area of advanced directives this means discussing patients' wishes well before they become an issue. Logic, realistic thinking, and reliance on lifelong value systems are more likely involved in decision-making that is not forced by the passions of crisis, anxiety, guilt, or fear. Time for meaningful discussion is often seen as a barrier by doctors. However, in the long run time is saved by avoiding problems, not to mention preventing psychological discomfort. This also preserves patient autonomy even after incapacitation, an important goal of physicians.

In this chapter we discuss a process for developing advanced directives as part of routine health care maintenance visits, and we then turn to resolving problems related to end-of-life decision-making. It is assumed that the physician already has a working knowledge of ethical principles that form the basis for such discussions, including such issues as autonomy (including informed consent), beneficence and nonmaleficence, sanctity of life, and quality of life including related functional status. It is beyond the scope of this chapter to discuss ethical principles in much detail. Two American Academy of Family Physician (AAFP) monographs (Brody, 1993; Fleetwood and Lipsky, 1998) have excellent discussions of these issues.

Legal issues including definitions of "informed consent" and the difference between "power of attorney" and a "living will" are also important. In general, informed consent requires that the patient understand the usual course of their illness, treatment options, and the likely outcome of their decision. This does require cognitive higher executive functions, so if the patient's mental status is compromised in the area of abstract thinking they likely cannot understand the outcome of their decision. Therefore they are not competent to make health care decisions. A "living will" spells out both generally and specifically what patients would want for treatment under certain circumstances. They may request a do not resuscitate (DNR) order if their functional status declines to a certain level (e.g., comatose). If they are in a permanent vegetative state they may request that they not be given artificial nutrition. The "durable power of attorney for health care" (DPOA) appoints individuals who patients believe know their desires and can interpret their overall preference for treatment in keeping with their general desires. In general, a DPOA is considered most important, as a knowledgeable person then can respond to specific circumstances often not anticipated in a living will. Appointing a DPOA also ensures that the patient's wishes are considered by doctors, who otherwise might not have access to the living will. Having both is considered ideal. The living will gives philosophic guides to the DPOA. Although in certain circumstances, such as when there is a great deal of family conflict, it may be useful to have the aid of legal counsel when drawing up a living will or DPOA, it is not a good idea to recommend a lawyer's assistance universally. To do so would present a barrier to many patients in being able to establish advanced directives. If physicians include in their progress notes a thorough description of issues that have been discussed related to advanced directives, it suffices if it becomes necessary to use this information. There are standard forms and computer programs that are excellent as well.

Communicating this information to the right people is essential to the outcome. That is, make sure the information gets to a nursing home or hospital in a timely fashion. Studies have shown this to be a significant barrier to implementation, although the situation has improved. The Patient Self-determination Act of 1991 requires that every facility that receives Medicare or Medicaid funds ask the patient on admission if they have advanced directives. This act was aimed at motivating this process to occur. Still only about 40% of patients have this on their record upon admission, and the acute situation is a poor time to have a rational discussion of these issues (Aitken, 1999). Obviously, an admission clerk is in no position to discuss these issues with the patient or family. They can at best give them a handout to read. Even if they note that the patient has advanced directives on the chart, it is up to the family doctor and family to make sure they are used.

An effective approach to timely discussion is for the physician to make it part of their routine to have a discussion of advanced directives with every patient over the age of 60 or 65 who has a health care maintenance visit. It is also beneficial to bring up advanced directives to the patient who has been diagnosed with an illness that could be terminal once the illness has been accepted. Some doctors are uncomfortable bringing up this issue with the patient, but most patients in these situations have thought about it long before the physician has and, in fact, are relieved when the physician makes it an acceptable topic. Not discussing death with dying patients isolates them and adds to their suffering. Bringing it up in a way that emphasizes one's desire to maintain the patient's control is often comforting for the patient. For example, the physician might say, "Because it is important to me as your doctor to have you remain in control of your health care, I routinely talk to patients and their families about advanced directives." To save time it is often helpful to give them a handout to read and share with their families that outlines common living wills and DPOAs. Handouts should describe various care options such as CPR, respirators, dialysis, and tube feeding so they can make more informed decisions. Asking them to mail back to the doctor what they want put in their record after discussion with their family or suggesting that at their next visit they have something prepared to discuss with you is an efficient way to implement advanced directives effectively.

It would be nice to believe that when it came to such critical issues such as advanced directives families would set aside other issues and rationally and realistically deal with the issues at hand. Unfortunately, families often deal with advanced directives in the same way they resolve all their other issues. This means that highly conflicted or guilt-ridden families consistently bring these issues into advanced directives as well. Although problems with advanced directives are uncommon, when they do occur it is often painful for everyone involved including the physician. Red flags that advanced directives could become problematic are high conflict families, excessive denial of terminal illness, and excessive guilt. When these situations are apparent, it is useful to call a family meeting to obtain advanced directives.

In families with high conflict, it is helpful if the physician or the health care staff contact the family. All significant others should be invited. Rather than avoiding people who are disagreeable in the family, it is usually advantageous to include them, often neutralizing their power. For some reason (perhaps guilt) the person who is farthest away and least involved in the day-to-day activities and decision-making often wants to have the most input into decisions. It is important to have these people at the meeting even if it is via teleconference. Having a speakerphone at the meeting is easily arranged. If the meeting takes place at the hospital or nursing home where care providers have gotten to know the patient quite well, it is helpful to include them in the meeting as well. These personnel likely have feelings for the patient and have an impact on how decisions are carried out.

The structure of the care conference is usually most effective when it follows the process described for brief therapy (see Chapter 1). The physician should start by requesting each person present make a brief statement of his or her concerns and views regarding the patient and the advanced directives. It is usually best to put the patient in the powerful position of going last, if mental status allows. If there are professionals present, such as nursing staff or a nursing home social worker, they might go last so the family is uninfluenced by their views. It is also usually best to have the most powerful people in the family go later, as again their views might inhibit the less assertive members from stating their true beliefs or concerns. During these opening statements it is important to not allow interruptions as it undermines people's comfort level when stating their position.

Once everyone has spoken the physician can proceed with education, knowing the family members' views. This helps physicians target the discussion most appropriately. If the patient has a disease with a poor prognosis, even though the illness has already been discussed it is best to get an understanding from the patient and family of what they know about the illness and treatment, as misconceptions sometimes linger. It is then helpful to provide general education regarding alternatives to terminal treatment such as a description of CPR, the use of respirators, dialysis, tube feeding, and palliative care. The doctor does not have to give these explanations in much detail but should provide a basic understanding, including likely outcomes of treatment in relation to the patient's goals of functional status. Also it is useful to provide education about the different circumstances that might lead to different levels of treatment. For example, permanent coma, irreversible loss of cognitive ability, whole body paralysis, and terminal illness are usually worthwhile covering in at least an elementary way.

At this point in the meeting the patient and family are usually in a position to make decisions. If the patient is present he or she should speak first, thus being in the position of ultimate authority. Family members can then respond as to how they believe this decision will affect them. It is helpful at this point if the physician can clarify who would be the DPOA in the event patients are unable to make decisions for themselves. It is important to make clear that the role of the DPOA is to carry out the wishes of the patient, not the desires of other family members or themselves.

If the patient is unable to speak for himself or herself at this meeting, it should first be decided what the patient would want and then who should speak for the patient. Although a DPOA cannot be appointed after a patient has become incapacitated, most state statues allow next of kin to function as a surrogate decision-maker.

If resolution of advanced directives is problematic, issues such as family conflict, denial, or unresolved guilt should be explored more directly. If the problem is denial, it should have become apparent during discussion of the illness course and prognosis. One approach to denial is to use an "as if" approach (see Chapter 1). The physician can tell the family that sometimes it is useful to practice difficult tasks in case they become necessary. Ask the family to discuss what the patient's wishes might be "as if" the illness was life-threatening. "As if" allows people to rehearse their response to a problem they are not yet ready to face. This exercise mirrors the natural process that occurs in response to difficult situations. If this maneuver does not lead to successful resolution, the approach taken to denial in Chapter 28 may be useful.

If guilt is interfering with decisions, and education on the illness has not helped, the next step might be to frame making ethical choices as *painful* to the family but *caring* to the patient. Pointing out all the positive ways the decision could help the patient (e.g., relief from pain or other suffering) can be reassuring and helps relieve guilt. When the doctor knows the family is too overwhelmed by guilt to make a decision, the doctor may offer a specific recommendation, taking a more paternalistic role but which under these circumstances provides noticeable relief. The key is for the doctor to assess accurately that if the family was relieved of guilt this is what they would want. By the doctor taking on some responsibility, the family can be relieved of some guilt. Input of a hospital ethics committee can also help some move past this hurdle. Clergy at times can be helpful with these dynamics. If an ethics committee or clergy recommends an action, people feel less guilt carrying it through. The physician almost never should offer futile treatment (e.g., CPR to a mottled patient in the emergency room or placing a feeding tube in an end-stage cancer patient). To do so places an unnecessary burden on the family. It is asking them to make a decision that is really not a decision.

Regarding power struggles, rather than trying to decide who is right or wrong (which is the usual approach in struggling families) it is more helpful to offer alternatives that are compromises between the two positions. Usually if the family is given such a choice, they relinquish the need to be victorious. In this case, the family may need to believe the suggestion came from the doctor and not a family member.

If these attempts to resolve problems still fail, another approach is to elicit the help of a hospital ethics committee. Often after discussing the issues with an ethics committee, their recommendations resolve the issues of denial, guilt, and power struggles. Many hospital ethics committees are open to case discussions even if the patient is an outpatient at the time of the discussion.

References

Aitken PVJ (1999) Incorporating advance care planning into family practice. Am Fam Physician 59:605–614, 617–620.

Brody H (1993) Medical Ethics Monograph, 166/167th ed. Kansas City, MO: American Academy of Family Physicians.

Duffield P, Podzamsky JE (1996) The completion of advance directives in primary care. J Fam Pract 42:378–384.

Fleetwood J, Lipsky M (1998) Medical Ethics Monograph, 231st ed. Kansas City, MO: American Academy of Family Physicians.

Siwek J (1994) Decision-making in terminal care: four common pitfalls. Am Fam Physician 50:1207–1208, 1211.

Index